CEREBRAL HEMISPHERE ASYMMETRY

Method, Theory, and Application

Edited by
Joseph B. Hellige
University of Southern California

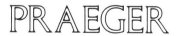

PRAEGER SPECIAL STUDIES • PRAEGER SCIENTIFIC

Library of Congress Cataloging in Publication Data

Main entry under title:

Cerebral hemisphere asymmetry.

   Includes bibliographies and index.
   1. Cerebral dominance. I. Hellige, Joseph B.
QP385.5.C47   1983   612'.825   82-16655
ISBN 0-03-058638-0

Published in 1983 by Praeger Publishers
CBS Educational and Professional Publishing
a Division of CBS Inc.
521 Fifth Avenue, New York, New York 10175 U.S.A.

3456789   052   987654321

Printed in the United States of America
on acid-free paper

Contents

Contributors

M. P. Bryden
Department of Psychology
University of Waterloo
Waterloo, Ontario
Canada

Alfonso Caramazza
Department of Psychology
The Johns Hopkins University
Baltimore, Maryland 21218

Michael S. Gazzaniga
Division of Cognitive Neuroscience
Department of Neurology
Cornell University Medical College
1300 York Avenue
New York, New York 10021

Alan S. Gevins
EEG Systems Laboratory
1855 Folsom
San Francisco, California 94103

Curtis Hardyck
Institute of Human Learning
University of California
Berkeley, California 94720

Joseph B. Hellige
Department of Psychology
University of Southern California
Los Angeles, California 90089

Merrill Hiscock
Psychology Division
University Hospital
University of Saskatchewan
Saskatoon, Saskatchewan
Canada

Larry F. Hughes
Kresge Hearing Research Laboratory
Department of Otorhinolaryngology
    and Biocommunication
Louisiana State University Medical Center
1100 Florida Avenue
New Orleans, Louisiana 70119
                and
Department of Psychology
University of New Orleans

George W. Hynd
Department of Educational Psychology
University of Georgia
Athens, Georgia 30602

Marcel Kinsbourne
Behavioral Neurology Department
Eunice Kennedy Shriver Center for
    Mental Retardation, Inc.
200 Trapelo Road
Waltham, Massachusetts 02254

Jerre Levy
Committee on Biopsychology
Department of Behavioral Sciences
University of Chicago
Chicago, Illinois 60637

Randi C. Martin
Department of Psychology
The Johns Hopkins University
Baltimore, Maryland 21218

Manfred J. Meier
University of Minnesota
Neuropsychology Laboratory
Department of Neurosurgery
Minneapolis, Minnesota 55455

Francis J. Pirozzolo
Department of Neurology
Baylor College of Medicine
Texas Medical Center
Houston, Texas 77030

Robert J. Porter, Jr.
Department of Psychology
University of New Orleans
and
Kresge Hearing Research Laboratory
Department of Otorhinolaryngology
   and Biocommunication
Louisiana State University Medical Center
New Orleans, Louisiana 70119

Keith Rayner
Department of Psychology
University of Massachusetts
Amherst, Massachusetts 01003

John J. Sidtis
Division of Cognitive Neuroscience
Department of Neurology
Cornell University Medical Center
1300 York Avenue
New York, New York 10021

D. A. Sprott
Department of Statistics
University of Waterloo
Waterloo, Ontario
Canada

W. Gary Thompson
University of Minnesota
Neuropsychology Laboratory
Department of Neurosurgery
Minneapolis, Minnesota 55455

Frank Wood
Section of Neuropsychology
Bowman Gray School of Medicine
Wake Forest University
Winston-Salem, North Carolina 27103

Eran Zaidel
Department of Psychology
University of California, Los Angeles
Los Angeles, California 90024

The Study of
Cerebral Hemisphere Differences:
Introduction and Overview

Joseph B. Hellige

There is now a large body of clinical and experimental evidence indicating that the left and right cerebral hemispheres in humans process information somewhat differently from each other. Evidence for cerebral hemisphere asymmetry comes from an unusually wide variety of sources. For example, studies are conducted using such varied populations as patients with unilateral brain damage, patients with the corpus callosum and other connective tissue surgically severed (the "split-brain" patients), neurologically normal adults, and children of various ages and levels of reading ability. Experimental techniques include such things as the investigation of auditory, visual, and tactile perceptual asymmetries and the study of response asymmetries, including lateralized motor activity, electrophysiological activity measured at the scalp, and regional cerebral blood flow. To adequately digest and understand this vast literature, it is critical to appreciate the methods used in the scientific investigation of cerebral asymmetry.

The use of many subject populations and experimental paradigms in order to converge upon a common set of conceptual issues is a very positive aspect of the scientific investigation of cerebral laterality. However, this variety also creates some difficulty. Ultimately, theories about cerebral laterality must account for the findings from each of the subject populations investigated and from each of the experimental paradigms employed. Integrating information across the various approaches demands the ability to evaluate the quality of research, using several rather different techniques. It has become increasingly obvious that each of the approaches taken to study cerebral laterality requires careful consideration of methodological and inferential issues in order to systematically rule out alternative explanations of phenomena intended to reflect hemispheric specialization. Even researchers who actively investigate cerebral hemisphere asymmetry are typically expert for only a small subset of the techniques used. Because it is impossible to consider theoretical and conceptual issues intelligently without adequate appreciation of the principles that serve to identify methodologically adequate laterality studies, this chapter briefly reviews the approaches most commonly used, considers some of the advantages and disadvantages of each, and outlines critical issues that remain to be determined. The remaining chapters in this volume provide a more detailed discussion of the various approaches, focusing on both important methodological considerations and critical theoretical issues.

For convenience of exposition, this chapter divides the techniques used to study cerebral laterality into several categories and discusses the categories separately. Although the division is somewhat arbitrary, it is intended to emphasize certain common characteristics among methods within the same category and to highlight important differences among categories. The categories are: the study of brain-damaged individuals, the study of split-brain individuals, perceptual laterality in neurological normals, and lateralized responses in neurological normals. For all of these methods, the emphasis is on the interaction of experimental variables with left versus right cerebral hemispheres. Consequently, a subsequent section of this chapter considers issues related to the interpretation of interaction patterns and issues surrounding the computation of a laterality index. Following this is a brief discussion of additional issues involved in the study of individual differences in the magnitude and direction of hemispheric asymmetry. The final section of the chapter points out some of the important theoretical issues that cut across all of the various research methods and considers possible directions for future research.

METHODS OF INVESTIGATION

Study of Brain-damaged Individuals

The earliest evidence of cerebral hemisphere asymmetry came from observations of the disorders produced by unilateral brain damage. For example, the tendency for various language disorders to be more severe after left hemisphere damage than after right hemisphere damage has been explicitly noted at least since the important observations published by Broca (1865). The study of patients with various types of brain damage continues to be an important technique for learning more about the cerebral bases of perceptual and cognitive functions in humans. One advantage of studying brain-damaged individuals is that the deficits are often quite striking, even though it is sometimes challenging to pinpoint the precise cognitive nature of the impairment. Problems of interpretation can and do arise, and it is important to consider various sources of difficulty and techniques to deal with them.

It is instructive to briefly consider what an idealized study of brain-damaged individuals would be like because the idealized situation provides an illustration of this approach at its very best. In many ways, brain-ablation studies with animals serve as a prototype for this idealized research.

One would probably want to begin with a reasonably large sample of neurologically normal subjects and randomly divide them into as many groups as needed for the research at hand. Having selected certain areas to be ablated, it would be necessary that the ablation be precise, involving only the relevant tissue. In most cases it would be advisable to include one or more placebo groups, perhaps undergoing sham operations. At the appropriate times after ablation, the subjects would be tested on specific behavioral tasks chosen to examine the cognitive processes deemed most interesting. By comparing the performance of various groups, one could piece together a coherent story about brain-behavior relationships. Finally it would be necessary to double-check the accuracy of the ablation procedure, perhaps by doing detailed postmortem examinations.

Even under these highly idealized circumstances, it is often difficult to make strong inferences about the function of an anatomical structure by observing how the organism behaves after the ablation of that structure. What is actually observed in such studies is what the remaining, intact tissue can still do, and it is from this that we must infer the function of the damaged tissue. This is tricky business under the best of circumstances. It is rather obvious that, even though a particular behavior is impaired by damage to a particular brain area, it cannot be automatically assumed that the function is "housed" in that anatomical location. An analogy proposed by Gardner (1978) is that the functioning of a radio can be completely terminated by destroying the plug; but it would be misleading to infer that the functioning of the radio was "housed" in the plug. Still, it could be concluded that the plug is necessary for normal functioning of the radio, so something of potential importance would have been learned.

Also consider the case in which a particular behavior is not impaired after damage to a particular area of the brain. It certainly cannot be assumed that the damaged region normally plays no role in the behavior. It is possible that the task has been neurologically reorganized or that is is now performed with a different strategy that does not depend upon the damaged area, even though the damaged area is normally involved in performing that task. Making inferences about these possibilities and others is extremely important when evaluating studies of brain-damaged patients. Additional discussion is provided by Caramazza and Martin in Chapter 2 of this volume, in the context of studying language disorders after left hemisphere brain damage. The group/ case study approach that they outline is a particularly promising way to use the performance of brain-damaged patients for the study of cerebral laterality.

The issues considered thus far apply to interpreting the results from brain-damaged patients under highly idealized conditions that can never be met and may seldom be approached. Additional problems arise in actual research of this sort. For example, there is often less certainty about the precise locus of brain damage than is desirable, and the damage is rarely so specific as that that can be induced experimentally in animals. Furthermore, homogenous groups of human beings are not randomly arranged into various experimental and control groups; thus, many individual difference characteristics may influence the results. Characteristics such as age, general physical and mental health, sex, and so forth must be taken into account when interpreting the results from left- and right-hemisphere damaged groups. While the problems are great, they are not insurmountable. Chapter 3 in this volume by Meier and Thompson provides a detailed discussion of many of these individual difference issues in the context of studying individuals with right-hemisphere brain damage and indicates steps that can be taken to deal with potential problems.

Study of Split-Brain Individuals

In many ways, the most dramatic evidence for hemispheric asymmetry comes from the study of patients who have had the corpus callosum severed in order to control severe epilepsy. As Zaidel (Chapter 4 of this volume) argues, it is the study of such split-brain patients and the often dramatic asymmetries that they exhibit that created the contemporary zeitgeist in which the study of cerebral laterality flourishes. In these patients, the left and right cerebral hemispheres are disconnected and no longer communicate with each other. It is possible, therefore, to examine the functioning of each cerebral hemisphere in isolation.

It is instructive to digress for a moment and again to consider an idealized split-brain preparation for studying hemispheric asymmetry and the important functions of the corpus callosum. In many ways, the work of Myers and Sperry (1953), using split-brain animals, provides an animal prototype for an idealized preparation to study cerebral laterality in humans. Once again, consideration of the idealized situation provides a look at the optimal split-brain case study.

Were it not for ethical and practical reasons, it would be desirable to take healthy adults who have probably developed typical hemispheric specializations and to surgically disconnect the two cerebral hemispheres. By using lateralized presentation and response techniques, it would be possible to test each hemisphere separately on a variety of tasks. There is no doubt that the study of such individuals would provide a great deal of important information about the abilities of the left and right hemispheres. Studying such individuals avoids the problems of inferring the function of one brain region from observations of what the remaining tissue can do. Instead, the observation of what Zaidel has called the "positive competence" of each hemisphere provides a direct observation of what each cerebal hemisphere can do. While there is no doubt that the information collected from such patients would be invaluable, it is important not to overlook issues involved in generalizing to functional asymmetry in the intact brain.

Even in the idealized case, there is no guarantee that all of the asymmetries discovered in split-brain patients operate similarly in the intact brain with the labyrinth of interhemispheric communication. For example, it is possible that, for some tasks, the efficiency of interhemispheric communication is so great that the functional significance of hemispheric asymmetry for that task is obscured or of only minimal importance. It is also possible that, in the intact brain, activity in one cerebral hemisphere inhibits activity in corresponding regions of the other cerebral hemisphere. This inhibition could conceiveably serve to magnify the functional cerebral hemisphere asymmetry relative to that found in the idealized split-brain individual. For these reasons and others, it is obviously important to develop techniques for studying hemispheric asymmetry in neurologically intact individuals (a topic that will be considered later) and to systematically compare the effects obtained with various split-brain patients to the corresponding effects obtained with neurologically normal individuals. Exactly these types of comparisons have recently been made, and two independent lines of such research are discussed by Zaidel in Chapter 4 and by Sidtis and Gazzaniga in Chapter 5 of this volume.

Thus far, the discussion of split-brain research has assumed a highly idealized case. In practice, the surgical procedures resulting in complete or partial commissurotomy are not considered lightly. The patients typically suffer from severe epilepsy and almost certain neurological abnormality of varying type and degree. If these patients have developed atypical patterns of hemispheric asymmetry because of previous disease, it is obviously critical that this be taken into account when generalizing to the neurologically normal population. The problem is compounded by the fact that there are rather large individual differences among split-brain patients in the nature of prior neurological disorders, with each individual being a unique case study.

While the existence of neurological abnormalities and large individual differences increases the difficulty of making inferences from the split-brain patients, the difficulties do not seem overwhelming. The fact that there are large individual differences in prior neurological disorders makes it that much more impressive when a group of these patients all shows the same laterality effect. For example, Zaidel reports a dichotic listening experiment with consonant-vowel syllables for which each of six split-brain patients shows a large left-hemisphere advantage, despite individual differences on a number of variables. When individual differences in laterality pattern occur (and they certainly do), they not only constitute a challenge for interpretation but also provide a unique opportunity to observe the potential of each cerebral hemisphere to develop various cognitive functions. The systematic case study of individual patients has recently been aided by the opportunity to test patients both before and after partial and complete commissurotomy, clarifying the functions of the connecting fibers as well as shedding light on hemispheric asymmetry (see Sidtis & Gazzaniga in this volume).

In summary, while the split-brain patients are not the highly idealized population described earlier, they have provided a unique opportunity to observe the competence of each cerebral hemisphere acting alone. The careful study of these individuals serves as a rich source of hypotheses about brain-behavior relationships that can be tested in a variety of ways.

Perceptual Laterality in Neurological Normals

In the intact brain, it is not possible to test each cerebral hemisphere in isolation. However, it is possible to examine various aspects of task performance as a function of which hemisphere receives a stimulus directly and must, therefore, initiate processing. Such examinations of perceptual laterality are possible, using various stimulus presentation modalities. For example, when two different auditory stimuli are presented simultaneously to the left and right ears (i.e., dichotic listening), the input from each ear projects primarily to the contralateral cerebral hemisphere. It is the case in the human visual system that all information from one side of the visual field projects directly to the contralateral cerebral hemisphere. In addition, tactile information from the fingers of each hand projects to the contralateral cerebral hemisphere. Given the multidisciplinary nature of interest in hemispheric asymmetry and the noninvasive nature of the perceptual laterality techniques, an incredibly large number of studies have taken advantage of these anatomical arrangements to investigate cerebral hemisphere asymmetry in the intact brain.

If perceptual asymmetries are going to be used to make inferences about hemispheric asymmetry, it is important to understand exactly how hemispheric asymmetries produce perceptual asymmetries. In addition, it is important to consider how factors having nothing to do with hemispheric asymmetry can also influence perceptual laterality. These two points will be considered in turn.

As discussed elsewhere in this volume (e.g., Zaidel, Chapter 4; Porter & Hughes, Chapter 6; Hardyck, Chapter 7), Kimura (1966) originally advanced what has been called the "direct access model" to account for perceptual asymmetries on the basis of hemispheric asymmetries. According to this model, performance on a task will be better when the stimuli traverse an anatomical pathway directly to the hemisphere specialized for that task than when the stimuli project directly to the less efficient hemisphere. For example, according to this model, verbal stimuli are recognized better from the right ear than from the left ear because the stimuli from the right ear project directly to the left cerebral hemisphere, which is most often more efficient for processing verbal stimuli.

In contrast, Kinsbourne (1973, 1975) has advanced an attention-bias explanation that emphasizes the balance of activation between the two cerebral hemispheres. According to this hypothesis, performance on a task is better if the stimuli are presented to the side of space contralateral to the hemisphere that is more activated by the task being performed. According to this model, the right ear advantage for recognizing verbal stimuli occurs because the left hemisphere is more activated than the right by a verbal recognition task, thereby permitting attention to be directed more easily to the right side of space.

A detailed review of the status of these theoretical approaches is beyond the scope of this chapter, but it does not seem that either of the two explanations, in their orginal form, can account for the entire body of perceptual laterality results. Consequently, both approaches have undergone a great deal of revision, and it has become very difficult to test between them. Still, the controversy has been very useful because it has focused attention upon the manner in which hemispheric asymmetry acts to produce perceptual laterality. Ultimately, the mechanism must become well understood for perceptual laterality to realize its full potential as a tool for the study of hemispheric asymmetry in the intact brain.

There is no doubt that many variables unrelated to hemispheric asymmetry can influence the magnitude and even the direction of perceptual laterality. Such variables include voluntary changes in attention to the two sides of space, order of reporting multiple stimuli, peripheral pathway asymmetries, postexposure scanning habits in vision, and so forth. (For further discussion, see the chapters by Porter & Hughes and by Hardyck in this volume and also Bertelson, 1982; Bryden, 1978; Hellige, in press.) If explanations of specific perceptual laterality results, in terms of these types of variables, cannot be ruled out, the results must be considered uninformative with respect to hemispheric asymmetry. In recent years a great deal of effort has been spent to refine dichotic listening and visual half-field methodology so that the effects of these variables can be minimized or eliminated. It is important to evaluate existing studies and to design future studies with the important methodological as well as theoretical issues in mind. Methodological and theoretical issues are often intertwined in the study of perceptual laterality.

For example, it has become apparent in perceptual laterality research that understanding the effect of input parameters is as important for theoretical as for methodological reasons. Consider recent work indicating that visual laterality effects for tasks involving letters depends in a systematic way upon a variety of input parameters such as size and perceptual quality (e.g., Bryden & Allard, 1976; Hellige, 1976, 1980; O'Boyle & Hellige, 1982; and Sergent, 1982). The fact that conditions of reduced perceptibility often shift the visual laterality pattern toward a left visual field (right-hemisphere) advantage is not only an important methodological concern when various studies are compared with each other; there are also important theoretical implications. For example, Sergent (1982) has recently used these effects to suggest that the right and left cerebral hemispheres are differentially efficient for processing low- and high-spatial frequencies, respectively. Had she and others not done a careful analysis of input parameters, this theoretical idea might not have emerged (see Hardyck, this volume, for further discussion of Sergent's theoretical position).

Lateralized Responses in Neurological Normals

Just as input from each side of space generally projects to the contralateral cerebral hemisphere, many measureable responses are produced by only one cerebral hemisphere or indicate the level and perhaps type of activity in specific regions of the cerebral cortex. The presence of response asymmetries can, therefore, provide important converging information about hemispheric asymmetry. The general approach has been to search for response asymmetry while individuals perform a variety of tasks in an effort to determine whether some tasks involve one cerebral hemisphere rather than the other.

Some research of this type takes advantage of the fact that movements of the distal musculature (e.g., finger movements) are controlled by the contralateral cerebral hemisphere. In prototypical experiments of this type, neurologically normal individuals are asked to perform manual tasks with the left or right hand while sometimes performing a concurrent task. The primary interest is on the extent to which concurrent activity of various sorts interferes with the manual activity of the right and left hands. It now seems clear that concurrent verbal tasks of various types (especially if verbal output is required) interfere more with activity of the right hand than with activity of the left hand whereas certain nonverbal spatial tasks (such as solving a block-design problem) interfere more with activity of the left hand (see Hellige & Longstreth, 1981; Hiscock, 1982; Kinsbourne & Cook, 1971).

Such results shed light on the nature of hemispheric asymmetry and also indicate that, in information processing terms, each hemisphere has a limited processing capacity that is at least partially separate from the capacity of the other hemisphere. Kinsbourne and colleagues have advanced the principle of functional cerebral distance to explain these interference effects on a physiological level; this principle as well as several methodological issues are reviewed in Chapter 8 of this volume by Kinsbourne and Hiscock.

During the last decade, a number of studies have been published using electrophysiological activity recorded at the scalp as evidence for the cerebral lateralization of higher cognitive functions. The use of such measurements has a great deal of popular appeal, possibly because there is a temptation to suppose that the closer to the brain the dependent measures are obtained, the less chance there is for artifact. Despite the initial enthusiasm for the use of electrophysiological measures and the apparent simplicity of early results, there has been a growing awareness that many of these studies are methodologically flawed. In many experiments, conclusions have been reached about the lateralization of higher cognitive functions (e.g., spatial reasoning), but there were inadequate controls to rule out explanations in terms of simpler processes involving perception, response programming, overall task difficulty, and so forth. In some cases, there has been either no appropriate baseline measure of electrophysiological activity or the baseline conditions have been inadequately specified. These points and many others are discussed in detail by Gevins in Chapter 9 of this volume, and guidelines are offered about the conduct of future studies of scalp potentials. Of special importance is a relatively new procedure developed by Gevins and his colleagues that is designed to permit dynamic spatiotemporal brain potential patterns to be discovered. Such techniques may allow the flow of physiological activity to be traced among neural areas that are functionally interrelated. To date, the results indicate that even very simple tasks involve a dynamically changing pattern of activity involving many different brain areas from both cerebral hemispheres. Such results suggest that it may be too simplistic to think of overall left versus right hemisphere specialization for higher cognitive activities without being precise about specific stages of processing and their temporal characteristics.

During the last few years, additional techniques for monitoring the level of neural activity in subareas of the cerebral cortex have been used. For example, it has become possible to monitor the amount of blood flow to different cortical regions and to obtain other measures of localized metabolic activity. These new technologies appear to be very promising ways of learning more about brain-behavior relationships in the intact brain, but, like all new technologies, there are many issues that need to be considered in the design and evaluated in the interpretation of experiments. Some of the techniques allow very precise spatial resolution (i.e., can monitor small areas of the cerebral cortex) but have a rather poor temporal resolution (e.g., it may take 30 minutes or longer for the measures to be obtained). Other techniques have poorer spatial but better temporal resolution. Issues related to spatiotemporal resolution and additional issues involved in using some of this new technology are discussed by Wood in Chapter 10 of this volume. There is every reason to believe that the appropriate combination of response measures will lead to important advances during the next few years.

HEMISPHERE X TASK INTERACTION AND LATERALITY INDEXES

Among the most interesting findings in the literature on cerebral hemisphere asymmetry are indications that the direction and magnitude of hemispheric asymmetry change with task demands. Indeed, such findings are the very reason for the development of the concept of hemispheric asymmetry. Conceptually, such results involve the investigation of what might be called Hemisphere X Task interactions. An interaction is said to occur whenever the effect of one variable is not the same at all levels of a second variable. For example, in a study of hemispheric asymmetry, an interaction occurs when the differences between the right and left hemispheres (using one of the techniques described earlier) is not the same for different tasks or under different experimental conditions. When two tasks or experimental conditions produce hemisphere advantages in opposite directions (i.e., one task shows left hemisphere superiority and the other shows right hemisphere superiority), interpretation of the interaction is relatively straightforward. In many cases, however, two tasks produce a hemisphere advantage in the same direction (e.g., both show a left hemisphere superiority), but the magnitudes of the advantages are not equal. In these cases, the Hemisphere X Task interaction can be quite difficult to interpret.

The interpretation of interaction patterns has been considered for many areas of psychological research, and Hellige (Chapter 11 of this volume) discusses the implications for research on hemispheric specialization. Several recommendations can be made for the design of laterality experiments with a view toward producing more interpretable interactions. For example, it is necessary to avoid ceiling and floor effects, and it is highly desirable to choose dependent measures that are known to be related in specific ways to the psychological process of interest. This can best be accomplished by embedding studies of hemispheric asymmetry in a larger information-processing context. It is also important to remain cautious about certain problematic interaction patterns unless the dependent variables possess known scale properties.

The consideration of issues related to the interpretation of certain Hemisphere X Task interaction patterns has also led to an extensive discussion in the literature of laterality indexes. A laterality index is intended to provide a single value that reflects the magnitude as well as the direction of hemispheric asymmetry for a particular task performed by a particular individual or group of individuals. If an index actually provides such a value, virtually any Hemisphere X Task interaction would become interpretable. There has been considerable debate about the criteria that should be employed in choosing the best laterality index (e.g., whether an index should be independent of overall accuracy) and about the extent to which various indexes satisfy the criteria. Because the choice of measures can, in some circumstances, have important consequences for the interpretation of laterality studies, the laterality index issue is important for virtually all of the techniques used to study hemispheric asymmetry. Consequently, several chapters in the present volume consider the choice of an index, with the most extensive treatments being provided by Hellige, Chapter 11; Sprott and Bryden, Chapter 12; and Levy, Chapter 13. Although it is not obvious whether there can be a truly "atheoretical" laterality index that is to be preferred for all situations, it is obvious that careful thought must be given to the interpretation of certain Hemisphere X Task interaction patterns. In situations where different ways of scaling the results (i.e., different laterality indexes) lead to vastly different conceptual conclusions, it is necessary to be very cautious.

THE STUDY OF INDIVIDUAL DIFFERENCES

Consideration of the methodological issues discussed earlier and of the problems of interpreting Hemisphere X Task interactions is particularly important when attempting to identify individual differences in cerebral hemisphere asymmetry. This is true for several reasons. For any single individual, there are likely to be a number of factors that contribute to observed laterality effects, many of which are related only indirectly or not at all to cerebral hemisphere asymmetry. For example, asymmetry in peripheral pathways can influence side-of-presentation effects in perceptual laterality experiments, and such factors as asymmetry in skull thickness can influence certain responses measured at the scalp. Furthermore, different individuals may bring vastly different strategies to bear upon the same task, and there is reason to believe that the strategy used is one important determinant of measured laterality. Many of these things might be expected to "average out" in a relatively homogenous group of subjects, but they cannot do so at the level of an individual subject. Consequently, in order to make strong statements about the direction and magnitude of hemispheric asymmetry in a single individual, it is especially important to systematically rule out other possibilities. Because different individuals often have different overall levels of performance on the same task, it can also be particularly difficult to determine when they have hemispheric specializations in the same direction but of different magnitudes.

In many studies of individual differences, subjects are classified into subgroups using some dimension such as handedness, sex, age, overall level of task performance, and so forth, and the goal is to determine whether the subgroups differ in cerebral hemisphere asymmetry. Even though the emphasis is on the average performance of each group (rather than explicity on each individual), it is still possible that the groups are systematically different in areas such as preferred processing strategy. Consequently, the same concerns apply as when focusing on a single individual.

Many of the potential problems with the study of individual differences and several ways of dealing with them are discussed by Levy in Chapter 13 of this volume. Despite potential problems, it is clear that individuals do differ in the direction and magnitude of hemispheric asymmetry for a variety of tasks and such differences may occur even within the adult right-handed population (see Levy, this volume). It is important, therefore, to consider whether individual differences of this sort are related to important cognitive processes.

One complex cognitive task that might be related to the magnitude and direction of hemispheric asymmetry is reading, which requires the interplay between rather demanding visuospatial processing and a variety of syntactic, semantic, and pragmatic processing stages. For some time, there have been suggestions that children with specific reading disabilities suffer from subtle neurological abnormalities. More specific suggestions include the possibility that reading-disabled children have an incomplete lateralization of function or have impaired transfer of information from one cerebral hemisphere to the other. Only in recent years have many of the noninvasive techniques described earlier been used to compare various reading-disabled populations with appropriate control groups who read normally. Chapter 14 in this volume by Pirozzolo, Rayner, and Hynd reviews this literature and provides at least some separation of adequate studies from those with various methodological problems. In so doing, this chapter provides an example of how the various methods outlined here can be applied to the study of specific individual differences in cognition. The nature of the problem is important, and investigation is almost certain to continue.

THEORETICAL ISSUES AND FUTURE RESEARCH

As the preceding sections indicate, many different techniques have been used to study cerebral hemisphere asymmetry and its consequences for information processing in the intact brain. Each technique requires careful consideration of methodological details and provides, at best, only a modest amount of information about cerebral laterality and its implications. However, when the major results from the various types of research are considered together, there can be little doubt that the human cerebral hemispheres process information differently. Furthermore, whatever the precise differences may be, they lead to left hemisphere superiority for many types of tasks demanding verbal processing and to right hemisphere superiority for many nonverbal, spatially demanding perceptual tasks.

Much more careful work is necessary before the details of cerebral laterality are completely understood. Given the complexity of laterality results and the need for methodological sophistication, it is not likely that the important issues will be resolved by single experiments that happen to find some interesting laterality effect. Instead, progress will depend upon the programmatic use of each of the techniques outlined here, converging on a common set of conceptual issues. It may be especially useful to conjoin two or more of the techniques, for example, comparing split-brain patients and normals on the same set of perceptual laterality tasks (see Sidtis and Gazzaniga, Chapter 5; and Zaidel, Chapter 4) or monitoring brain potentials while subjects engage in perceptual laterality tasks.

It is always difficult to identify the most important conceptual issues for future research, and there are probably as many ideas about the relative importance of different issues as there are active investigators. Nevertheless, a few common themes run through the chapters in this volume and through the contemporary laterality literature and cut across the various research techniques. Some of these themes are briefly considered in the remainder of this chapter.

There has come to be a general concensus that no simple dichotomy is likely to characterize adequately the differences between the two cerebral hemispheres. In the past, the left and right hemispheres, respectively, have been characterized as verbal versus nonverbal, serial versus parallel, analytic versus holistic, digital versus analog, and so forth. To date, no single, well-defined dichotomy has been shown to be the basis for all laterality results (see Bertelson, 1982; Bradshaw & Nettleton and commentary on their article, 1981). Most suggested dichotomies have been so poorly defined that it is impossible to provide strong empirical tests to choose among them; consequently, there is little remaining enthusiasm for debate about which pair of dichotomous labels is most appropriate.

Instead of debate about dichotomous labels, the last few years have seen a growing interest in localizing hemispheric asymmetries more precisely within a sequence of information-processing stages. In order to do this, many relatively well-developed tasks have been borrowed from cognitive psychology and psycholinguistics and adapted for use in laterality experiments. In addition, new tasks have been designed with a processing-stage analysis in mind. Examples can be found for most of the techniques outlined in this chapter.

For example, process-oriented tasks indicate that damage to Broca's area of the left hemisphere interferes primarily with processing syntactic information while damage to Wernicke's area interferes more with semantic processing (see Caramazza & Berndt, 1978; and Caramazza & Martin, this volume). In split-brain studies, tasks have been developed to distinguish between right hemisphere superiority for visuospatial analysis and what Sidtis and Gazzaniga (this volume) refer to as manipulospatial analysis. Zaidel (this volume) has developed different versions of a dichotic listening task to separate phonetic processing from semantic processing. In the preceptual laterality literature, tasks such as short-term memory scanning have been used to separate perceptual encoding from serial memory comparison and to suggest different hemispheric asymmetry for different stages in the processing sequence (e.g., Hellige, 1980; O'Boyle & Hellige, 1982). In his studies of electrophysiological asymmetry, Gevins (this volume) has paid close attention to the variety of processes involved in the task given to the subjects. This refinement of behavioral tasks is likely to continue, as it seems quite possible that hemispheric asymmetries vary from stage to stage in a processing task and that the results observed depend upon such things as the relative difficulty of the various processing stages in a particular task at a particular level of practice.

Another important trend in contemporary studies is a growing emphasis on the cooperation between the two cerebral hemispheres in the performance of both simple and complex cognitive tasks. In part, this trend among serious scientists may have developed to counteract gross overgeneralizations and misstatements in the popular press abut such things as "logic," "art," and "creativity" being carried out exclusively in one hemisphere or the other. More important is the fact that recent data demands that the extent of cooperation in the intact brain be recognized. As already noted, new electrophysiological procedures described by Gevins (this volume) indicate the involvement of many cortical regions in relatively simple tasks. In addition, perceptual laterality experiments and lateralized motor interference experiments demonstrate that performance suffers when one cerebral hemisphere is overloaded, compared with the case in which the processing load is distributed more evenly across both hemispheres (e.g., Friedman & Polson, 1981; Friedman, Polson, Dafoe, & Gaskill, 1982; Hellige, Cox & Litvac, 1979; Kinsbourne & Hiscock, this volume). The continued investigation of such issues related to the cooperation of the left and right hemispheres is likely to be important for cognitive psychology in general as well as for the study of cerebral hemisphere asymmetry in particular.

CONCLUDING COMMENT

As in any area of investigation, advances in knowledge about cerebral hemisphere asymmetry are only as sound as the methods used to gather relevant data. Appreciating the important conceptual conclusions is difficult unless a good deal is understood about the techniques actually used. With this in mind, the present chapter has given an overview of the methods used to make inferences about cerebral hemisphere asymmetry, considering some of the advantages and limitations of each technique. Together, these techniques provide a strong arsenal for increasing our understanding of brain-behavior relationships. The remainder of this volume provides expert discussion of each of the various techniques: consideration of how research is most properly conducted, critical evaluation of empirical studies that are encountered, and the theoretical conclusions that are justified on the basis of well-done studies using these techniques.

REFERENCES

Bertelson, P. Lateral differences in normal man and laterization of brain function. *International Journal of Psychology*, 1982, *17*, 173–210.

Bradshaw, J.L., & Nettleton, N.C. The nature of hemispheric specialization in man. *The Behavioral and Brain Sciences*, 1981, *4*, 51–91.

Broca, P. Sur la faculté de language articulé. *Bulletin Societé Anthroplogia*, 1865, *6*, 493–494.

Bryden, M.P. Strategy effects in the assessment of hemispheric asymmetry. In G. Underwood (Ed.), *Strategies of information processing*. London: Academic Press, 1978.

Bryden, M.P., & Allard, F. Visual hemifield differences depend on typeface. *Brain and Language*, 1976, *3*, 191–200.

Caramazza, A., & Berndt, R.S. Semantic and syntactic processes and aphasia: A review of the literature. *Psychological Bulletin*, 1978, *85*, 898–918.

Friedman, A., & Polson, M.C. The hemispheres as independent resource sytems: Limited-capacity processing and cerebral specialization. *Journal of Experimental Psychology: Human Perception and Performance*, 1981, *7* 1031–1058.

Friedman, A., Polson, M.C., Dafoe, C.G., & Gaskill, S.J. Dividing attention within and between hemispheres: Testing a multiple resources approach to limited capacity information processing. *Journal of Experimental Psychology: Human Perception and Performance*, 1982, *8*, 625–650.

Gardner, H. What we know (and don't know) about the two halves of the brain. *Harvard Magazine*, 1978, *80*, 24–27.

Hellige, J.B. Changes in same-different laterality patterns as a function of practice and stimulus quality. *Perception & Psychophysics*, 1976, *20*, 267–273.

Hellige, J.B. Effects of perceptual quality and visual field of probe stimulus presentation on memory search for letters. *Journal of Experimental Psychology: Human Perception and Performance*, 1980, *6*, 639–651.

Hellige, J.B. Visual laterality and cerebral hemisphere specialization: Methodological and theoretical considerations. In J.B. Sidowski (Ed.), *Conditioning, cognition, and methodology: Contempory issues in experimental psychology*. Hillsdale, N.J.: Erlbaum, in press.

Hellige, J.B., Cox, P.J., & Litvac, L. Information processing in the cerebral hemispheres: Selective hemispheric activation and capacity limitations. *Journal of Experimental Psychology: General*, 1979, *108*, 251–279.

Hellige, J.B., & Longstreth, L.E. Effects of concurrent hemisphere-specific activity on unimanual tapping rate. *Neuropsychologia*, 1981, *19*, 395–405.

Hiscock, M. Verbal-manual time sharing in children as a function of task priority. *Brain and Cognition*, 1982, *1*, 119–131.

Kimura, D. Dual functional asymmetry of the brain in visual perception. *Neuropsychologia*, 1966, *4*, 275–385.

Kinsbourne, M. The control of attention by interaction between the hemispheres. In S. Kornblum (Ed.), *Attention and performance IV*. New York: Academic Press, 1973.

Kinsbourne, M. The mechanism of hemispheric control of the lateral gradient of attention. In P.M.A. Rabbitt & S. Dornic (Eds.), *Attention and performance V*. New York: Academic Press, 1975.

Kinsbourne, M., & Cook, J. Generalized and lateralized effects of concurrent verbalization on a unimanual skill. *Quarterly Journal of Experimental Psychology*, 1971, *23*, 341–345.

Myers, R.E., & Sperry, R.W. Interocular transfer of a visual form discrimination habit in cats after section of the optic chiasma and corpus callosum. *Anatomical Record 115*, 1953, 351–352.

O'Boyle, M.W., & Hellige, J.B. Hemispheric asymmetry, early visual processes, and serial memory comparison. *Brain and Cognition*, 1982, *1*, 224–243.

Sergent, J. The cerebral balance of power: Confrontation or cooperation? *Journal of Experimental Psychology: Human Perception and Performance*, 1982, *8*, 253–272.

2

Theoretical and Methodological Issues in the Study of Aphasia

Alfonso Caramazza
Randi C. Martin

Long-standing, well-documented observations have confirmed that cerebral insult to the left hemisphere results in differentiated patterns of language disturbance, depending upon the particular area damaged. Damage to homologous areas of the right hemisphere does not result in readily detectable language impairments. These facts, first clearly described by Broca and Wernicke, allow the conclusion that the two cerebral hemispheres are asymmetric with respect to language representation; the left hemisphere is specialized for language processing while the right has no language competence.

Recently it has been argued that the right hemisphere has at least some minimal language capacity (see Zaidel, this volume). However, given the overwhelming evidence that the left hemisphere subserves language processing (Luria, 1947/1970; Geschwind, 1965), most research on language impairments has focused on patients with unilateral damage to the left hemisphere.

Although it is clear that the left hemisphere does sustain normal language competence, what remains unclear are the processing mechanisms that underlie language and how these mechanisms can be localized within the left hemisphere. The method for studying these questions has been reliance on data from pathological cases, looking at the differential patterns of spared and impaired functions resulting from lesions to specific areas within the left hemisphere. This method has the advantage not found in research with normals of allowing one to look at the functioning of language components independent of the component that has been impaired and, thus, of allowing one to make inferences about the role of the missing component in normal language.

Although research with brain-damaged populations has its advantages, it also raises theoretical and methodological problems, some of which are also encountered in research with normals but some of which are unique to the study of pathological cases. This chapter will discuss the theoretical and methodological problems associated with research on unilaterally brain-damaged populations as well as possible solutions to those problems. While the issues raised are relevant to any research on cognitive function, be it memory, perception, or mathematical thinking, the focus here will be on the formulation of the processing mechanisms that underlie language and the localization of these functions, using data from aphasia. The discussion of these issues will be organized in relation to the following topics: neuropsychological theory and the study of aphasia, group research methodology and the problem of patient classification in aphasia, the case study approach, and the group/case study approach. The chapter is concluded with the discussion of an example: the difficulties encountered in attempts to formulate the mechanisms that underlie poor comprehension in aphasia.

NEUROPSYCHOLOGICAL THEORY AND THE STUDY OF APHASIA

Two sets of basic data underlie a neuropsychological theory of language: a set of neuroanatomical information specifying the locus and extent of cerebral damage and a set of associated behavioral symptoms. These data pairs constitute the basis from which inferences are made about the linguistic and other cognitive processes that characterize normal language use and about the cerebral localization of the hypothesized processes. Since neuropsychological theory is a formulation of the organization of psychological processes in the brain, the range of facts that must be accounted for by this theory include (or must not be inconsistent with) those that form the basis for normal cognitive theory. Stated differently, neuropsychological theory is that subset of cognitive theory that is consistent with neurological data.

This view of neuropsychological theory makes the strong assumption that neuropsychological data can be used as a basis from which to draw inferences about normal processes. This assumption could be false. If this were to be the case, one could not use data obtained with aphasic patients to study normal language process, and the study of aphasic patients would have only clinical value. Unfortunately, it is not possible to assess the validity of the assumption at the present time. Neither cognitive theory nor the current understanding of aphasia is sufficiently well developed to allow a resolution of the issue. In the cases of data with both aphasic and normal subjects, there are complex and poorly explicated assumptions that underlie the use of the data in theory construction. Thus, the discussion that follows on the relationship between aphasia data and neuropsychological theory should not be construed as assigning a more problematical status to data obtained with aphasic patients than in the analogous situation with normal subjects.

How does one draw inferences about normal processes from aphasia data? The inferential process is based upon observations of patterns of impaired and spared functions. In the ideal situation, one is able to show that a patient's performance is normal in tasks that do not require the functioning of a particular process but that performance is impaired when that process is necessarily implicated in some task. Furthermore, one is able to show that the impaired performance can reasonably be considered to reflect the functioning of the residual, unimpaired process. In other words, it is assumed that aphasia data represents the working of the normal cognitive system after the removal (subtraction) of a hypothesized impaired linguistic (cognitive) process. To accept the logic of this inferential process, one must assume that cognitive processes are represented as independent components that can be selectively disrupted, consequent to brain damage. Aphasia would represent, then, the fractionation along natural boundaries of the normal language-processing system.

Even if one were to assume that, on occasion, brain damage produces the total and selective disturbance of a single processing component, one cannot assume that the patient's performance would directly reflect the absence of that processing component. Compensatory, "nonnormal" operations could come into play in such situations, leading to complex, indirect relationships between performance and the disrupted processing component. Thus, if cognitive components $x_1, x_2, \ldots x_i \ldots x_n$ were to be normally implicated in the performance of some task and component x_i were to be selectively impaired, the new operations implicated in the task would not necessarily be $(x_1, x_2, \ldots x_i \ldots x_n) - x_i$ but could be $[(x_1, x_2, \ldots x_i \ldots x_n) - x_i] + Y$, where Y represents either pathologically induced operations or suboptimal normal processing strategies, activated to compensate for the absence of x_i. However, it is assumed that, even if complex, the relationship between residual performance after brain damage and impaired processing components is, in principle, discoverable.

The assumption that one can discover the role of a processing component by looking at performance in its absence is one that has often been made in research with normals. For example, to examine the role of phonological coding in reading comprehension, researchers have required subjects to perform a secondary task that presumably occupies their phonological system while performing a main task involving reading comprehension (e.g., Baddeley & Hitch, 1974; Kleiman, 1975; Levy, 1975, 1977; Slowiaczek & Clifton, 1980). Even if one assumes that this secondary task effectively eliminates a processing component, the question of compensatory mechanisms coming into play for the main task could be raised in this research with normals. However, as in aphasia research, the relative contributions of components normally involved in a language function and compensatory strategies coming into play in a particular task are potentially discernible.

Unlike research with normals, however, the cognitive processing components revealed through the analysis of brain-damaged patients' performance can be correlated to the locus of insult in an attempt to localize processing mechanisms. In this case, the objective is to produce a neuroanatomical mapping of the individual processing components assumed to characterize a complex function such as language. For example, it could be hypothesized that the anterior regions of the language area (Broca's area and regions extending slightly posteriorly) subserve syntactic processing (Berndt & Caramazza, 1980). It is assumed here that the localized functions consist of basic processing components that have an independent status in cognitive theory (e.g., syntactic processes, auditory-verbal short-term memory storage, etc).

In the ideal case of localization of function, it is assumed that one can show a one-to-one correspondence between an impaired processing component and an associated locus of cerebral insult (e.g. Geschwind, 1965). This formulation of localization of function presupposes the entire inferential machinery assumed for the disruption of independent processing components from aphasic performance. In addition, however, one must assume that psychological processes are discretely represented in clearly defined regions of the brain. This classical, strong localizationist hypothesis, first proposed by Wernicke (1872; see Eggert, 1977), is not universally accepted and has been subjected to repeated criticism almost from the time it was first proposed (Freud, 1891/1953; Jackson, 1874/1958).

One extreme criticism of the localizationist hypothesis challenges the most basic assumptions of neuropsychological theory. It is argued that brain damage may disrupt one or more independent processing components (although the issue of independence is not critical for this argument) but that the behavioral consequences of the damage cannot be considered in terms of the normal functioning of the unimpaired components. Instead, it is assumed that the residual performance represents the functioning of a de novo reorganization of the unimpaired components that does not bear a transparent relationship to the original functioning of those components when they formed part of a normal system (Jackson, 1874/1958). It is clear that the assumed opacity between aphasic performance and normal cognitive operations not only makes localization of function impossible but also undermines the possibility of using pathological data to draw inferences about normal process. While this view may ultimately prove to be correct, it has little heuristic value as an alternative to the strong localizationist hypothesis. A more reasonable hypothesis is the position that brain damage may induce some compensatory operations that reflect suboptimal strategies available to the normal system. In this way the pathological performance continues to have a discoverable, albeit complex, relationship to the normal system.

A less extreme criticism of the strong localizationist hypothesis maintains that, even in the ideal situation where one-to-one relationship can be established between locus of insult and hypothesized processing component, one cannot draw the inference that brain tissue constitutes the neuroanatomical substrate for the correlated process (e.g., Luria, 1973). Proponents of this criticism point out that the damaged area is necessary for the hypothesized process and not that the damaged area actually carries out the process. However, since the strong (necessary and sufficient) and the weak (necessary) hypotheses are empirically indistinguishable, the localization hypothesis will be stated here in its stronger form.

The goal of neuropsychological theory of language, as presented here, is to propose a set of statements about the processing components that underlie normal language use and about the neuroanatomical realization of these processes in the normal brain. Several possible problems that may undermine the enterprise have been indicated, but it is also argued that there are no compelling logical grounds on which to base an a priori refutation of neuropsychological theory. The sections that follow will consider the methodological problems that are encountered in developing the empirical basis for neuropsychological theory.

GROUP RESEARCH METHODOLOGY AND THE PROBLEM OF PATIENT CLASSIFICATION

Psychological research with normal subjects makes extensive and almost exclusive use of group research methodology. The procedure and rationale for the use of this methodology are relatively straightforward. A hypothesis, usually stated in terms of the characteristics of some hypothesized process, is formulated for experimental assessment. For example, it could be hypothesized that information stored in short-term memory (STM) is retrieved in serial order. A task assumed to require storage and subsequent retrieval of information from STM is chosen. Continuing with this example, one could choose a task — the probe recognition paradigm — in which a subject is presented from trial to trial with to-be-remembered word sets of different size and then must decide whether a probe word is or is not a member of the memory set. The STM serial scanning and comparison hypothesis predicts that positive and negative trial reaction times (RT) should be parallel, linear functions of memory-set size. This hypothesis can be tested experimentally by having a group of subjects perform the task described, averaging the subjects' RTs, and testing the mean RT of different set sizes for linearity and the absence of interactions between negative and positive trial performance.

The advantage of the group research method is that findings from the group can be generalized by statistical means to the population from which the group was presumably drawn. The validity of the generalization from the average results of a group to normal psychological processing in general rests upon the assumption that cognitive processes function similarly in all normal individuals. Corollaries of this assumption are that people normally scan information stored in STM serially and that variation among subjects in deviations from parallelism between positive and negative trials and variations in scanning rates are distributed randomly about true values among members of the population (ignore for the moment within-subject error variation).

The assumptions that subjects in group research are drawn from a homogeneous population and that subject variation in performance can be considered to be a random factor irrelevant of the theoretical issues investigated are not strongly challenged in scientific practice. For the most part, acceptance of these assumptions has not led to strange conclusions about cognitive theory. There are, however, situations in which variations in performance among subjects cannot be considered simply as a random factor of no theoretical relevance. In such cases, averaging performance across subjects can lead to grossly distorted conclusions about cognitive processing. However, there are statistical procedures that can be used to assess the degree of group heterogeneity, and steps can be taken to analyze separately homogeneous subgroups to reveal alternative processing strategies available to subjects (see Martin & Caramazza, 1980). The example used here, memory scanning, is an instance of a situation in which individual differences have been assumed to reflect important cognitive processing differences and not just irrelevant random variation (Hunt, Frost, & Lunneborg, 1974).

The group research method became the major methodological paradigm in neuropsychological research in the mid-1950s (e.g., the work of Teuber and Weinstein). Performance of groups of aphasic patients is compared with the performance of appropriate control groups in an effort to describe both qualitatively and quantitatively the nature of language impairments produced by brain damage. If this research method is to generate valid conclusions about language disorders and neuropsychological theory, one must be able to defend some form of the assumption of homogeneity of target populations (e.g., aphasics). However, the assumption of group homogeneity is extremely difficult to defend in aphasia research, and special precautions are needed for the use of group research methodology in neuropsychological research.

There are several different types of criteria that have been used to define target populations in aphasia research. One distinction is based strictly upon considerations of locus of brain damage. In this case, the target populations can be defined by the presence of unilateral brain damage to either the right or left hemisphere. The performance of groups thus defined is compared across a wide range of tasks implicating various psychological functions (e.g., auditory and visual perception, speech comprehension, object naming, etc.). Performance can also be compared for more narrowly defined groups. The definition of group membership can be specified not just in terms of damage to left or right hemisphere but in terms of damage to gross anatomical hemispheric landmarks such as left parietal region, right temporal region, and so on. There is a considerable body of published research with this methodology that has provided important information about gross localization of function, for example, the left temporoparietal area is important for language comprehension (see Boller, Kim, & Mack, 1977). The use of new, sophisticated, lesion-localization techniques continues to provide important function-localization information (e.g., Naeser & Hayward, 1978).

Although, in principle, the logic of defining groups in terms of lesion site provides an important method for the development of neuropsychological theory, in practice it has not led to remarkable results concerning the localization of cognitive processes (as opposed to localization of gross psychological functions such as "comprehension"). Furthermore, even with new, relatively precise lesion-localizing techniques, it is not obvious what criteria should be applied to safeguard against violation of the group homogeneity assumption and, therefore, whether this methodology would allow valid conclusions about localization of processing components.

Essentially, there are two related issues that must be resolved for the valid application of lesion-site grouping criteria to group research. One concerns the degree of variability in localization of function in normal brains; the other concerns the feasibility of having any reasonable degree of lesion site and size overlap for accidentally produced lesions. Unfortunately, there is no simple way of answering these questions at this time. However, even if one could assume that there are only small individual differences in function localization and that it is practical to consider the testing of groups of patients with lesion site and size that are approximately the same, small quantitative differences could have important, qualititive consequences upon performance. In other words, one could group together functionally heterogeneous subjects because of the differential involvement of various processing components in different patients.

Another criterion used to group patients, also used extensively since the mid-1950s (e.g., the work of Goodglass), is syndrome type. In this case, the emphasis is primarily on behavior. Patients are grouped together on the basis of co-occurring patterns of symptoms. For example, aphasic patients who speak effortfully, misarticulate words, and have a reduced spontaneous output and relatively good comprehension are classified as Broca's aphasics and could be grouped together for comparison with other patient types. However, grouping by syndrome type is no less problematical than grouping by lesion site and, in fact, there are practical reasons that make it easier to misuse the syndrome-criterion grouping procedure.

Presumably, the basic motivation for using a syndrome-criterion grouping procedure is the assumption that patients thus grouped share an impairment to a common processing system. Comparison of different patient types would allow inferences about the functioning of different patient-type processing components. Logically, this grouping procedure is a valid one, and its use has led to important results concerning the nature of language impairments (e.g., Goodglass, 1968). Nonetheless, there are serious theoretical and practical problems associated with the use of this grouping procedure, specifically with regard to the violation of the assumption of group homogeneity.

The theoretical problem concerns the definition of syndrome types. Syndromes are empirically derived concepts that have been defined in terms of patterns of co-occurrence of symptoms as, for example, the definition of Broca's aphasia. The symptoms, in turn, consist of gross behavioral features such as comprehension, repetition, articulation, and so forth. While the notion of syndrome presented here may have heuristic value in a clinical setting, it is much too poorly specified to play the role of defining group membership in neuropsychological research. Several factors support this contention.

One factor is the question of what constitutes impaired performance such that it may qualify as a symptom. There are certainly many cases in which it is clear that a patient does or does not have an impairment in a particular aspect of language, but there are also cases where it is uncertain that a patient has a sufficient degree of difficulty such that one would confidently attribute a particular symptom to that individual. This problem is magnified when there are several conditions that must be satisfied for inclusion in the patient category. The intrinsic vagueness in the definition of a syndrome cannot be avoided nor can it be ignored. Consequently, if one is to continue doing group research where groups are defined by syndrome type, one must develop unambiguous inclusion criteria that take into consideration the problem of syndrome vagueness.

A more serious problem concerns the choice of gross behavioral features to define symptoms. The original choices of identifying symptoms in terms of functions, such as comprehension, were made before there had been much progress delineating the psychological components of those gross functions. These choices may have historical value, but it is doubtful that they have current scientific merit. It is now obvious that functions such as comprehension or repetition are complex and involve a number of different cognitive/linguistic processes for normal execution. Such functions could be disrupted at several different levels of processing. Performance relevant to a gross function, such as comprehension, depends critically upon the choice of test material. This point is clarified by considering an example.

Consider the case of Broca's aphasia. The classical definition of this syndrome included the feature, "relatively good" or "near-normal" comprehension, as part of the syndrome description. Recent research has shown, however, that patients classified as Broca's aphasics by the classical definition have a severe comprehension impairment when syntactic analysis is required for a normal level of comprehension performance (e.g., Caramazza & Zurif, 1976). Thus, depending upon the type of comprehension test administered, one could show that Broca's aphasics have "near-normal" comprehension or that they have severely impaired comprehension.

A further complication that arises as a result of using performance of ill-specified complex functions to define syndromes is that patients with different underlying defects will be classified as belonging to the same syndrome type. A concrete example of this situation is the classification of patients as conduction aphasics. The major feature of this syndrome is the "disproportionate inability to repeat words," co-occurring with the relative preservation of other language functions. It has been argued, however, that poor performance of the complex function, "repetition," could arise from at least two different sources — a deficit in storage capacity of auditory-verbal STM or a deficit in the output encoding mechanism (Shallice & Warrington, 1977). Thus, classifying patients as conduction aphasics on the basis of poor performance in a repetition task could lead a researcher to include both types of patients in the experimental group, thus violating the homogeneity assumption of group research methodology. Further, different researchers could have different proportions of the two types in their samples. Consequently, the findings of one study may not replicate those of another simply because the researchers are testing groups that differ in the predominant underlying deficit.

A final consideration of the theoretical problems associated with syndrome-based grouping concerns the question of whether a single- or multiple-deficit explanation is required to account for the co-occurrence of symptoms within a given syndrome. A positive feature of this grouping method is the assumption that a single processing mechanism is disrupted in patients of a given syndrome type. However, it is becoming increasingly clear that the classical syndrome types cannot be explicated on the basis of single-deficit hypotheses. Complex syndromes such as Wernicke's aphasia, a syndrome defined by poor comprehension and fluent, paragrammatic speech, almost certainly involve impairments in phonological processing and lexical-semantic processing, and Broca's aphasia involves the disruption of syntactic processing and articulatory mechanisms (Berndt & Caramazza, 1980).

The theoretical difficulties that characterize the syndrome-criterion method for patient grouping are considerable. However, assuming that one wished to investigate a classically described syndrome to determine if global behavioral symptoms can be analyzed in terms of one or more specific processing impairments, one then encounters the practical problems associated with identifying members of a classically defined syndrome. There are two ways in which a patient could be classified—through clinical judgment or by performance on a standard aphasia battery. The clinical judgment approach is certainly inadequate for research purposes. Different investigators have different criteria for defining the presence of a symptom and different criteria for the definition of a syndrome. In this situation, results obtained by an investigator can be generalized only to patients who meet that investigator's subjective classification criteria.

The reasonable alternative is to use a standardized test battery; unfortunately, there is no test battery that is agreed upon by all investigators. In the United States the most widely used test battery for research purposes is the Boston Diagnostic Aphasia Examination (BDAE) (Goodglass & Kaplan, 1972). However, a substantial proportion of group research has used other test batteries, and comparisons between this latter research and that carried out with patients classified by the BDAE are difficult to make. It is impossible to provide prescriptive criteria for patient classification to the research community, but unless a common classification device is adopted, the problem of nongeneralizability across studies will remain. Similarly, the basic process of replication to confirm important results will be thwarted unless a common classification device is used in group research.

This discussion of group research has focused upon the validity of the assumption of group homogeneity in aphasia research. This assumption can be defended neither on theoretical nor on practical grounds. Unlike the case of research with normal subjects, when evaluating group performance of aphasic patients, one cannot consider the within-group variance as consisting primarily of random error variance but must seriously consider the possibility that a large part of this variance is caused by theoretically important individual differences. Consequently, special precautions should be taken when designing and interpreting aphasia research based upon group methodology.

THE CASE STUDY APPROACH

One way to solve the problem of group heterogeneity in aphasia research is to adopt the method of single case study. The single case study approach has a time-honored place in aphasia research. Research with this methodology formed the original basis for the classical syndrome typology in aphasia and has continued to play an important role in more recent times (e.g., Marshall & Newcombe, 1966). Furthermore, most if not all research in aphasia prior to the 1950s used the case study approach. This methodology was strongly criticized on the grounds that arbitrary decisions were taken with regard to the patients selected for study (e.g., Weisenberg & McBride, 1935). The factor that most likely contributed to the shift in methodology was not the criticism of the case study method but the increasingly more important role played by researchers trained as experimental psychologists in neuropsychological research. These researchers were able to introduce into neuropsychology the methodologically sophisticated experimental approach that had been developed in experimental psychology, where the assumption of group homogeneity is more likely to be valid. However, the case study method did not simply disappear; it continued to be used in reports of unusual neuropsychological cases, and over the past decade it has reacquired considerable favor as an "experimental" method in neuropsychological research.

Shallice (1979), in a thoughtful and comprehensive assessment of the case study approach, has considered several potential problems but concluded that the case study method offers "...the most promising neuropsychological technique for providing information on the functional organization of cognitive subsystems" (p. 183). This method does have an important positive feature; it allows extensive analysis of clear syndrome cases without the contaminating factor of heterogeneous variation. This property of the case study method is sufficiently important to warrant its more extensive use in neuropsychological research.

There are two possible uses for the case study method in neuropsychological research: the classical use of describing new or unusual dissociations of functions and its use as an experimental methodology to expand on or test already described patterns of dissociations within syndrome types. There is clearly no alternative to the case study method for describing new patterns of dissociations. This use is unchallenged and does not require extensive justification; it assumes that component parts of the cognitive system can be disrupted selectively and that individual cases that manifest patterns of functional dissociations, explicable by assuming the disruption of some cognitive processing component, will exist.

Leaving aside the problem of how to determine that performance in some task constitutes an impaired level of performance and is, therefore, a candidate for consideration as a symptom (see Shallice, 1979, for a clear discussion of this problem), there is the issue of how to test the claim that a set of symptoms necessarily co-occurs and thus constitutes the basis for defining a single processing-component deficit. In the simplest case, the existence of a counterexample—a patient in whom the set of symptoms is dissociated—is sufficient to falsify the single-deficit hypothesis. (Incidentally, it should be noted that, in the case of rare syndrome types, the likelihood of finding dissociations of symptoms is greater than the probability of finding co-occurrences if, in fact, the symptoms do not arise from a single deficit. This would be the case no matter what the probabilities of the individual symptoms, unless anatomical proximity of the brain areas subserving the different psychological mechanisms made it likely that, if one locus were damaged, another would be as well.)

There are, however, more complicated cases where dissociation of symptoms does not automatically imply a falsification of a single component-deficit hypothesis. In these cases, the dissociated symptom(s) can co-occur with other symptoms not found in the defining set of the original case, and the dissociated symptom can be assumed to result from an impairment to a different processing mechanism. One example of such a situation is the reported dissociation of asyntactic comprehension from agrammatic speech production (Caramazza, Basili, Koller, & Berndt, 1981). Given that the syntactic-deficit hypothesis of Broca's aphasia assumes the co-occurrence of agrammatism and asyntactic comprehension, the demonstrated dissociation of these two symptoms could be interpreted as a falsification of the syntactic-deficit hypothesis. However, the dissociation of asyntactic comprehension from agrammatism is accompanied by a deficit in auditory-verbal short-term memory. It has been argued that the asyntactic comprehension in this latter patient type results from a disruption of the auditory-verbal STM component and that asyntactic comprehension is necessarily associated with agrammatism (Caramazza, Basili, Koller & Berndt, 1981).

Unfortunately, the inductive approach discussed here does not guarantee that there is a one-to-one correspondence between patterns of dissociations and theoretical explanation. Thus, there will first be a need to confirm through "replication" that the obtained pattern of dissociations is not the fortuitous result of some accidental combination of factors (e.g., "abnormal" localization, premorbid "anomaly," etc.) but that it reflects universal cognitive properties. Furthermore, there is the need to systematically explore these patients' performance in order to help choose among competing explanations for the syndrome. An analysis of the logic underlying the use of case study methodology in replicating and extending earlier results reveals that this methodology is subject to the same type of difficulties, although possibly to a lesser extent, that have been discussed for the group study methodology.

Consider first the problem of replication of single case studies. What constitutes replication? One way to replicate a single case study is to find another patient who manifests all, and no more than, the behavioral features used to define the original case reported. In other words, replication is simply the successful classification of a new case as a member of a previously defined syndrome. Consider next the problem of testing specific predictions, based upon alternative hypotheses of the underlying deficit in a particular patient. The research is essential for demonstrating generalizability across different patients presumed to be of the same type. For generalization to be accurate, one must be able to defend the assumption that the patients studied share a disruption of a common processing component. Here too, the critical issue concerns the possibility of unambiguous syndrome-type classification, albeit over an extended period of time, as opposed to the temporally concentrated case of group research. Consequently, at least at a theoretical level, the single case study method encounters similar problems to that of the group research method, with respect to the difficult issue of classification by patient type for the purpose of generalization.

It could be argued that a major difference of theoretical importance between the single case and group research methods concerns the fact that data are averaged over subjects in the latter method. This averaging procedure could lead to serious errors of interpretation if the patient population is heterogeneous; in the single case study, this danger is avoided. However, this argument is only valid if one does not intend to generalize from the single case study to a patient population of the type represented by the single case studied. To the extent that generalization is desired, the presumed disadvantage of averaging is no longer defensible. Assuming that the criteria employed to define membership in a syndrome type are the same for the single case and group research studies, the degree of error introduced by group averaging is directly comparable to the degree of generalization error for comparisons across single case studies. Furthermore, it cannot be argued that, in the single case study approach, differences among patients are more easily detectable since individual differences analyses can be carried out with the group research method.

The problems of averaging have been minimized in this discussion in order to reveal a common difficulty shared by the single case and group research methods. In practice, however, it could very well turn out that group research encourages a greater degree of error, relative to single case studies. The reason for this difference is strictly practical in nature; whereas case studies are typically carried out with those rare patients who present relatively clear dissociations, group research methodology encourages grouping the more frequently occurring patients who generally present a more complicated pattern of impairments. A practical consequence of choice of methodology is that stricter classification criteria may be employed in single case studies than in group research studies.

Another practical advantage typically associated with single case studies is the extensive and detailed nature of these studies. Single case studies usually report a patient's performance on a wide range of tasks, allowing a greater possibility of detailed analysis of the cognitive mechanisms implicated in the disorders. However, the fact that case studies look at performance on a number of tasks relevant to specific processing mechanisms rather than at gross behavioral systems leads to the use of nonstandardized tests. At present, there is no set of tasks that researchers will agree tests for the presence or absence of single psychological components. However, there is, in principle, no reason that standardized tests could not be developed to test for specific psychological components such as syntactic processing or phonological coding.

The preceding discussion has fostered the impression that, at least on practical grounds, the case study method is to be preferred to the group research method. However, while the case study method plays a crucial role in identifying new patterns of dissociations, and, more generally, in generating hypotheses about the fractionation of the cognitive system, it is not to be preferred to the group research method for testing hypotheses. The reason for this conclusion concerns the problem of interpreting performance variation among patients in single case studies. Specifically, working with single cases does not allow any reasonable, quantitative procedure for assessing the degree of variation across patients. Thus, interpretation of differences in level of performance among patients remains problematical.

Is a difference sufficiently large and important enough to justify the classification of the patients in different syndrome types, or is the difference within the range of random variation for that patient type? The only way one can estimate within-type random variation is to perform group studies. Thus, group studies are to be preferred to single case studies in testing hypotheses about patient types. However, this conclusion is equally problematical; the only way that group studies could be used to assess within-group variation is to accept the assumption that patients included within the group are members of the same class. If there are any doubts about the classification procedures, and there may be grave doubts, specific guidelines must be developed for assessing the within-group variation for possible violations of group homogeneity. Thus, it would appear that the appropriate methodological paradigm is one that allows individual difference analyses within a group research paradigm.

TOWARD A PARTIAL RESOLUTION OF THE PROBLEM OF PATIENT HOMOGENEITY

The previous two sections have presented a rather pessimistic account of the methodological problems associated with research of brain-damaged patient populations. The point has been made that performance variation among patients putatively considered to belong to the same syndrome type may, in fact, consist of important differences that reflect the differential involvement of mechanisms other than the assumed impaired processing component. Paradoxically, the very source of difficulty that underlies the development of adequate methodological paradigms for research with brain-damaged patients also provides a major motivation for the use of pathological cases to understand normal function. The fact that the normal cognitive system can be disrupted in various ways allows us to explore systematically in experiments-of-nature the rich network of interactions among cognitive subsystems. Thus, if it were to turn out that performance variation among patients classified as belonging to the same syndrome type resulted from the differential involvement of diverse mechanisms and if one could develop a methodological paradigm that permitted a systematic analysis of the observed differences, one would, in principle, be able to explicate the contribution of various processing components in complex functions, such as language comprehension.

What is suggested in effect, is that methodological paradigms for the study of aphasia must not only be designed to explore the major patterns of associations and dissociations of symptoms but must also be sufficiently powerful to permit the quantification of within-syndrome variations and the subsequent systematic analysis of any observed variations. Over the past several years we have been developing a methodological paradigm that we have called, unimaginatively, the *group/case study method.* This method was developed in response to the need for quantifying potentially important within-syndrome variation.

As indicated by the name, the method consists of a series of case studies carried out concurrently. The procedure is as follows:

1. Patient's language abilities are assessed through standardized aphasia and neuropsychological batteries as well as other specialized tests to determine an initial classification of patients. Patients who fall into the target syndrome category and control syndrome categories are selected for study. For example, if we were interested in the analysis of syntactic processing in various language functions, we would choose as our target population Broca's aphasics because of their hypothesized syntactic processing deficit, and as control patients conduction aphasics, who show asyntactic comprehension but not agrammatic speech;

Wernicke's aphasics, who presumably have a lexical processing defect; and a normal control group.

2. The patients selected for study are then tested on a wide range of experimental tasks. The tasks are designed to satisfy at least the following criteria: the tasks should assess a wide range of performances implicating the syndrome's defining symptoms as well as the presumed intact functions; and each functional component (e.g., comprehension) is assessed through several tasks such that together they implicate, in addition to the critical processing component assumed to be disrupted, various other processing components.

3. Individual patient's performance in the experimental tasks is evaluated, focusing especially on patterns of systematic similarities and differences among patients of the same syndrome type. Variation in performance is not automatically assumed to be random noise. Instead, specific new experimental tasks are designed to explore further the observed variation in order to determine whether or not it reflects the influence of other impaired mechanisms. Differences in performance within a group are pursued until a motivated account can be given for the noted variation. Averaging among patients is performed once group homogeneity has been satisfactorily determined.

The advantages of this approach are substantial and obvious. Equally obvious, however, are the limitations and problems. One problem is concerned with restricted usefulness. The group/case study method can be used with patients with commonly occurring syndromes. However, some patient types occur so rarely (e.g., pure word deafness) that it is extremely unlikely that one could form a group of such patients for study. Another problem concerns the cost of this type of research. To be able to test a group of patients in the extensive fashion proposed requires considerable investment of both time and money. This approach can be used only by large research groups that will be able to generate the extensive testing material and devote the time to test many subjects with the experimental battery.

While the group/case study method requires a considerable investment and seems impractical for use with rare syndromes, it may be necessary to use it in order to establish a clear and unambiguous empirical foundation for the development of neuropsychological theory. These types of problems are not uncommon in other scientific disciplines, but those scientists have adapted to the problems and managed to overcome them. For example, the problem of high cost and rarity of events is solved by astrophysicists by forming research consortia, through which research groups and individual researchers can pool resources. In a similar fashion, one could develop research consortia for the study of particular rare syndromes; rare patient-type groups could be formed by grouping patients available to consortium members. The practical problems associated with the formation of consortia are not inconsiderable, but neither are they irresolvable.

MECHANISMS OF COMPREHENSION REVEALED THROUGH THE STUDY OF APHASIA

The discussion of the methodological problems associated with research in aphasia has focused upon the problem of patient heterogeneity and its consequences for the validity of strong inferences about brain/function relations based upon data from aphasics. It has been concluded that extreme caution must be exercised when using either the group or case study approaches in drawing general conclusions about the processing mechanisms revealed by pathological performance. These difficulties are an inherent part of the research area, and there is no simple methodological solution to them. Nonetheless, despite these problems, there is now a rich data base on language and related cognitive disorders that allows important conclusions about cognitive and neuropsychological theory. These conclusions must be considered as preliminary since they are based upon experimental results and observations that have not received extensive verification. However, even in these circumstances, it is possible to outline some general conclusions about cognitive mechanisms. The following discussion will focus upon the problem of comprehension.

Language comprehension is a complex function that implicates a wide range of processing mechanisms. Even a simple, intuitive analysis of this function suggests that one must distinguish among perceptual, lexical, and syntactic processes. Linguistic and psycholinguistic evidence can be adduced to motivate and support a more rigorous analysis of the comprehension process in terms of distinct levels of linguistic analysis—phonological, lexical, and syntactic. In addition to these more linguistically motivated components, various theorists have assumed that a working memory component is necessary to support normal comprehension of sentences.

An aphasic patient's failure to comprehend a sentence could be caused by an impairment at any or any combination of these levels. Consequently, an analysis of language comprehension disorders must be sensitive to distinctions in patterns of failures that may reflect differential involvement of diverse processing components. Recent neuropsychological investigations have made considerable progress in identifying the factors that contribute to different patterns of aphasic performance.

A historically and theoretically important contrast in patterns of language impairments is that between Broca's and Wernicke's aphasics. Clinically, Broca's aphasics are patients who manifest a distinctive language production disorder that appears disproportionate to their language comprehension ability. The output of these patients consists of awkwardly articulated, agrammatic word sequences. That is, these patients tend to omit syntactically important grammatical morphemes such as auxiliary verbs, modals, prepositions, verb tenses, and number markers. In contrast, Wernicke's aphasics are clinically judged to have poor comprehension at both the word and sentence level, but their speech output is fluent although paragrammatic. The distinctive characteristic of paragrammatic speech is the clear presence of grammatical morphemes in sentencelike ungrammatical sequences.

If one bases the explanations of the two syndrome types on the clinical descriptions, the most reasonable conclusion would be that comprehension and production mechanisms of sentence analysis are independent processes that can be disrupted selectively. However, recent experimental evidence suggests that those deficits seen in Broca's aphasics' production are mirrored in their comprehension. That is, it appears that patients of this type fail to comprehend sentences in those tasks in which correct performance depends upon a normal ability to carry out syntactic analysis of the sentences (Caramazza, Berndt, Basili & Koller, 1981; Caramazza & Zurif, 1976; Deloche & Seron, 1981; Goodglass, Blumstein, Gleason et al., 1979; Heilman & Scholes, 1976; Schwartz, Saffran, & Marin, 1980). In light of this latter result, a natural reinterpretation of the Broca syndrome is in terms of the co-occurrence of agrammatic speech and asyntactic comprehension (see Berndt & Caramazza, 1980, for an extensive discussion of this point), which, in turn, motivates the theoretical inference that the underlying mechanism affected in this syndrome type is the syntactic-processing system.

It is important at this point to make explicit the logic motivating the inference of a syntactic-processing defect in Broca's aphasia. As discussed earlier, the assumption is made that a minimal requirement for inferring that linguistic processing is impaired is that the patient perfᵒᵣm poorly on all tasks requiring this component. In the case of Broca's aphasia, it has thus far been shown that patients of this type not only are agrammatic and have asyntactic comprehension but also perform "agrammatically" in tasks requiring judgments of within-sentence relatedness (Zurif, Caramazza, & Myerson, 1972; Zurif, Green, Caramazza, & Goodenough, 1976) and in sentence anagram tasks (Caramazza, Berndt, Basili, & Koller, 1981; von Stockert & Bader, 1976). Thus, there appears to be a coherent set of results that permits the conclusion that the syntactic-processing component is an independent processing mechanism that can be selectively disrupted in aphasia. This issue is far from settled, however. Several different types of objections have been raised against the syntactic-processing-deficit hypothesis of Broca's aphasia.

Two types of problems are directly relevant to the issues under consideration in this chapter. One of these concerns the general question of falsification of a hypothesis and, specifically, whether or not Broca's aphasics have a syntactic-processing comprehension impairment. Two recent reports have concluded that Broca's aphasics do not have a comprehension defect resulting specifically from an inability to carry out syntactic processing (Heeschen, 1980; Mack, 1981). Both Heeschen and Mack report that Broca's aphasics do not differ qualitatively from Wernicke's aphasics in sentence comprehension performance. Unfortunately, these studies do not present fair tests of the syntactic-deficit hypothesis, so it is difficult to assess their value with respect to the question of the nature of the impairment underlying Broca's aphasia.

In the case of the report by Mack, the comprehension performance of three groups of aphasic patients — nonfluent, mixed anteriors (nonfluent with poor comprehension), and fluents — were tested, using a modified version of the Token Test (DeRenzi & Vignolo, 1962). The original Token Test tested comprehension of increasingly more complex commands of the sort, "Touch the red circle" or "Touch the blue square with the red triangle." The modified version was constructed presumably to allow for independent assessment of syntactic and semantic comprehension. Nonfluent patients, which Mack equates with Broca's aphasics, were found to be no more impaired than the fluents on those items assumed to test for syntactic comprehension. Thus, he concluded that the syntactic-comprehension deficit is a generalized aphasic deficit and not one specific to Broca's aphasics. This conclusion is unwarranted on two grounds. The first is that, for many of his items where an error was judged to be syntactic, good performance required only comprehension of a locative preposition and a reference token. Since Broca's aphasics do not have difficulty with assigning references to concrete nouns and appear to understand the semantic content of locative prepositions (Schwartz, Saffran, & Marin, 1980), Broca's aphasics would not have been expected to be particularly impaired on these items. Leaving aside the issue of whether Mack's task tested syntactic comprehension, the second objection to his conclusion, and the objection relevant to the issue of classification, concerns his use of patients characterized as nonfluent to test the hypothesis of a syntactic impairment in Broca's aphasia. No mention is made of whether the patients were agrammatic as well as nonfluent; this is a critical component since the syntactic-deficit hypothesis links agrammatic speech with asyntactic comprehension.

A similar objection can be made to the work of Heeschen (1980). Here the test materials were adequate to test for syntactic comprehension, although it is not clear that his method of data analysis allows one to distinguish between difficulties due to semantic or to syntactic impairments (Caramazza, in press). He also does not state whether the Broca's aphasics whom he tested were agrammatic. Without this information, it is impossible to assess the relevance of the work of either Heeschen or Mack to the syntactic-deficit hypothesis. More generally, future work must specify unambiguously the defining features of the classification scheme employed and the extent to which patients satisfy those criteria.

The other issue to be considered here is also the most difficult one. It has been stated that the syntactic-deficit hypothesis of Broca's aphasia requires that these patients present performance difficulties in all tasks that implicate syntactic processing in some form. The logic motivating this argument is self-evident; one can only assume that a component of processing is impaired if it malfunctions in all possible implementations of the component. Thus, if cases exist that show a dissociation of the defining symptoms of a syndrome (e.g., an ability to perform some tasks that require syntactic processing but not others), it could mean either that there is no necessary unifying factor underlying the symptom complex and hence no need to postulate upon impairment to a single processing component or that the dissociated symptom results from an impairment to some mechanism crucial to the normal function of the target component of processing (syntactic processor in this case). For example, in the case of patients with impaired auditory-verbal STM, who show asyntactic comprehension impairments but not agrammatic production, it has been assumed that the comprehension deficit results from the inefficient use of syntactic processes in the face of an impaired working memory (Caramazza, Basili, Koller, & Berndt, 1981). This conclusion, based on a single case report, must be replicated and extended. However, it can be seen that the dissociation of symptoms from a symptom complex does not necessarily mean that any dissociation automatically falsifies single-component explanations of syndromes.

Not all dissociations can be accounted for in terms of deficits to supporting (necessary but not sufficient) mechanisms. An example of a dissociation that would undermine the syntactic-deficit hypothesis of Broca's aphasia would be a case presenting asyntactic comprehension for visually but not aurally presented sentences, or a case of a patient who is agrammatic in oral production but not in written production. We are not aware of published cases that show such remarkable dissociations. Should such cases exist, however, it would be critical to fully document the patients' cognitive and linguistic processing abilities to rule out unlikely, but possible, explanations based upon assumptions of deficits to support mechanisms.

The dearth of clear information on patterns of dissociations in Broca's aphasia probably results from a combination of theoretical and methodological lack of sophistication. The poverty of theory is indicated by the conspicuous absence of detailed accounts of how features of agrammatism and asyntactic comprehension might result from an impairment to a common processing component. Similarly, on the empirical side, it is still necessary to provide a detailed description of the co-occurrence of agrammatism and asyntactic comprehension, which is necessary to defend a well-articulated hypothesis of a syntactic-processing defect in Broca's aphasia. Current claims about the co-occurrence of symptoms in Broca's aphasia are based upon suggestive but vague notions of both agrammatism and asyntactic comprehension. This is especially the case for the evidence from those group studies that have considered production and comprehension impairments separately. For example, in those cases for which the primary focus was on comprehension, no direct assessment of agrammatism was undertaken. Instead, Broca's aphasics were considered to be agrammatic without further specification of the nature of agrammatism and certainly not the specific form of agrammatic productions of the patients whose comprehension performance was being tested. There are several papers that have presented data on speech production and comprehension for the same patients (Caramazza, Berndt, Basili, & Koller, 1981; Saffran, Schwartz, & Marin, 1980; Schwartz, Saffran, & Marin, 1980); however, even in these latter cases, the level of analysis is far from satisfactory. Neither of these groups of researchers provides a detailed analysis of the agrammatism of their Broca's aphasics. It is clear that one must move beyond the vague level of description that characterizes much of the current work in this area. This step will necessarily entail serious considerations of methodology as well as theory.

The issues considered thus far concern the analysis of comprehension defects in terms of a syntactic-processing impairment and of an auditory-verbal STM limitation. However, the comprehension defect in Wernicke's aphasia cannot be explained in terms of impairments to either the syntactic component or to memory. It has been assumed, instead, that for at least a subset of the Wernicke-type aphasic, a lexical-semantic deficit underlies poor sentence comprehension (e.g., Caramazza & Berndt, 1978). However, this latter claim is not based upon detailed experimental evidence. Given the complexity and possible heterogeneity of the Wernicke syndrome, it is unclear at this time what the bases are for the poor sentence comprehension in these patients. It is premature to exclude the possibility that some Wernicke's aphasics may have poor comprehension because of a phonological processing defect, as suggested by Luria (1947/1970). Blumstein, Baker, and Goodglass (1977) have shown that there is no direct relationship between phonemic processing impairments and sentence comprehension performance. However, in a later paper, these same authors (Baker, Blumstein, & Goodglass, 1981) concluded that both phonological and lexical-semantic processing impairments contribute to the poor sentence comprehension performance in Wernicke's aphasics. It appears, then, that Wernicke's aphasia is a heterogeneous syndrome that includes patients with lexical-semantic defects and with phonological processing defects. These two processing mechanisms are independent and can be dissociated. We have recently documented a clear dissociation of these two processing mechanisms in a patient with a pure phonological processing defect and have assessed the consequences of this impairment for sentence comprehension (Caramazza, Berndt, & Basili, 1981).

Patient J.S. could not be classified easily. He could not understand aurally presented words and sentences but seemed to be able to understand visually presented words and sentences quite well. His speech output was fluent and paragrammatic with occasional neologisms. An extensive investigation of this patient's phonological processing ability revealed that he could not discriminate syllables at a phonetic level and could not discriminate words from nonwords when presented aurally, but performed comparably to normal controls with visually presented stimuli. In tasks that required phonological recoding of visually presented stimuli, he performed at chance level. In contrast with his poor performance in phonological processing, J.S. performed normally in lexical and lexical-semantic processing, as assessed by his comprehension of single words. Careful testing of his comprehension of written sentences showed that he understood such sentences only when semantic plausibility could be used to assign grammatical role relations. With reversible sentences (e.g., "the dog was chased by the cat") that require an analysis of syntax for their comprehension, he performed poorly. Thus, J.S.'s comprehension of visually presented sentences was asyntactic. We have interpreted this pattern of results as indicating that normal comprehension of visually presented sentences requires a phonological recoding process. It is assumed here that syntactic processes require the support of a phonologically based working memory. Since J.S. could not recode visually presented words into a phonological format, he could use only the lexical-semantic information in a sentence and thus comprehend asyntactically (see Caramazza, Berndt, & Basili, 1981; Martin & Caramazza, 1982; for further discussion).

We have included this case here for several reasons: first, because at face value, his performance would suggest a dissociation between asyntactic comprehension and agrammatic speech, but, as was the case for the conduction aphasic, his asyntactic comprehension can be shown to derive from a disruption of the STM system used to support syntactic analysis. Secondly, the case is interesting from a theoretical viewpoint because it suggests the possibility that a component of processing involved in normal comprehension of both aurally and visually presented sentences is a phonologically based memory. (This position is consistent with the earlier discussion of comprehension in patients with auditory-verbal STM defects). The final reason concerns the heuristic value of this case for the earlier discussion of methodological problems in case studies. We will now focus upon the problem of classification of our patient as pure word deaf and generally upon the problems of classification in single case studies.

J.S.'s performance is, in many respects, similar to that of pure word-deaf patients. A dissociation between visual and auditory language processing is the characteristic feature of pure word deafness. However, J.S.'s comprehension of visually presented sentences was not normal but asyntactic, and his speech was paraphasic and paragrammatic. These aphasic symptoms are not generally considered to be part of the pure word-deafness syndrome. Are we justified, then, in calling our patient pure word deaf? A simple solution would be to classify our patient as a *phonological processing defect* patient. This "solution" avoids classifying the patient in terms of the classical syndrome but, at a more general level, does not solve the problem of classification. Thus, we are left with three choices. We could assume that other pure word-deaf patients had aphasic symptoms similar to our patient's that were not noted because of "inadequate" testing; or we might assume that, given our patient's paraphasic and paragrammatic speech, he should be classified as a Wernicke's aphasic; or we might consider the possibility that the patient type we have described forms a distinct, new syndrome type. Let us consider first the classification of our patient as pure word deaf. The discordant features in this classification are the asyntactic comprehension and paragrammatic speech. A review of the literature on pure word deafness reveals that a number of investigators have noted that this patient type does have subtle comprehension difficulties for visually presented sentences as well as speech problems (e.g., Goldstein, 1974). However, this does not mean that all the patients who have been classified as pure word deaf had aphasic symptoms. If we assume that there are cases that have all the symptoms of pure word deafness at the level of phonological processing described for our patient plus intact comprehension, the explanation that we have offered for J.S.'s comprehension failure would be incorrect. We would then have to assume that our patient's performance results from two independent processing defects — one that is responsible for the phonological processing impairments and another that is responsible for asyntactic comprehension.

Another way to illustrate this issue of classification is to compare our case with that reported by Saffran, Marin, & Yeni-Komshian (1976). Saffran and colleagues reported an extensive investigation of a single case of pure word deafness, focusing on the patient's ability to process auditory information. They concluded that their patient had a defect at the level of prephonetic auditory processing. However, these authors did not systematically assess their patient's ability to phonologically recode visually presented material, as we had done in our case study. It is possible, then, that their patient may have had a phonological processing defect and not one restricted to a prephonetic level of processing. Alternatively, it is possible that their patient would have performed normally in the recoding tasks and thus have demonstrated a dissociation that suggests that a prephonetic level of processing can be disrupted independently of a more central phonological processing system.

An alternative classification of J.S. would be as a Wernicke's aphasic. This classification is no less problematical, however. Although classifying J.S. as a Wernicke is consistent with his speech problems, it does not easily accommodate the dissociation of visual and auditory language-processing ability that was noted. J.S. had no demonstrable lexical-semantic problems when stimuli were presented visually, and he could understand visually presented sentences quite well when the meaning of the sentence was consistent with the most plausible reading, given the major lexical items of the sentence. In contrast, he performed at chance on all tasks that required processing on auditory input. This remarkable dissociation is not characteristic of Wernicke's aphasics. Consequently, if we are to maintain Wernicke's aphasia as a coherent syndrome, we must exclude patients such as J.S. from this classification (see Hier & Mohr, 1977, for a different position).

At this point it would appear that the most reasonable conclusion is to define our patient's performance as a rare, new syndrome type. However, it must be emphasized that, if other "Wernicke" and "pure word-deaf" patients were tested in as detailed a manner as we have used, many such patients might have shown patterns of performance similar to that of J.S.

This discussion on the classification of J.S. demonstrates the problems involved in classification of even single cases. Some of the problems are obvious — vague classification schemes; the difficulty of comparing different cases; and the lack of detailed, exhaustive testing even in single case studies. A less clear but equally important problem concerns the possibility of falsifying hypotheses formulated on such cases. Specifically, depending upon the particular theoretical interests of the investigator(s), patients will be assessed on different language and cognitive functions, making it difficult (if not impossible) to provide an undisputed data base from which theoretical issues can be resolved in a systematic, analytical fashion.

By focusing upon the problems that characterize single case study research, we do not wish to convey the impression that this methodology is to be avoided. On the contrary, we think that the logic of case study research should form the core of research on language pathology. This classical approach does, after all, provide the richest source of data on symptom co-occurrence and symptom dissociation. Extensive data are now available on many important syndromes (for information on deep dyslexia, see Coltheart, 1980), making it possible to formulate increasingly sophisticated hypotheses about the structure of neuropsychological theory. It is hoped that more researchers will adopt the group/case study approach in order to overcome some of the problems inherent in single case study methodology.

In conclusion, returning briefly to the discussion of language comprehension mechanisms, it appears that, although many issues remain unsettled, the study of aphasia allows systematic exploration of the interaction of various processing components implicated in normal language comprehension. Specifically, there are data from aphasia that suggest that, despite the caveats noted above, syntactic processes are an autonomous set of operations (and thus can be disrupted selectively), that these syntactic processes are dependent upon a normal working memory for their execution, and that the code of working memory for normal syntactic analysis may be phonological in nature. While these conclusions may ultimately prove to be false, they do provide a coherent framework for understanding language processing and for guiding research in the pathology of language.

ACKNOWLEDGMENTS

The preparation of this manuscript was supported by NIH Grant Nos. 16155 and 14099 to The Johns Hopkins University. We would like to thank Rita Sloan Berndt for her incisive comments on an earlier version of this chapter, and would also like to acknowledge her contribution in the development of many of the ideas discussed in this chapter.

REFERENCES

Baddeley, A.D., & Hitch, G. Working memory. In G.H. Bower (Ed.), *The psychology of learning and motivation: Advances in research and theory* (Vol. 8). New York: Academic Press, 1974.

Baker, E., Blumstein, S.E., & Goodglass, H. Interaction between phonological and semantic factors in auditory comprehension. *Neuropsychology*, 1981, *19*, 1–15.

Berndt, R.S., & Caramazza, A. A redefinition of Broca's aphasia: Implications for a neuropsychological model of language. *Applied Psycholinguistics*, 1980, *1*, 225–278.

Blumstein, S.E., Baker, E., & Goodglass, H. Phonological factors in auditory comprehension in aphasia. *Neuropsychologia*, 1977, *15*, 19–30.

Boller, F., Kim, Y., & Mack, J. Auditory comprehension in aphasia. In H. Whitaker & H.A. Whitaker (Eds.), *Studies in Neurolinguistics* (Vol. 3), New York: Academic Press, 1977.

Caramazza, A. A comment on Heeschen's "Strategies of decoding actor-object relations by aphasic patients." *Cortex*, in press.

Caramazza, A., Basili, A., Koller, J., & Berndt, R. An investigation of repetition and language processing in a case of conduction aphasia. *Brain and Language*, 1981, *14*, 235–271.

Caramazza, A., & Berndt, R.S. Semantic and syntactic processes in aphasia: A review of the literature. *Psychological Bulletin*, 1978, *85*, 898–918.

Caramazza, A., Berndt, R.S., & Basili, A. The selective impairment of phonological processing. Unpublished manuscript. The Johns Hopkins University, 1981.

Caramazza, A., Berndt, R.S., Basili, A., & Koller, J.J. Syntactic processing deficits in aphasia. *Cortex*, 1981, *17*, 333–348.

Caramazza, A., & Zurif, E.B. Dissociation of algorithmic and heuristic processes in language comprehension: Evidence from aphasia. *Brain and Language*, 1976, *3*, 572–582.

Coltheart, M. Deep dyslexia: A right-hemisphere hypothesis. In M. Coltheart, K. Patterson, & J.C. Marshall (Eds.), *Deep dyslexia*. London: Routledge and Kegan Paul, 1980.

Deloche, G., & Seron, X. Sentence understanding and knowledge of the world: Evidence from a sentence-picture matching task performed by aphasic patients. *Brain and Language*, 1981, *14*, 57–69.

DeRenzi, E., & Vignolo, L.A. The token test: A sensitive test to detect receptive disturbances in aphasics. *Brain*, 1962, *85*, 665–678.

Eggert, G.H. *Wernicke's works on aphasia*. The Hague: Mouton, 1977.

Freud, S. [*On aphasia*] (E. Stendle, trans.). London: Imago, 1953. (Originally published, 1891).

Geschwind, N. Disconnection syndromes in animals and man. *Brain*, 1965, *88*, 237–294; 585–644.

Goldstein, M.N. Auditory agnosia for speech ("pure word-deafness"): A historical review with current implications. *Brain and Language*, 1974, *1*, 195–204.

Goodglass, H. Studies on the grammar of aphasics. In S. Rosenberg and K. Joplin (Eds.), *Developments in applied psycholinguistics research*. New York: Macmillan, 1968.

Goodglass, H., Blumstein, S.E., Gleason, J.B., et al. The effect of syntactic encoding of sentence comprehension in aphasia. *Brain and Language*, 1979, *7*, 201–209.

Goodglass, H., & Kaplan, E. *The assessment of aphasia and related disorders*. Philadelphia: Lea & Febiger, 1972.

Heeschen, C. Strategies of decoding actor-object relations by aphasic patients. *Cortex*, 1980, *16*, 5–19.

Heilman, K.M., & Scholes, R.J. The nature of comprehension errors in Broca's conduction and Wernicke's aphasics. *Cortex*, 1976, *12*, 258–265.

Hier, D.B., & Mohr, J.P. Incongrous oral and written naming: Evidence for a subdivision of the syndrome of Wernicke's aphasia. *Brain and Language*, 1977, *4*, 115–126.

Hunt, E., Frost, N., & Lunneborg, C. Individual differences in cognition: A new approach to intelligence. In G. Bower (Ed.), *The psychology of learning and motivation* (Vol. 7). New York: Academic Press, 1974.

Jackson, J.H. On the nature of the duality of the brain. *Medical Press and Circular*, 1874, *1*, 19, 41, 63. (Reprinted in J. Taylor (Ed.), *Selected writings of John Hugling Jackson*. New York: Basic Books, 1958.)

Kleiman, G. Speech recoding in reading. *Journal of Verbal Learning and Verbal Behavior*, 1975, *14*, 323–339.

Levy, B.A. Vocalization and suppression effects in sentence memory. *Journal of Verbal Learning and Verbal Behavior*, 1975, *14*, 304–316.

Levy, B.A. Reading: Speech and meaning processes. *Journal of Verbal Learning and Verbal Behavior*, 1977, *16*, 623–638.

Luria, A.R. [*Traumatic aphasia*] (English translation). The Hague: Mouton, 1970. (Originally published, 1947).

Luria, A.R. [*The working brain: An introduction to neuropsychology*] (English translation by Basil Haigh). New York: Basic Books, 1973.

Mack, J. The comprehension of locative prepositions in nonfluent and fluent aphasia. *Brain and Language*, 1981, *14*, 81–92.

Marshall, J.C., & Newcombe, F. Syntactic and semantic errors in paralexia. *Neuropsychologia*, 1966, *4*, 169–176.

Martin, R.C., & Caramazza, A. Classification in well-defined and ill-defined categories: Evidence for common processing strategies. *Journal of Experimental Psychology: General*. 1980, *109*, 320–353.

Martin, R.C., & Caramazza, A. Short term memory performance in the absence of phonological coding. *Brain and Cognition*, 1982, *1*, 50–70.

Naeser, M.A., & Hayward, R.W. Lesion localization in aphasia with cranial computed tomography and the Boston Diagnostic Aphasia Exam. *Neurology*, 1978, *28*, 545–551.

Saffran, E.M., Marin, O.S.M., & Yeni-Komshian, G. An analysis of speech perception in word deafness. *Brain and Language*, 1976, *3*, 209–228.

Saffran, E.M., Schwartz, M.F., & Marin, O.S.M. The word order problem in agrammatism: II. Production. *Brain and Language*, 1980, *10*, 263–280.

Schwartz, M.F., Saffran, E.M., & Marin, O.S.M. The word order problem in agrammatism: I. Comprehension. *Brain and Language*, 1980, *10*, 249–262.

Shallice, T. Case study approach in neuropsychological research. *Journal of Clinical Neuropsychology*, 1979, *1*, 183–211.

Shallice, T., & Warrington, E.K. Auditory-verbal short-term memory impairment and conduction aphasia. *Brain and Language*, 1977, *4*, 479–491.

Slowiaczek, M.L., & Clifton, C. Subvocalization and reading for meaning. *Journal of Verbal Learning and Verbal Behavior*, 1980, *19*, 573–582.

von Stockert, T.R., & Bader, L. Some relations of grammar and lexicon in aphasia. *Cortex*, 1976, *12*, 49–60.

Weisenberg, T. & McBride, K. *Aphasia*. New York: Commonwealth Fund, 1935.

Zurif, E.B., Caramazza, A., & Myerson, R. Grammatical judgments of agrammatic aphasics. *Neuropsychologia*, 1972, *10*, 405–417.

Zurif, E.B., Green, E., Caramazza, A., & Goodenough, C. Grammatical intuitions of aphasic patients: Sensitivity to functors. *Cortex*, 1976, *12*, 183–186.

3

Methodological Issues in Clinical Studies of Right Cerebral Hemisphere Dysfunction

Manfred J. Meier
W. Gary Thompson

This chapter attempts to identify the methological issues that need to be addressed when conducting clinical research for the neuropsychological correlates of right cerebral hemisphere involvement. This requires a review of many independent variables that can affect neuropsychological outcomes of revelance to right hemisphere dysfunction in clinical populations. For the neuropsychologist interested in isolating behavioral deficits directly attributable to right hemisphere involvement, such factors may be regarded as nuisance variables that distort the direct effects of intrinsic neuropathological changes. As with other areas of experimental research, the effects of these variables are treated as individual differences and are incorporated into the error term in statistical comparisons. The focus of the research then becomes reductionistic in nature and is designed to isolate that portion of the variance that can be attributed to lesion laterality. Clinical research into right hemisphere dysfunction has shown, however, that recognition of the influence of such correlated factors may increase one's understanding of the functions of the right hemisphere and lead to the formulation of new hypotheses and tasks for investigating lateral asymmetries of hemispheric function.

No attempt will be made to review the vast clinical literature on right hemisphere dysfunction since substantial reviews are available (Benton, 1979; Heilman, 1979; Joynt & Goldstein, 1975). Since some of the determinants to be discussed involve subsets of the literature that will be reviewed in other chapters in this volume (e.g., see Caramazza & Martin), they will not all be examined in equal detail. This discussion is intended to explore the factors that may be confounded with laterality and localization variables in clinical studies, to examine possible interactions among those variables to produce a wide range of individual differences on dependent neuropsychological variables, and to identify how these variables have been controlled or considered in representative clinical studies. These studies will be selected on the basis of their frequent citation in the literature or their generally accepted role as being significant for the understanding of right hemisphere dysfunction. Following this analysis, independent variables that are more directly manipulated in the design of specific assessment procedures or tasks will be outlined, with selected examples from the literature.

COVARIATES OF NEUROPATHOLOGICAL FACTORS

Lateral asymmetries of function in normals can be explored without a great deal of attention to individual differences since the neuropsychological outcomes are subject to a narrower range of extraneous influences. In the conduct of clinical neuropsychological research, special consideration must be given to these factors as well as to the neuroanatomical determinants of behavioral differences. In a review of the methodological considerations in clinical neuropsychological research, Parsons and Prigatano (1978) provide a basis from which this analysis may proceed.

Before attempting a clinical investigation, adequate background in the traditional areas of psychological measurement, psychopathology, and the clinical neurosciences is essential. It is also helpful to proceed from some model used for identifying the sources of individual differences in outcome measurements. An example of such a model is provided by Jarvik (1975), as applied to individual differences in normal aging. Such differences are determined by different classes of variables that cut across genetic, environmental, social, and biologic processes. The wide range of possible interactions among these variables may produce an almost infinite variation in individual outcomes in addition to the effects of focal or diffuse central nervous system (CNS) disease factors. Neuropsychological deficits, considered descriptively as deviations from some ideal norm, are found in may different clinical populations with and without known CNS involvement; thus, the entire range of psychopathological variables must be considered when designing clinical studies. Most neuropsychological research into right hemisphere dysfunction does not incorporate psychiatric controls such as depressives or schizophrenics. More typically controlled are independent variables such as age, sex, education, socioeconomic status, and handedness. However, equating subgroups to be compared on these variables may not take into account possible interactions among these variables and between these variables and the diverse etiological conditions encountered in neurological populations. Differing etiologies, in turn, are associated with varying rates of disease progression and recovery potential as well as response limitations introduced by primary sensorimotor, attentional, and emotional disturbances associated with the lesion. Adequate control of the wide range of variables that affect the neuroanatomical substrate and the behaviors under consideration, in the absence of a lateralized lesion, constitutes a formidable challenge and an ideal that is rarely met even in the most rigorous clinical studies.

Age

Although age is widely acknowledged as a variable to be controlled, there is a surprising disregard of this factor in clinical studies (Heaton, Baade, & Johnson, 1978). Right hemisphere-dependent functions are correlated especially with age and show the earliest indications of decline with age in normal populations (Schaie & Schaie, 1977). There are striking parallels between normal age-related changes in function and diffuse CNS changes, which, when superficially interpreted, may lead to the conclusion that the right cerebral hemisphere is more affected than the left in the aging process (Goldstein & Shelly, 1981).

An appreciation of the parallels between a normal age change and the effects of right cerebral hemisphere disease requires appreciation of both the detrimental and facilitative correlates of change in normal aging. There is extensive literature that implicates a host of factors in the determination of the functional age gradients for the declines in visuospatial, visuoconstructional, and memory functioning with age. Individuals of higher initial ability levels tend to survive longer and to achieve higher performance levels in old age (Botwinick, 1977; Schaie, 1970). Similarly, people of higher education may survive longer to achieve the same result. Older individuals may vary in motivation, interest, and effort, particularly when processing novel stimuli of little relevance. When utilizing older individuals as volunteer controls, values and motivational considerations may introduce sampling biases. A given measure of function may not be equally valid at each chronological age level and the instrument yielding the measure may not be of equal relevance throughout the life span. Biological survival conditions may be associated with behavioral trait variations. If a neuropsychological function is positively correlated with survival, it may contribute a positive change component to the functional age gradient. If a right hemisphere-dependent function shows a selectively greater decline with chronological age, it is reasonable to expect that survivors may perform higher than the norm and, when compared with patients with right cerebral disease and lower survival potential, lead to an accentuation of intergroup differences and to exaggerated conclusions regarding right hemisphere-specific effects. Similarly, if a correlated detrimental factor (such as diet/weight) is negatively correlated with survival, it could contribute a negative component to functional age gradients in normal aging and lead to underestimates of the effects of right cerebral hemisphere disease in intergoup comparisons involving a normal control group that happened to differ on that factor. There is evidence of selectively greater declines in cognitive functioning in some clinical populations shortly before death (Jarvik & Falek, 1963). Therefore, if clinical samples are drawn from relatively acute or subacute disease samples or from nursing homes and other institutional settings, such terminal changes may accentuate the relative degree of impairment between control and experimental samples and lead to exaggerated conclusions regarding specific right cerebral hemisphere effects.

The life-span developmental psychology literature identifies deficiencies of the norms for tests in clinical and general use, including many standardized tests of right cerebral dysfunction. The performance subtests of the Wechsler Adult Intelligence Scale are a striking example of measures for which the norms are incomplete or inaccurate. Careful control of age would remove such deficiences, to a large extent. Ideally, age norms should be established for a new test being developed. An appreciation of the difficulties involved in estimating functional age gradients for a proposed right hemisphere test may lead to fewer interpretive errors in generalizing from the data. The major difficulty in establishing age norms relates to the confounding of age (ontogenetic), cohort-related (generational), and historical (time of measurement) factors.

Cross-sectional norms are most readily obtained and are frequently the only norms available for the neuropsychological tests used as dependent variables in right hemisphere research. They involve the relative status on a given measure of different cohorts tested in the same year. Such norms confound age and cohort-related factors and yield an estimate of earlier and steeper decline of function in people in their 60s and 70s (Schaie, 1977). In normal aging studies, such declines are seen especially on speeded psychomotor and nonverbal functions, the latter overlapping considerably with the known psychological changes associated with right cerebral hemisphere involvement. Cross-sectional norms overestimate the degree of normal age change, but they do show how impaired some normal older people can be on tests of right cerebral hemisphere dysfunction.

Longitudinal norms require the assessment of change in the same cohort monitored over decades. Such norms confound age and historical factors and yield an estimate of more gradual and milder decline after age 50, with no sharp decline noted until the 80s on tests that are sensitive to age and, by implication, to right hemisphere involvement. They show how preserved some people remain into their 80s, even on tests that show remarkable changes when comparisons are made by means of cross-sectional norms. The methodological solution to the establishment of normative changes with age is the development of the cross-sequential design in which different cohorts are monitored over shorter periods (Schaie and Labouvie-Vief, 1974). This procedure combines the cross-sectional and longitudinal approaches and results in a reduction in the confounding of nondevelopmental determining factors. Cross-sequential norms yield a more moderate picture of decline and are considered to reveal more accurately the changes that occur in aging.

One approach to dealing with the dilemma posed by longitudinal, as contrasted with cross-sectional, designs in controlling age effects in right cerebral hemisphere research was introduced by Goldstein and Shelly (1981). They defend the use of cross-sectional designs despite the confounding of age and disease-related effects on the assumption that biasing effects associated with terminal changes in longitudinal studies can distort the data as much as the cohort-related biases associated with cross-sectional studies (Reitan, 1964). Russell, Neuringer, and Goldstein (1970) developed a taxonomically organized decision system that generates predictions of lesions laterality on the basis of a set of quantitative rules derived from the literature on dysfunctions associated with right cerebral hemisphere involvement. They hypothesized that the right cerebral hemisphere may age more rapidly than the left but acknowledged that the specific cognitive functions of the right hemisphere are not well understood and, therefore, changes in cognitive ability in cross-sectional studies should be qualified if interpreted as attributable to right hemisphere changes with age. However, the methodological requirement of equating verbal and nonverbal tests for degree of novelty, familiarity, and relevance for the older individual is not met by empirically isolating the patterns of right hemisphere-dependent functions. The resolution of this methodological problem depends upon the establishment of a taxonomy of functions that may be affected by right hemisphere lesions (Gardner, 1977, 1978).

Accurate norms are necessary for longitudinal studies of dementing illness, head injury, and cerebrovascular disease. The growing interest in recovery of higher cortical functions associated with focal cerebral disease is prompting increased considerations of longitudinal factors. Age-related determinants of change and recovery of function will be necessary to identify, describe, and quantify neuropsychological deficits associated with right cerebral hemisphere disease and for the design of appropriate intervention strategies to reverse, slow, or compensate for these deficits. The anticipated direction of right cerebral hemisphere research over the next decade calls for more careful consideration of age-related determinants of change, not only for the purpose of improving the rigor of clinical study design but also as an independent variable to be manipulated for the purposes of determining the contribution of age to neuropsychological outcomes, either as a main effect or in interaction with other independent variables.

Although the literature implicating right cerebral hemisphere-dependent functions and age is not extensive, it is interesting to note that virtually all age-related changes reported to date involve deficits in visuospatial and visuoconstructional behavior in addition to nonspecific (verbal and nonverbal) changes in memory functioning (Craik, 1977; Schaie & Schaie, 1977). These changes have been interpreted as a selective decline in fluid abilities involving the processing of new information and the solving of problems requiring the application of new principles or assumptions (Cattell, 1963; Horn & Cattell, 1967). Such deficits may appear to be due to lateralized cerebral changes since they appear to be specific to figural stimuli of an essentially nonverbal nature. Since most verbal functions are relatively more overlearned and involve more familiar stimuli, it is difficult to design tasks of a verbal nature that are equivalent to nonverbal tasks in novelty and relevance. Learning and memory tasks are the most notable exception to this general expectation. Although they involve familiar stimuli, they often require higher information loads and the introduction of phased processes such as the organization, storage, and retrieval of information. Most verbal tests designed for use in laterality research on clinical populations are not constructed deliberately for dimensions such as novelty and familiarity. Thus, studies that attempt to relate the laterality dimension to aging may not be utilizing tests with equal factor loadings on the fluid ability dimensions.

Sex

There is evidence that sex may interact in subtle ways with hemispheric location of the lesion to produce differences in function (Inglis & Lawson, 1981; Lansdell, 1964; McGlone, 1980; McGlone & Kertesz, 1973). Sex differences in the normal population have been documented to reveal relatively greater superiority of verbal processing skills in females with correspondingly greater visuospatial integration in males. Such differences have been demonstrated even in children and may be associated with lateral asymmetries in hemispheric structure (Wada, 1976; Witelson & Pallie, 1973). While such differences are not striking in the general population, they are sufficiently important to warrant control in clinical studies. As Parsons and Prigatano (1978) point out, groups should be equated for number of males and females and, if this is not feasible, the study should focus on one sex and generalize to that sex only.

Direct effects are relatively amenable to control by equating samples to be compared, but the effect of sex may be sufficiently complex to warrant detailed analysis. For example, Seidman and Mirsky (1980) found an interaction between sex and side of lesion in determing personality differences between right and left temporal lobe epileptics. Further, they reported interactions between personality and cognitive factors, which are discussed in a subsequent section of this chapter. While such effects may become confounded when the investigator is attempting to isolate right cerebral hemisphere correlates, they may raise more questions than can be answered. This is particularly true when the study design addresses a set of hypotheses that differs from the hypotheses derived from higher order interactions in the data. The latter may be uninterpretable on the basis of the inital study design.

Psychosocial Influences

There is a set of demographic characteristics that may introduce sampling biases and related incremental or detrimental effects on neuropsychological outcomes. These include education, socioeconomic level, vocational choice, ethnicity, and race. These factors rarely function independently of one another and, in turn, interact with age and sex, thus rendering them difficult to control precisely in clinical studies. Education and vocational choice have particular relevance to right hemisphere-dependent functions where knowledge, skills, and competencies may emphasize visuospatial and visuoconstructional abilities. Skilled and semiskilled manual trades and certain professions may favor greater superiority in nonverbal functions and introduce variation in initial ability in lesioned samples. Similarly, initial superiority in verbal functions may be present at the higher educational levels. Higher initial verbal abilities may be associated with lower visuospatial abilities, although individual differences in the relationships between verbal and visuospatial processes are not well understood. Ethnic and racial factors are highly confounded with environmental deprivation, economic opportunity, and early language learning, including bilingualism. At the individual level, the confounding of such factors may produce advantages or disadvantages in verbal and nonverbal abilities.

Virtually, all of these variables have effects on crystallized (overlearned and heavily reinforced) abilities that may be redundantly represented in the cerebral hemispheres. They may also accentuate impairment of fluid abilities and, depending upon the hemisphere that may subserve the particular ability, render the function more vulnerable to the effects of focal lesion. Thus, a college professor who suffers a right cerebral hemisphere infarction may experience more profound losses of visuospatial ability than will a mechanic with a similar lesion. Correspondingly, a mechanic who suffers a dominant cerebral hemisphere infarction may evidence greater impairment of verbal abilities than will an English professor. Clinicians are well aware of such differences and incorporate them into interpretive reports. However, they have not been extensively investigated and may operate only within fairly narrow limits of severity of the disorder since larger lesions may override such subtle effects. Larger lesions may introduce a wider range of sensorimotor impairments that complicate the selection of manipulanda for measuring responses to test items.

Interactions between these variables and age are implied in the evidence for a greater maintenance of higher cognitive functions in older individuals of higher education and socioeconomic status (Benton, 1981). While racial factors involving the less educated and more disadvantaged typically introduce detrimental influences, they may also have incremental effects. For example, a Japanese stroke sample matched for age, education, intelligence, lesion laterality, severity, and time since lesion onset was superior to a corresponding U.S. sample when compared on the Porteus Maze Test (Meier, 1970; Meier & Okayama, 1969). Such cross-cultural differences may reflect both environmental and hereditary factors and related differences in the organization of function within and between the cerebral hemispheres. The latter may be amenable to control through the assessment of cerebral dominance.

Cerebral Dominance

Most clinical studies utilize handedness, as assessed by self-report, as a means of controlling individual differences in cerebral dominance. It is widely acknowledged that at least 95% of dextrals are left-cerebral dominant for language and, by implication, right-cerebral "dominant" for visuospatial and visuoconstructional functioning. Even among dextrals, however, there are notable exceptions, as evidenced by scattered reports of right-hemisphere representation of speech in right-handers (Kinsbourne, 1971; Smith, 1966, 1981; Zangwill, 1960). Self-report of handedness is generally regarded as the best single measure of lateral dominance (Geschwind, 1974). However, sinistrality, defined on the basis of self-report, introduces a less consistent estimate of hemispheric dominance for language since leftsided preferences are not as consistent across the wide range of lateralized activities that are included in self-reported inventories (Benton, 1962). Thus, left-handers tend toward ambilaterality in actual usage. The neural substrate underlying handedness differences may be organized less precisely for material-specific information processing so that the usual functions of the cerebral hemispheres may be bilaterally represented with a considerable degree of variation in left-handers. Further variation in dominance relationships between the hemispheres may be introduced by differences between acquired and familial left-sided preferences. Variations in cerebral dominance among dextrals as well as sinistrals are probably much greater than is generally recognized and require more attention in research design.

For most clinical research purposes, limitation of the sample to dextrals serves as the typical control. Even with such a restriction to sample selection, a comprehensive self-report inventory of lateral preferences may provide a basis for estimating possible differences in dominance patterns between a given right cerebral hemisphere group and comparision or control groups. Individuals can then be paired to make them more comparable for lateral preferences. A number of such inventories are available (Annett, 1967, 1972; Fennell, Satz, Van den Abell et al., 1978; Oldfield, 1971; Satz, 1973; Varney & Benton, 1975).

The dichotic listening, visual half-field, and hand-posture testing paradigms utilized in experimental research on cerebral dominance in normals may be of significantly less value than preference inventories for assessing lateral dominance in lesion samples, due to the contralateral effects that may become confounded with premorbid hemispheric asymmetries after focal cerebral involvement. The reliability and validity of such measures in the normal population is yet to be fully established although, as shown in other chapters of this volume (see Porter & Hughes; Hardyck), they do yield consistent and often robust data with respect to the normal functioning of the cerebral hemispheres and may prove useful in clinical research (Bryden, 1965, 1975; Kimura, 1973; Levy & Reid, 1976, 1978; Satz, Achenback, Pattishall, & Fennel, 1965).

While self-report still constitutes a reasonable basis for inferring cerebral dominance relationships at the hemispheric level, lateral preference measures should be extended to include at least an inventory of activities for the sensory or response modality used in determining behavioral outcomes. This suggestion would apply especially to sinistrals who can be expected to manifest considerable within-group variation in activity and sensory preference patterns (Herron, 1980).

ETIOLOGY AND CHARACTERIZATION OF THE LESION

While the development of specialized neurological diagnostic procedures has made it possible to characterize the lesion in specific anatomical terms under differing etiological conditions, the correlation between the resulting lesion-localization classifications and neuropsychological outcomes is not very high (Kaszniak, Garron, Fox, et al., 1979). Even computerized axial tomography, the most direct anatomical localizing technique available, may not yield complete neuroanatomical information in all cases. This is more characteristic of some etiological circumstances than others; thus, an understanding of the neuropathological heterogeneity that may exist within a given etiology is essential for the effective selection of patients and for the isolation of independent variables of relevance in studies of the effects of lesion lateralization and the recovery and plasticity of CNS functioning. Etiological considerations may impose constraints upon the use of external diagnostic criteria and the selection of independent variables for clinical investigation.

The neurological examination and the various specialized diagnostic procedures are extremely helpful in localizing lesions but are not completely valid, even under the most optimal clinical assessment conditions. The criterion problems for validating behavioral tests and for classifying lesions are better understood by examining the etiologies that are most frequently represented in lesioned samples. This section of the chapter addresses the range of variation in the neuroanatomical changes that occur under varying etiological conditions in patient populations used for clinical studies of right hemisphere dysfunction. Most prevalent among these are head trauma; cerebrovascular infarction; cerebral neoplasms in the generation of focal cerebral lesions; and the degenerative, infectious, inflammatory, and metabolic diseases in diffuse neuropathological changes.

Head Trauma

Closed head injury provides a useful point of departure for examining individual differences in neuroanatomical change within a particular etiological category. Difficulties involved in lesion classification are highlighted by neuropathological findings in nonsurviving cases (Courville and Ames, 1952; Strich, 1961). In pure cases of sudden death in closed head injury, there are frequently no indications of contusions, lacerations, or hemmorhage. However, there may be an interesting and peculiar distribution of changes in the white matter, leaving the gray matter relatively unaffected. Normal in appearance, such brains evidence widespread shearing and tearing of the white matter of the cerebral hemispheres and the long tracts, both ascending and descending, especially in the reticular activating system of the brain. Such changes are expected to be present in surviving cases, although perhaps not to the same degree and depth as that seen in nonsurvivors. These changes may not be evident on CT scans during the first year following injury, but they may later be associated with ventricular enlargement, including lateralized asymmetries in ventricular size.

Animal research on the direct and indirect concussive effects of closed head injury (Ommaya and Gennarelli, 1974) has shown that the shearing and tearing of the white matter may be seen even at subconcussive levels and that the effects may extend beyond the hemispheres to involve deeper thalamic and subthalamic structures. More severe impact results in longer durations of coma and posttraumatic amnesia (Smith, 1981).

Due to the large size and compressible nature of the brain, the resulting changes in velocity of the head produce marked lateral dislocations of the brain and variations in the rotational forces that shear and tear the white matter at deeper levels as the force levels increase in magnitude. Secondary effects of a more localized nature may occur in the form of contusions, lacerations, and hemorrhages. These changes may be similar to those seen in penetrating head injuries but emphasize locations immediately beneath the point of impact (coup) or directly opposite the point of impact (contrecoup), depending upon the circumstances of contact (Courville, 1944).

Less well understood are the vascular changes that may add to an already wide range of individual differences in clinical status. When designing clinical studies, these changes usually will not be directly identifiable, although they may be expressed indirectly through such variables as duration of coma, retrograde and anterograde amnesia, and subtest pattern on batteries of neuropsychological tests (Levin, Grossman, Rose, & Teasdale, 1979; Russell, 1971; Russell & Smith, 1961). For the purpose of characterizing the lesion, it is necessary to take CT scan data, focal neurological findings (with or without CT verification), and neuropsychological deficits (other than those under investigation) into account. Table 3-1 shows the neuropsychological correlates expected for involvements at progressively deeper levels of the CNS in closed head injury. Table 3-2 summarizes the focal correlates of open head injury that may also be seen as epiphenomena in more severe instances of surviving closed head injuries. Thus, severity has been shown to be a strong limiting factor in estimating the likelihood of focal disturbances in closed head injury (Fahey, Irving, & Miller, 1967). In addition, natural history studies have shown that age is a primary determinant of the course of restitution of function and that deficits are more severe as a combined function of age and severity (Carlsson, von Essen, & Lofgren, 1968). Failure to control for age can, therefore, distort the outcomes for a given dependent variable in head trauma quite remarkably.

TABLE 3-1.

Approximate Relations between Neuroanatomical and Neuropsychological Variables in Closed Head (Acceleration Concussion) Injury

Neuroanatomical	Neuropsychological
Longitudinal tracts (brain stem RAS)	Attention, vigilance, concentration
Brain stem/limbic system or deep fronto-temporal connections	Learning, memory, personality disturbances
Fiber systems within hemispheres	Subtle subjective complaints
Interhemispheric commissures	Possible disconnexion phenomena
Secondary focal involvement	Superimposed focal deficits

TABLE 3-2.

Approximate Relationships between Neuroanatomical and Neuropsychological Variables in Open Head (Penetrating) Injury

Neuroanatomical	Neuropsychological
Direct and indirect focal involvement	Wide range of possible deficits
Superficial and/or deep penetration	Admixture of cortical/subcortical deficits
Prefrontal	Abstract reasoning, fluency
Frontothalamic	Planning, anxiety deficits
Anterior temporal	Perception, learning
Mesial temporal/diencephalic	Learning, memory, personality
Temporoparietal	Complex perception/comprehension
Deeper parietal	Cognitive and perceptual integration
Occipital	Primary and secondary visual processes

Cerebrovascular Infarction

Of all localized cerebral lesions seen clinically, cerebrovascular accidents produce the most sharply localized changes. While these may be multifocal in patients who have a history of repeated strokes, they more characteristically occur on a single unilateral basis, predominately in the distribution of the middle cerebral artery. For this reason, the resulting lesions are found largely on the lateral convexity of one or the other cerebral hemisphere. More rarely, cerebrovascular infarctions occur in the distribution of the posterior cerebral artery with related involvement of the posterior and medial portions of the hemisphere. Equally rarely, occlusion of the anterior cerebral artery may produce infarctions in the anterior and superior portions of the medial wall of the hemisphere. CT scans have been shown to be quite sensitive to isolating the area of involvement, although a period of 14 to 21 days is usually necessary for the scan to show the infarction, even with special contrast enhancement procedures (New, Scott, Schnur et al., 1975; Paxton & Ambrose, 1974). The behavioral status of such patients is quite variable during the acute and subacute periods before well-defined CT scan findings may appear. Sensorimotor functions show the earliest recovery changes and plateau first in the recovery process (Twitchell, 1951); the highest functions of the affected hemisphere may show recovery changes as late as three years (Geschwind, 1974). These longitudinal changes are characterized by wide differences among patients within a given localization category and require careful control of time since symptom onset and of the confounding effects of unilateral sensorimotor deficits when research interest lies in higher cognitive functions involved with stimulus processing, organization, retention, and abstract reasoning.

Recovery changes may be predictable, at least in part, from neuropsychological test patterns (Meier, 1980). These are limited primarily by the severity or extent of the lesion and its location but may also be affected by extraneous premorbid factors over which it is difficult to obtain exact control, such as individual differences in age-related cognitive decline, premorbid exposure to toxins and associated diffuse underlying changes, and degree to which the function being assessed by the dependent variable was overlearned or crystallized in the ability repertoire.

Cerebral Neoplasms

In contrast to head trauma and cerebrovascular infarction, which have an abrupt onset and a significant probability of progressive improvement over time, cerebral neoplasms are typically of gradual onset and produce progressively detrimental changes in neurological status and neuropsychological functioning. Time since symptom onset is a critical variable since the target-dependent variables are likely to show more rather than less deviation from the norm or from an appropriate control group with time. Neoplasms also introduce remote effects throughout the hemisphere or bilaterally as a function of the nature and progression of the neoplastic process. Growth of the tumor may involve infiltration of the hemisphere from a primary site, as seen in astrocytoma. Glioblastomas, by contrast, are space-occupying lesions that often produce extensive remote effects within and between the hemispheres. Patients with such tumors are not suitable subjects for research until after neurosurgical intervention, when estimates of the severity of the lesion can be obtained. Meningiomas do not affect the brain parenchyma directly, although they may produce secondary neurological and neuropsychological impairments before removal by irritating the cortex. Age may be an important interacting factor that will produce variation in effects; however, the most important factor to be controlled may be the rate of progression of the disease process, which is quite variable from patient to patient and extends over a relatively longer period of time with the astrocytomas than with the gliomas. Meningiomas carry a better prognosis and often do not recur after surgery. Such patients may completely recover higher functions after surgery and do not then constitute suitable subjects for laterality and localization research unless CT scans of neurosurgical reports reveal structural changes in the brain parenchyma.

Diffuse Cerebral Neoplasms

It has been shown that relatively diffuse neuropathological changes are associated with declines in many of the functions that become impaired in focal right cerebral hemisphere disease and, to a lesser extent, in the older normal population. Therefore, it is appropriate to include such representative samples of nonfocal etiology for comparison in clinical studies. The most frequently considered disorders involve the degenerative and toxic encephalopathies. Among the degenerative disorders, Alzheimer's-like dementia, multiinfarct dementia, and the alcoholic encephalopathies are of greatest interest. Diffuse cerebral involvement and related dysfunction can be verified by CT scans and electroencephalograms (EEGs). Time since symptom onset is an important variable to control. Alzheimer's dementia is an untreatable progressive process with varying rates of progression in different individuals. In advanced stages, even highly overlearned and verbal abilities become impaired, and the patient eventually becomes unsuitable for formal assessment; therefore, only patients in the early stages of the disease provide a comparison group of significant empirical and theoretical interest. The toxic encephalopathies, such as alcoholism, progress over much longer periods of time and are potentially treatable. Impairments may be at least partially reversible so that the degree of remission and control of the problem is an important factor in the selection of subjects. Where diffuse cerebral changes have occurred, these patients may perform at significantly higher levels than a comparable sample of Alzheimer's dementia cases, equated for ventricular enlargement on the CT scan. Impairment of functions subserved by the frontal and temporal regions is most common in patients with a long history of alcohol abuse. The Wernicke-Korsakoff's syndrome is associated with more circumscribed bilateral CNS changes in the periventricular region, particularly the dorsomedial nucleus of the thalamus and the mammilary bodies of the hypothalamus (Victor, Adams, & Collins, 1971). When utilizing such a comparison group in right hemisphere research, consideration should be given to the possibility that one hemisphere may become involved more extensively than the other at a given point in time and that fluid abilities may be more represented in right hemisphere-related measures. Some rare forms of diffuse degenerative disease, such as Pick's disease, involve changes in the frontotemporal regions bilaterally whereas in Alzheimer's dementia, the changes may be even more widespread at a given point in the course of the disease. Anatomical variations are seen in other forms of diffuse disease such as herpes encephalopathy, in which there may be selectively more involvement of the periventricular region (Brain, 1962). When combining instances of the differing etiologies and possible anatomical variations into a control or comparison sample, it cannot be concluded that the sample is neuropathologically homogeneous.

Symptomatic Status in Relation to Etiology: Seizure Disorders

Many patients used as subjects in localization research have seizure disorders. Presence of a seizure disorder has no implications with respect to the etiological conditions that may be producing the pathophysiological changes underlying the disorder (Baker, 1958). Focal seizures are classified on the basis of focal neurological manifestations in the seizure and may have localizing value. Such patients may be candidates for neurosurgical ablation of the pathophysiologically abnormal tissue, as confirmed by in-depth electroencephalography performed at the operation. This group has provided the basis for much of the research into the effects of regional ablations within the right hemisphere; the direct anatomical control provided by a well-documented resection makes this a desirable group for research purposes. However, even this group must be carefully classified to control for individual differences in age at which the original lesion occurred, any relative differences in cerebral dominance resulting from a very early lesion, genetic predisposition to seizures that may be present even in focal lesion disorders, and anticonvulsant medication effects.

Since seizure disorders arise primarily from early atrophic lesions, they may be associated with varying degrees of subcortical as well as cortical involvement. For this reason, seizure disorders are often mixed between focal and centrencephalic sources. The latter are often associated with deficits in attention, which may be confounded by deficits of cortical origin (Penry, 1973). Since these lesions occur early in life, ontogenetic factors may have altered the course of not only the establishment of cerebral dominance and intrahemispheric relations but also the organization of function within the affected cerebral hemisphere. Recent electrocorticographic studies have shown that such early injuries may alter the topographic representation of higher functions remarkably (Ojemann & Whitaker, 1978). Therefore, seizure classification alone, even if it carries specific implications for lateralized cerebral involvement, may reflect etiological heterogeneity and individual variations in the developmental course. Attendant organization and representation of function may not be equivalent to that seen with focal cerebral disease of adult onset.

Pseudoneurologic Disorders

There is no neuropsychological deficit that may not appear in the comprehensive assessment of higher cortical functions in the psychiatric disorders. Ostensibly, these do not reflect specific underlying neuropathological changes, although neurochemical influences may provide a biological basis for the fluctuations in motivation and attention believed to be responsible for impaired functions in psychiatric populations. These may be characterized as functional in efficiencies rather than neuropsychological impairments and may be elicited by tests of right hemisphere-dependent functions (Matthews, Shaw, & Kløve, 1966). For this reason, the functional disorders may make a useful control insofar as they may help to establish the boundary conditions within which variability across functions may be related to focal rather than general state disturbances. In addition, if the investigator wishes to manipulate procedure-based independent variables, the role of strategy and style in information processing and retention may be more easily isolated for both lesioned and functional disorder samples. As knowledge of the anatomical, neurochemical, and physiological correlates of neurological and psychiatric disorders becomes more established, research in these two general domains may converge. This expectation is reinforced by evidence of emotional responsivity as a lateralized phenomenon, either as a direct consequence of the lesion or in interaction with the cognitive deficits produced by a lesion (Gainotti, 1972; Valenstein & Heilman, 1979).

TASK REQUIREMENTS AND SPECIALIZATION

Examination of the task requirements and conditions of individual tests that are sensitive to lesions in different regions of the right cerebral hemisphere is essential to an understanding of the problems to be addressed in designing tests for experimental and clinical research. It is beyond the scope of this chapter to review the extensive literature relating to quantitative outcomes, as measured by neuropsychological tests, in clinical studies of nonlocalized right cerebral hemisphere involvement. A number of excellent reviews provide entry into this literature and deal with the characteristic correlates of right hemisphere disease in clinical populations (Benton, 1979; Joynt & Goldstein, 1975; Smith, 1975). Much of this literature focuses upon the visuoperceptive, visuospatial, and visuoconstructional deficits associated with larger lesions involving much of the hemisphere, particularly those that are located more posteriorly. These lesions characteristically produce conspicuous clinical phenomena such as hemispatial neglect, spatial confusion, constructional apraxia, and a wide range of deficits involving the perception, learning, and recall of nonverbal stimuli. Task variables have included animate and inanimate objects, the localization of objects in space, perceptual closure of imcompletely presented objects, figure-ground differentiation, integration of disparate figural elements into a meaningful whole, color recognition and association, judgment of distance and direction, topographical orientation, unilateral spatial neglect, and the manipulation of materials that are not readily subject to verbal coding or subvocal verbal mediation. Much of the clinical literature involves comparisons between left and right hemisphere groups that are mixed for etiology, time since disease onset, age, age of onset, and other factors that may influence test outcomes. Since the samples have been characteristically selected on the basis of neurological classifications, before CT scan verification was available, there may be a preponderance of larger and more posterior lesions represented in earlier clinical research. Clinical criteria such as the presence of sensorimotor deficits and visual field cuts have been utilized for identifying the presence of right hemisphere involvement and for differentiating anterior from posterior lesions. Many studies do not differentiate among regional subgroupings within the right cerebral hemisphere. Some investigations differentiate between anterior and posterior lesions, thereby adding anatomical criterion refinements to the design.

Other investigations include samples that are relatively restricted to particular regions within the hemisphere. This last group is of greatest interest insofar as it represents the strongest neuroanatomical controls available in the clinical literature. Although relatively limited in number, such studies provide a basis for examining task construction issues in clinical research. Illustrative examples from this portion of the literature will be mentioned to identify the kinds of task requirements and variations that are likely to elicit those performance deficits of greatest relevance to an understanding of the functions of the right hemisphere. A review of the entire clinical literature could readily be the subject of a complete chapter, if not an entire volume. This section, therefore, is limited to a discussion of illustrative examples of studies that control for regional localization of the lesion and to other selected references germane to this discussion.

Right Prefrontal Region

The construction of tests that are likely to be sensitive to unilateral frontal lobe lesions may constitute the greatest challenge to the clinical investigator. Gross disturbances in intellectual functioning may not be present clinically and, in fact, general intellectual functioning may improve after extensive right anterior removals of cerebral neoplasms. This early observation (Hebb & Penfield, 1940) provided the basis for the development of theory and spurred further research, some of which has shed some light on the role of the frontal lobes in higher adaptive functioning (Luria, 1966; Milner, 1964; Teuber, 1964). Interest in the frontal lobes was also stimulated by observations of patients with bilateral involvement; the associated "frontal lobe syndrome" reflects changes in both personality and cognition. Early investigators focused on particular features of the syndrome in order to devise tasks of likely sensitivity to the underlying changes. Luria's work (1966, 1967) expanded our knowledge of the disintegration of serially organized, goal-directed behavior with frontal lobe involvement. Clinical descriptions emphasized impairments of abstract reasoning and categorical behavior as well as the inability to anticipate the consequences of actions and decisions in everyday problem-solving situations (Goldstein & Scheerer, 1941; Halstead, 1947; Hécaen, 1964). Prefrontal involvement was also associated with personality changes such as reduced anxiety and abbreviated response to failure and frustration (Goldstein, 1952; Rylander, 1939). These led to early psychosurgical interventions for the treatment of chronic anxiety states and schizophrenia.

A convenient point of departure for isolating outcomes of frontal lobe disease is provided by the early literature that identified the Porteus Maze Test as an effective instrument for assessing frontal lobe dysfunction (Porteus, 1959). The subsequent literature indicates that the component functions required for effective solution of tactually guided maze problems may be implicated even after unilateral lesion (Corkin, 1965). The Porteus maze is a serially organized, goal-directed task in which all the necessary information is available to the subject at all times during task execution. The effective solution of the problems requires relatively intact perceptual organization, inhibition of faulty alternative solutions at particular choice points, active visual scanning of the maze, and effective strategy formation. Failure can then be attributed to one or more impairments of this array of deficits. If emotional response to failure is brief and the patient is indifferent to negative outcomes, impulsive responding is more likely to occur. Like most complex tests, multidimensional processes are involved and task failures are not exclusively related to a single neuroanatomical region.

Another test that has demonstrated sensitivity to even unilateral involvement of the prefrontal regions, the Wisconsin Card Sorting Test (WCST), was applied by Milner (1964) in a series of studies suggesting that the dorsal lateral portions of the frontal lobes are more crucial in the mediation of abstract reasoning and categorical behavior. It is interesting that the reductions in abstract reasoning and increasingly perseverative responses on this task occur after removal of static atrophic lesions of very early origin. It seems reasonable to expect that such effects might be even more accentuated with removal of more recently involved or intact tissue. Partial replications have confirmed the detrimental effects of frontal lobe lesions on WCST performance, especially the increase in perseverative errors when shifting concepts (Robinson, Heaton, Lehman, & Stilson, 1980). Another study (Drewe, 1974) implicated the medial area of the frontal lobes more than the dorsolateral convexity, but the samples were not comparable to Milner's for etiology and rate of refusal to participate among nonfrontal controls. A repeated outcome of these studies is that lateralized asymmetries are not striking, although the left perform somewhat more poorly than the right frontal patients. Superficially, the WCST appears to be largely a nonverbal problem-solving task. However, examiner feedback with respect to correctness of response may encourage verbal mediation of strategies and selection of alternative sorting criteria on the part of the subject.

Except for the reduction in language fluency associated with involvement of Broca's area, lateral differences in higher functions are not striking on intellectual tests that include verbal and nonverbal components (Borkowski, Benton, & Spreen, 1967; Reitan, 1964). There are exceptions, however, suggesting that lateralization of function follows the known specialization of the hemispheres even anteriorly, although perhaps not to the striking degree seen posteriorly. For example, Milner and her associates earlier demonstrated a reduction in verbal associative fluency after anterior ablation; it was significantly greater after left-sided removals (Milner, 1964). Similarly, selectively greater impairment of nonverbal or figural associative fluency results from right frontal or frontocentral involvement (Jones-Gottman & Milner, 1977). The strength of their findings with a figural fluency task is accentuated by the inclusion of temporal-lobe-ablation comparison groups and the demonstration that this deficit is relatively limited to anterior lesions. This is a clear demonstration of an associative function of the right frontal lobe, a region of the hemisphere that does not produce any gross clinical changes when involvement spares the motor cortex. However, subtle disturbances of muscle tone, gait and posture, motor control, and orienting response and bradykinesia may contribute to deficits in associative functions and, therefore, require thorough neurological criterion specification in clinical research (Damasio, 1979). Clinical studies do not appear to have controlled for subtle variations in clinical neurological status, which may have introduced sampling biases between left and right lesion subsamples. In any case, damage to the right frontal lobe may result in a nonverbal analogue of the deficit in associative verbal fluency, seen following left frontal lobe damage. Verbal associative fluency deficits were confirmed by Borkowski, Benton, and Spreen (1967) in nonaphasic patients with left cerebral meningiomas. Benton (1968) also provided evidence of impairment with right frontal involvement with three-dimensional block constructions and design copying. Deficits on such tasks are often observed in patients with right posterior lesions, although design-copying abilities have been shown to be relatively intact, except for larger lesions, in patients undergoing temporal lobectomy (Milner, 1964). Thus, Benton's finding is somewhat suprising, although more complex forms of visuoconstructional behavior, such as three-dimensional assemblies, may require a sufficient degree of integrative, goal-directed behavior to elicit impairments even in right anterior lesion groups. Benton did not include a nonfrontal focal lesion control group but based his conclusions upon differences between focal and bilateral prefrontal disease groups.

A recent study examined differences between anterior and posterior lesion groups on a test of cognitive estimation (Shallice & Evans, 1978). The test requires the provision of a reasonable answer to a number of questions that tap general knowledge available to most people (e.g., What is the length of an average man's spine? How fast do race horses gallop? How tall is the average English woman?). A reasonably accurate and appropriate answer to the question requires the application of some evaluative strategy. Patients with anterior lesions proposed significantly more extreme responses when compared with a posterior lesion group. There was no lateralized discrepancy among the posteriors, but the left anteriors provided signficantly more bizarre responses than the right anteriors on many of the items. Since this is a verbally mediated task, this finding is not suprising, but it is noteworthy that the right anterior group also provided more bizarre responses than either posterior lesion group. This suggests that anterior lesions produce faulty assumptions about the premises underlying the question.

Another study demonstrating the efficacy of tasks requiring cognitive control and the inhibition of inappropriate or ineffectual responses (impulsivity) has shown promise for differentiating left from right frontal lobe lesion groups and evidence for a dissociation of function between anterior and posterior groups (Drewe, 1975). A go-no-go learning test derived from the animal literature on prefrontal dysfunction required that the subject switch off a light by pressing an appropriate key; 70 randomized trails were given,

35 to a red ("go") and 35 to a blue ("no-go") light. Reinforcement was asymmetric, with the light offset for correct positive responses only. Additional trials were given without reinforcement, with the patients required to respond "yes" if they thought the light would go off when the key was pressed and no if it would not. Anteriors differed from posteriors on mean trials to criterion, number of errors, number of false positive errors, and number of false negative errors. Right frontals did not differ from left frontals. This would be the expected finding since there is no disproportionately greater verbal or nonverbal component to the task, although some verbal mediation might well have been present. The authors report that patients with medial lesions made more false positive errors than did all other patients combined, which is consistent with animal studies (Mishkin, 1964; Rosvold & Mishkin, 1961). Positive responses were predominant in the anterior groups; thus, they showed a deficit when the preferred response tendency was incorrect. Posteriors made more nonpreferred, no-go responses. There were some subtle intergroup differences such as negative correlation between false positive error rate and the verbal factor in right frontals and a positive correlation between age and false positive error rate in the left frontal group. Chronicity of lesion was not a significant factor, nor did performances of patients with dorsal lateral and orbital lesions differ from the posterior group. The finding that medial lesions, irrespective of laterality, was an important correlate of high false positive error rate was consistent with Drewe's previous report (1974) that medial lesions produced greater impairment on the WCST. The number of categories obtained, total errors, and maximum classification scores on the WCST were correlated with the go-no-go false positive error rate in the total group. With lesions judged to be limited to the frontal lobes, on the basis of his criteria, only the WCST perseverative error score was associated with a false positive error rate. This raises the possibility that different deficits may be involved in the poor performances on each test and, by inference, that different parts of the frontal lobes could be involved in the determination of specific outcomes. However, it is also conceivable that some differences between dorsal-lateral and medial lesions would "wash-out" if factors such as age, intelligence, etiology, chronicity of lesion, time since symptom onset, differences in lateral dominance, and detrimental premorbid factors could be completely controlled.

The ineffective control of preferred response tendencies appears as a recurring correlate of frontal lobe pathology. This type of deficit raises questions with respect to the influence of personality factors upon performance. This is not to suggest that personality factors would account entirely for the deficit but that such factors could increase the magnitude of its expression in quantitative studies. Very little is known about frontal lobe pathology beyond the effects of frontal lobectomy and the clinical descriptions of personality change in patients with extensive prefrontal involvement. Earlier research involving the use of the Minnesota Multiphasic Personality Inventory (MMPI) suggests that patients with frontal lobe lesions are likely to produce "hysteroid" profiles, in which anxiety and other measures of affective discomfort fall well within the normal range, partly due to denial of emotional problems and personal shortcomings (Friedman, 1950; Williams, 1952). This is consistent with the effect of psychosurgery in the early studies of schizophrenics and chronic anxiety disorders. In both of these studies, there were no differences in personality measures between left and right hemisphere groups. However, some recent studies (Bear & Fedio, 1977; Seidman, 1980) have raised the question of lateralized effects on personality functioning in patients with focal temporal lobe lesions, the findings of which are discussed below.

An earlier study by Corkin (1965) provides a bridge in thinking about the functions of the right frontal lobe, as contrasted with the more posterior regions of the association cortex of the right hemisphere. This study was an extension of Milner's work that contrasted frontal and temporal lobe groups, in this case postoperatively. These studies are noteworthy for their attempts to control for individual differences in cerebral dominance by limiting samples to those patients who demonstrated representation of speech in the left hemisphere, as determined by the Sodium Amytal Test (Branch, Milner, & Rasmussen, 1964). The ablations were not equivalent from patient to patient, but there was considerable overlap among all four major subgroups. Broca's area was spared in the left frontal lobectomies, while the right frontal lobectomies extended onto the mesial surface, including either the anterior cingulate gyrus, the subcallosal gyrus, or both. Thus, the extent of ablation appears to have been more extensive in the right frontal subgroup, as contrasted with the left. Milner (1964) had already demonstrated that a stepping-stone visual stylus maze elicited selectively greater learning impairments after right temporal lobectomy, particularly with radical excision of the hippocampus. While preferred response tendencies may be operative in visual stylus mazes, the learning of the correct pathway through the maze is determined primarily by the ability to develop a cognitive map of the pathway and would not appear to elicit a preferred response as readily as a go-no-go learning situation. Hence, it does not seem too suprising that patients with right temporal lobe ablations perform more poorly on a visual stylus maze. Corkin (1965) set out to determine whether or not a tactual stylus maze would elicit a comparable deficit, thereby extending the generalizability of a maze learning deficit to the tactile modality. The type of maze and maze path is not identical in the two studies, although learning and memory factors would appear to enter into the type of performance more than they would, for example, in performing a visually guided maze in which all choice-point information is immediately available. The size of frontal samples was relatively small, however; thus, the significance of those results is somewhat uncertain. Nevertheless, it is of interest to note that the frontals, particularly the right frontals, performed significantly more poorly, making almost twice as many errors before reaching criterion as the right temporal group. An isolated frontotemporal patient performed at levels between the frontal and temporal groups, a somewhat paradoxal finding since the deficit should have been even more accentuated under such neuropathological conditions. Bilateral temporal lobe excisions, as in the case of the now famous patient, H. M., have been associated with profound impairments, consistent with performance on other learning and memory tasks (Milner, 1965). What is perhaps most significant about Corkin's data is the higher incidence of repetitive error scores in the right frontal group, similar to other reports of an inability to inhibit previously reinforced responses in serially organized problem-solving situations with frontal lobe involvement. A suprising finding was the relatively intact performance of patients with small parietal lobe excisions in either hemisphere, even in the presence of severe somatosensory losses. Earlier reports on route-finding tasks demonstrated a substantial parietal-lobe component (Semmes, Weinstein, Ghent, & Teuber, 1955), but those studies were performed on patients with penetrating missile wounds that may have produced larger lesions than the small parietal lobe excisions for intractible sensory seizures that made up the posterior subsample in Corkin's study.

A major implication of research on frontal lobe dysfunction in humans is that lateralized cognitive impairments are not as readily elicited with tests of demonstrable sensitivity to anterior involvement. Furthermore, the component functions required in the execution of the more sensitive tests need to be defined precisely and incorporated operationally into test procedures. The variation in outcomes seen on maze-solving tasks is probably due to differing requirements and corresponding variation in the degree to which planning, judgmental, learning, memory, and even personality factors participate in task execution. The separation of these processes through manipulation of task-related variables, combined with the need to control for demographic and lesion-related variables presents a continuing challenge to the clinical investigator. This is especially true for lateralization research that proceeds from a reductionistic theoretical orientation and attempts to design experiments that would isolate that portion of the variance to be attributed specifically to the lesion and its location. Since it is virtually impossible to control all these variables in a typical clinical research context, most investigators settle for some measure of each variable, if they consider them at all, and then search for interactions among selected independent variables. The growing theoretical and practical interest of these interactions, however, probably accounts for expansion of clinical neuropsychological research beyond the laterality question.

Right Anterior and Mesial Temporal Lobe Lesions

As in the case with the frontal lobes, unilateral lesions of the temporal lobes do not produce remarkable focal neurological deficits. Conspicuous clinical manifestations occur with bilateral involvement. Clinical descriptions emphasize personality changes and profound disturbances in recent memory when involvement includes the hippocampi (Milner & Teuber, 1968). The effects of temporal lobectomy reveal more consistent evidence of lateral specialization of the hemispheres, as contrasted with frontal lesions, at least when gross aphasic disturbances are not present. Thus, material-specific disturbances in learning and retention occur relatively independently of the mode of stimulus presentation or technique used for measuring learning and retention. Where tasks are designed to minimize verbal coding, lesions of the right anterior temporal lobe have been shown to produce clear impairments that are relatively independent of the modality through which the stimuli are presented (Milner & Teuber, 1968). Verbal and nonverbal learning and memory tasks consistently elicit evidence of dissociated impairments after unilateral temporal lobectomy. This double dissociation between the effects of lesions in these regions is now one of the most accepted principles of human neuropsychology.

Tasks that have effectively discriminated between right and left temporal lobectomized patients include recognition of unfamiliar photographed faces (Kimura, 1964; Milner, 1960); left ear advantage for dichotically presented musical patterns (Gordon, 1970; Kimura, 1964; Shankweiler, 1966); memory for recurring nonsense figures (Kimura, 1963); discrimination of complex concentric fragmented circle patterns (Meier & French, 1965a); and discrimination of tonal patterns and timbre (Milner, 1962). These findings are consistent with demonstrations of a half-field or contraear superiority for material-specific inputs of the visual and auditory stimuli utilized in research on hemispheric specialization in normals, which is discussed in greater detail elsewhere in this volume (e.g., see chapters by Zaidel, Porter & Hughes, and Hardyck). Of particular interest for right hemisphere specialization are demonstrations of a left-field superiority for recognition of faces (Rizzolatti, Umiltá, & Berlucchi, 1971), location of quantity of dots (Kimura, 1969), and slope discrimination in the perception of lines (Durnford & Kimura, 1971). Deficits in stereopsis (Benton & Hécaen, 1970; Carmon & Bechtoldt, 1969) have also been shown to have a corresponding right hemisphere superiority in normals, as evidenced by a lower threshold for binocular depth perception in the lower left as contrasted with the right visual field (Durnford & Kimura, 1971). The specific role of the temporal lobes in binocular depth perception is not known, since the clinical studies have not involved patients with lesions limited to that region.

An apparent conclusion to be drawn from this literature is that most perceptual tasks sensitive to lesions limited to the temporal lobes will show a deficit when the lesion is located more posteriorly. However, measures of learning and memory tend to be more sensitive than measures of perception to lesions of the temporal lobes so that if a perceptual deficit is demonstrated after temporal lobe excision, it is somewhat unusual, particularly if the deficit is of an equivalent magnitude to that observed with more posterior lesions. In any case, deficits in perception and perceptual organization are relatively more difficult to demonstrate with right temporal lobe lesions and ablations, while recall of recurring nonsense figures is more consistently impaired with such removals (Kimura, 1963; Milner, 1967). Moreover, recognition deficits appear to occur more often in response to unfamiliar faces, as contrasted with nonsense or complex geometric designs (Milner, 1968). Thus, not all nonverbal stimuli will elicit a perceptual deficit after right temporal lobectomy, and the prevalence of figural learning and memory deficits is much more readily demonstrable. Such material-specific learning and memory disturbances are accentuated by the degree of hippocampal removal.

Some interesting task variations have shown promise for identifying the role of the hippocampus in material-specific learning and recall. In a dissertation by Corsi, cited by Milner (1971), the role of hippocampus and related periventricular structures in the retention of simple verbal or nonverbal information was explored. Corsi's data suggested a relationship between the degree of impairment and the extent of hippocampal excision on a simplified version of the technique of Peterson and Peterson (1959). The task required recall of a group of three consonants after a brief interval, during which a distracting verbal activity is performed. Recall is a function of the length of interpolated activity but also of the extent of hippocampal removal. A dissociated defect was found on a nonverbal task requiring the subject to reproduce the position of a cross on a line after a period of interpolated activity with a distractor after right temporal lobectomy, a task designed by Posner (1966). The dissociated impairments were greater with extensive hippocampal removals.

Similarly, a double dissociation of the effects of frontal and temporal lobe ablations was demonstrated by means of sequential tasks in material-specific learning and retention. The Digit-Sequences Learning Task, a verbal learning test devised by Hebb (1961), involves the learning of a supraspan digit list that exceeds the patient's immediate memory span by one. On this task, the sequence recurs every third trial between nonrecurring and intervening sequences. This procedure elicited impairments in left temporal lobectomized patients in proportion to the extent of hippocampal removal. Similarly, Corsi is reported to have demonstrated an analogous deficit on a block-tapping task that required the patient to tap out a test pattern immediately after presentation (Milner, 1971). The test yields a measure of the maximum number of blocks tapped in correct order, as in the assessment of immediate auditory digit span. A set of supraspan sequences are then presented, with the target recurring sequence appearing on every third trial. Performance on this task remained intact even after left temporal lobectomy, irrespective of extent of hippocampal removal. Block-tapping span remained normal after right temporal lobectomy but reproduction of patterns exceeding this span was slightly impaired. A more severe learning deficit was inferred from poor learning of the recurring sequence. Again, the most impaired group was the right temporals with extensive hippocampal removals.

Dissociation of the Effects of Frontal and Temporal Lobe Lesions

Some interesting "hybrid" tasks of relevance to both frontal and temporal lobe dysfunction have yielded results that may relate to the differentiation of function of the frontal and temporal regions (Milner, 1971). Dissociated deficits appear on tasks of the delayed paired–comparison type developed by Konorski and applied by Prisko of the McGill group (Milner, 1964). On such tasks, different stimuli recur in different pairings throughout the sequence. In order to produce a correct response, the subject must compare the stimulus with one that immediately preceded it and ignore or suppress the pairings to stimuli earlier in the test. The required ability to differentiate among the trials in pairing the stimulus was impaired after frontal lobectomy. This finding prompted Corsi to explore the discriminability of recency in patients with frontal and temporal excisions (Milner, 1971). He devised a verbal form of the recency task requiring the subject to read two spondaic words on each of 184 cards. Aperiodically, a test card appeared bearing a question mark between the two words; the patient would then report which word had been seen most recently. Instead of words, paired reproductions of abstract art were provided on the nonverbal form of the test. A recognition condition was also introduced concerning which one of the words was new. The task again required the indication as to which picture had been seen most recently. Simple recognition of a previously seen work or figure was impaired only in patients with right temporal lobe excisions. However, the recency judgments of both the right and left temporal lobe groups were normal. Right frontal and right frontotemporal groups were superior to corresponding left removals on the verbal recency task, while the same group was more impaired on discrimination of recency of exposure to abstract art. The inferred impairment in the ability to maintain the temporal order of the stimuli may reflect disturbed inhibitory processes rather than a recent memory deficit, consistent with the literature on the effects of unilateral frontal lobectomy. These are illustrations of the kinds of tasks that are likely to yield doubly dissociated deficits and to increase our understanding of the relative contributions of the frontal and temporal regions to the deficits that have been demonstrated to occur relatively systematically with involvement of these clinically "silent" regions.

Personality Changes in the Temporal Lobes

Since the temporal regions are neurologically silent, much like the frontal lobes, discrete neurological changes are not present and, therefore, were not available for early observation as a guide in formulating clinical hypotheses or, more recently, clinical research questions. Etiologically, most of the early cases of frontal lobe involvement were head injuries or brain tumors, although in recent years some focal motor epileptics also have provided the case content for clinical research. The clinical changes in temporal lobe lesions are perhaps even less dramatic than those seen with frontal lobe lesions, but the most common form of seizure disorder seen clinically is related to temporal lobe dysfunction and accounts for the great clinical interest in the temporal lobes. This interest has been reinforced by neuroanatomical description of the limbic system and the complex symptomatology of partial complex (focal) seizures in humans. Clinical analysis of these seizures provides strong support for the conclusion that emotional changes are associated with epileptogenic foci in or near the limbic system, particularly the anterior and medial portions of the temporal lobes (Blumer & Benson, 1975; Meier & French, 1965b; Valenstein & Heilman, 1979). Confusion, restlessness, irritability, and combativeness may be present postictally. A high incidence of "schizophreniform psychosis" in patients with temporal lobe epilepsy has also been reported (Stater & Beard, 1963). Early descriptions attempted to establish an "epileptic personality," although major personality disorders are not a necessary consequence of even a relatively severe seizure disorder, temporal lobe in origin or otherwise (Guerrant, Anderson, Fischer et al., 1962). The changes seen in temporal lobe epilepsy are dissimilar from those seen in frontal lobe lesions and have been described extensively on a qualitative clinical basis.

Whether or not stable and predictable personality changes can be measured in such subgroups, it is necessary to establish the validity of these changes and to examine their relationship to the cognitive and memory disturbances reported in clinical studies of the effects of unilateral temporal lobectomy. Furthermore, there is a small but growing literature that implicates the cerebral hemispheres differentially in emotion and personality (Bear & Fedio, 1977; Gainotti, 1972; Gasparrini, Satz, Heilman, & Coolidge, 1977; Meier & French 1965a; Seidman, 1980; Valenstein & Heilman, 1979; see also Levy, this volume). Preliminary evidence suggests that lesions of the left cerebral hemisphere, particularly the left temporal lobes, are associated with higher incidence of ideational disturbances and schizoid features while lesions of the right cerebral hemisphere, especially the right temporal lobe, produce affective disturbances (Bear & Fedio, 1977). If valid, such interhemispheric differences could well be confounded with lesion laterality as a determinant of impairments on verbal and nonverbal tests. A brief review of some of the relevant work in this area may assist the clinical investigator in controlling for personality differences between left and right (temporal lobe) groups or investigating such changes as dependent variables in lesion localization research.

Confounding of cognitive and personality factors seems likely on the basis of the clinical descriptions of psychopathology in epileptic and particularly temporal lobe epileptic populations. Descriptions include reduced sexual arousal and response, deepening of emotional experiences and responses, episodic discharge of anger and rage, intensification of religious feelings and preoccupations, an increased ethical sense and preoccupation with trivia ("viscosity"), hypographia, pedantic speech, and reduced appreciation of humorous situations, especially those with sexual overtones (Blumer, 1975; Geschwind, 1975, 1977).

Quantitative studies of personality functioning have emphasized the use of the MMPI. Early work resulted in the development of an empirical scale that differentiated parietal from frontal subgroups of patients of mixed etiology (Friedman, 1950). This scale was modified with the addition of a temporal lobe group and was shown to be valid for differentiating focal anterior from focal posterior lesions (Williams, 1952). Group profiles of patients with left, as contrasted with right, cerebral lesions were not significantly different. However, differences between anterior and posterior lesion subgroups were reported, with the latter exhibiting more evidence of somatic preoccupation, depression, and ideational disturbances. Subsequent comparisons of large temporal lobe samples, before and after temporal lobe removals, again failed to demonstrate marked lateralized differences in personality change among right temporals (Meier, 1969; Meier & French, 1965a, 1965b). However, among patients with intractable seizure disorders, the most likely to be treated neurosurgically — those with left hemisphere lesions — scored higher on the paranoia scale while those with primarily right temporal lobe involvement scored higher on the manic scale. Both subgroups exhibited elevations on the schizophrenia scale. By far the most prominent pathophysiological correlate of personality changes on the MMPI was provided by the EEG, in which the presence of bilateral EEG abnormalities, particularly bitemporal independent spike foci, were associated with the most disturbed mean MMPI profiles. Thus, there was some suggestion of a subtle laterality effect, but this was relatively minimal when compared with a rather overriding effect of independent pathophysiological changes in the temporal lobes, as inferred from the EEG. Since such EEG changes tend to be associated with greater chronicity, more severe seizure disturbances, poorer occupational histories, and more prolonged exposure to the stigmata associated with the seizure disorder, it was concluded that personality changes reflected an interaction between intrinsic neuropathological and extrinsic environmental effects. Verbal learning deficits in left temporal lobe subjects might well be accentuated by suspiciousness, distrust, and other paranoid manifestations while the trend toward affective disturbance with right temporal lobe involvement might be influenced by deficits in facial recognition and recall and in the perception and recall of musical stimuli.

The question remains as to whether or not a lateralized effect might be present to which the MMPI is not sensitive. The MMPI was not constructed to measure the specific traits inferred from clinical observations. A recent study (Bear & Fedio, 1977) and a partial replication thereof (Seidman, 1980) attempt to isolate lateralized personality changes and to provide some interesting and provocative results. Bear and Fedio converted the clinical descriptions derived from the neurological and psychiatric literature on epileptics into quantitative terms by means of a trait-questionnaire approach. They devised 18 5-item scales designed to sample a wide range of traits; these were rationally devised scales supplemented by 10 items from the MMPI lie scale, selected as neutral items with low potential for discriminating the temporal lobe from other groups to be studied. These items might also provide indications of gross distortion due to denial and other invalidating response sets. They were relatively obvious items that might be readily distorted, as suggested by the extensive MMPI literature on validity scaling (Dahlstrom, Welsh, & Dahlstrom, 1975). Two forms were developed, a self-report inventory and a rating survey that could be completed by an observer. Small groups of right temporal and left temporal lobe patients were identified on the basis of clinical history and EEG criteria, but not on the basis of direct anatomical selection criteria. A control group of normals with peripheral neurological and neuromuscular problems of noncentral origin was also included. There were no centrencephalic or other focal cortical comparison groups. They also reported no cognitive data; thus, the possibility of an interaction between cognitive and personality factors could not be evaluated. On the basis of a stepwise discriminant function analysis of the left and right temporal lobe groups, it was shown that the left scored higher on anger, paranoia, dependence, and sense of personal destiny while the right scored higher on elation, professionalism, viscosity, emotionality, and sadness. Similar, although not identical, results were obtained on the basis of ratings by trained observers. The results were interpreted to reflect enhanced affective association of previously neutral stimuli; events or concepts with the side of lesion determined the particular emotional coloration in accord with the known lateral specialization of the hemispheres. This study is remarkable for the high degree of predictive accuracy attained in discriminating between left and right temporal lobe abnormalities on the EEG; hence, its relevance to the role of the right hemisphere in personality functioning. However, before concluding that the temporal lobes have a differential significance for personality, the limitations of this study and the findings of a subsequent partial replication require elaboration.

A number of methodological problems reduce the generalizability of the Bear-Fedio findings. The five-item scales seem too brief to be reliable; this expectation is based upon established psychometric principles (Cronbach, 1947). There is no provision for a cortical nontemporal lobe and subcortical comparison group. In addition, no attempt was made to control for interactions between cognitive and affective changes that may have determined the behavioral manifestations on which the ratings and self-report data were based.

A similar study (Seidman, 1980; Seidman & Mirsky, 1980) included the addition of a temporal lobe seizure group with bilateral EEG abnormalities. The trait scales again differentiated between left and right temporal lobe EEG groups beyond chance, although not to the high degree evidenced in the Bear-Fedio study. Some of the traits that had been more characteristic of right temporals (e.g., altered sexuality, viscosity, guilt, and emotionality) were now more elevated in the left temporals, and one trait that had been more characteristic of left temporals (anger) was now more characteristic of right temporals. Such shifting in patterns of personality correlates may be due to low reliability of brief trait scales. Six traits that had been hypothesized to differentiate between left and right temporals failed to reach significance, although the means were generally within the predicted direction. The MMPI was also included in this study and did not exhibit as much sensitivity to laterality of the EEG focus as did the temporal lobe inventory. Of greatest interest was the demonstration of interactions between cognitive and personality changes and the influence of sex as a covariate. Thus, laterality effects were greater in males with left temporal lobe foci, although the males in this sample were older, of lower socioeconomic status, and had a longer seizure history. Females with right temporal lobe foci and males with left temporal lobe foci tended to score higher on ideational and schizoid characteristics. A large number of correlations between cognitive and psychopathological traits reached significance, suggesting that personality disturbances may reflect pathological exaggerations of cognitive styles associated with changes in cognitive functioning. For example, ideational trait deviations were positively correlated with performance on the Boston Naming Test and negatively with trigram learning and retention. By contrast, anger (a right temporal lobe trait) was negatively correlated with naming error scores, as predicted. By far the greatest portion of the outcome variances could be attributed to the presence of bilateral, as contrasted with unilateral, EEG abnormalities; this is consistent with the earlier literature (Meier & French, 1965b, 1965c).

The need to control for personality disturbances as covariates of cognitive change in lateralized cerebral involvement is underscored further by other studies that implicate sex differences in cognitive style as a function of lesion laterality (Smokler & Shevrin, 1979). A higher incidence of schizophreniform psychoses in left-handed females with temporal lobe lesions has been reported (Taylor, 1975), while greater deficits in paired associate learning and retention under delayed conditions, fine manipulative dexterity, and vigilance have been elicited in temporal lobe seizure patients with depressive or schizoid features on the MMPI (Thomas, Hauser, Strauman et al., 1980). If not directly interested in such "extraneous" variables, the investigator would do well to control such factors as covariates. Far from extraneous, however, such covariates of cognitive change are worthy of incorporation into evolving theoretical models of brain-behavior relationships and are expected to determine the direction of future clinical research.

Right Frontoparietal Region

Since the emphasis of this chapter is on association cortex, discussion of frontoparietal changes will be limited and introduced mainly to highlight the need for consideration and control of motor and somatosensory deficits in clinical studies of right hemisphere dysfunction. Many of the visuoconstructional and visuospatial tests in the hemisphere literature involve manual operations. Motor and somatosensory deficits have been of direct interest to many investigators. This literature demonstrates that the measurement of such discrete changes is a difficult technological challenge (Corkin, 1964). Early evidence suggested that sensorimotor functions are more focally represented in the left hemisphere than the right (Semmes, 1968; Semmes, Weinstein, Ghent, & Teuber, 1960). The observed differences were reported across a wide range of such functions from simple to complex. Some subsequent research (Carmon, 1971) failed to confirm lateralized asymmetry in tactile sensitivity, although greater perceptual loads appear to require greater participation of right association cortex in order to produce lateral differences in tactile perception of direction and number (Carmon & Benton, 1969). The possibility remains that the cerebral hemispheres participate differentially in functions attributed to the primary sensorimotor region. In the meantime, such factors should be subject to greater control as covariates than has been characteristic of right cerebral hemisphere research. If introduced at all, control usually consists of equating left and right subgroups for the presence of rated focal neurological impairment. Psychomotor performance criteria have sometimes been used for laterality predictions or for monitoring function as a dependent variable rather than as a covariate (Costa, Vaughn, Levita, & Farber, 1963; Meier, Ettinger, & Arthur, in press). The degree to which sensorimotor deficits may be confounded with or become a central component of higher order functions such as visuospatial integration or visuoconstructional ability remains a question for further investigation.

Right Temporoparieto-Occipital Region

It is widely accepted that lesions of the right posterior association cortex are readily demonstrated by means of informal perceptual and visuoconstructional tests administered at the bedside. The clinical manifestations of a posterior lesion are often striking, as evidenced by a high incidence of hemispatial neglect, dressing apraxia, susceptibilty to a sensory extinction even with intact sensorimotor function, and impaired spatial orientation (Critchley, 1953; Hécaen, 1962). Static atrophic lesions of the kind that produce temporal and frontal lobe seizure disorders are found more posteriorly, although they are not frequently candidates for surgical ablation. Parietal lobe ablation group sizes, therefore, have been smaller in the human excision studies. Most studies of parietal lobe dysfunction involve patients of other etiologies, including cerebrovascular infarction, brain tumors, and trauma, with or without an operable epileptogenic focus. Cerebrovascular accidents have provided perhaps the most carefully studied etiological grouping, since such lesions occur abruptly and are more likely to produce striking behavioral consequences. Posterior lesions are more likely than either anterior temporal or prefrontal lesions to produce large discrepancies between verbal and spatial abilities on conventional intellectual tests and neuropsychological test batteries (Meier, 1970; Reitan, 1964). Verbal-visuospatial discrepancies may be present independently of somatosensory or motor deficits since posterior lesions may spare such functions, although they will frequently introduce visual field deficits. Where all sensory and motor functions are spared, careful neurological examination may elicit suppression in all sensory modalities, with bilateral stimulation. Since these lesions are among the most localizable on a clinical basis, much of the early research focused on the right posterior association cortex. Differentiation of anterior from posterior lesions, before the availability of the CT scan, was frequently determined by the relative distribution of sensory and motor deficits. However, owing to the remote effects of acute cerebrovascular lesions and advanced neoplasms, clinical criteria may not provide a precise basis for localizing underlying pathophysiological changes. This probably accounts for the wide range of individual differences within right hemisphere subsamples in clinical research. Nevertheless, posterior lesions may produce the most consistent and predictable changes on neurological and behavioral measurements of any region within the right hemisphere.

Many nonverbal functions that have been attributed to the right hemisphere, with the exception of the more subtle frontal and temporal lobe-related functions outlined above, are readily elicited with larger right posterior lesions. While facial memory is affected by right temporal lesions, facial recognition, particularly of unknown faces, has long been associated with right parietal lobe involvement (Warrington & James, 1967). Closure of incomplete figures, letters, and shapes is similarly impaired after parietal involvement (Kinsbourne & Warrington, 1963). Even simple dot and line-slope matching procedures may elicit impairments in right parietal lobe disease (DeRenzi, Faglioni, & Scotti, 1971; Taylor & Warrington, 1973; Warrington & Rabin, 1970). Impairment of memory for rod position is more severe in the presence of visual field effects and related posterior location of the lesion, although lesion laterality may not be a significant contributing factor (DeRenzi, Faglioni, & Scotti, 1969). As spatial judgments are increased in difficulty, differentiation of left from right hemisphere groups is more readily demonstrable, particularly with right posterior involvement (Taylor & Warrington, 1973). There is a trend toward greater impairment of function in the presence of visual field defects. However, visual field defects are not a necessary or sufficient condition for impairment on visuospatial tasks, not even for disruption of the simpler discriminations required in the initial processing of visuospatial information (DeRenzi, 1968). Indications that the addition of a memory component to a spatial task may elicit greater hemispheric asymmetries have been reported, although the absence of direct anatomical controls in these earlier studies may have obscured possible involvement of the temporal as well as the parietal regions. More complex visuospatial and visuoconstructional tasks have long been known to be affected by right posterior lesions. As the task requirements involve higher levels of cognitive processing, they may also introduce the possibility of verbal mediation and strategy setting and, thereby, also elicit disturbances in performance in patients with left posterior lesions (DeRenzi & Nichelli, 1975). An apparent contradiction within this literature is found in reports by Milner (1968) of greater impairment of facial recognition in right temporals, as contrasted with left temporals, frontals, and parietals. Facial recognition was tested without delay, with a brief delay during which an interpolated task was performed, and with a 90-minute delay that was unfilled. Without delay, only a slight inferiority of the right temporals was noted. The delay produced a major right temporal lobe effect. However, this study did not include many right parietal lobe cases for comparison. The few cases that were available also showed marked impairment of recognition of unfamiliar faces. These studies underscore the need for exact anatomical information and tasks that embrace difficulty level, meaningfulness, familiarity, sequential operations, and structural stimulus parameters.

Although it seems almost axiomatic to attribute a larger role of the right posterior region to visuospatial and visuoconstructional functions, the data have not always been consistent with this expectation. For example, Benson & Barton (1970) introduced a number of instructional and drawing tasks of right hemisphere relevance, including stick-pattern reversals, template matchings, token patterns, drawings by copy and by memory, and visual as well as auditory reaction times. While their right hemisphere group scored consistently poorer on these procedures, none of the tasks elicited selectively greater impairment of function in their right parietal lobe sample. In a related study, both left and right parietal lobe subgroups performed poorly on the Stick Test under both matching and rotational conditions as well as on the Village Scene Test, although there appeared to be an interaction between severity of clinical symptomatology and posterior involvement on the latter (Butters & Barton, 1970). The extent to which verbal encoding may be a factor in strategies or in selecting solutions may also have contributed to bilateral equivalence in this study.

Ratcliff and Newcombe (1973) reported some findings that appear to contradict evidence of the primacy of the right temporal and frontal lobes in visually guided stylus maze performances. Penetrating missile wounds of the right posterior region were associated with more severe deficits than was a small group with nonposterior lesions, although bilateral posterior lesions produced the poorest performances.

Visually guided stylus maze performances have also been investigated in right posterior lesion groups, defined on the basis of presence of defects in the left visual half-field. The task was modified from Milner's (1964) version to allow assessment of ipsilateral and contralateral errors. Right hemisphere-involved patients were more impaired than those without visual field defects and those with left hemisphere lesions, with or without field defects. This pattern of impairment contrasted with the equal impairment of left and right posterior lesion groups on Corsi's motor-tapping sequence recall procedure (DeRenzi & Nichelli, 1975). Milner had de-emphasized the role of the right posterior association cortex in visually guided maze learning performance, but her conclusion was based upon a relatively small right parietal lobe ablation sample in which a static atrophic lesion had been removed. Such removals might well be associated with milder impairments than would be found, for example, in the acute cerebrovascular infarction and neoplasm group used by DeRenzi, Faglioni, and Villa (1977). Their study revealed remarkably poorer performances of patients with right posterior lesions with visual field defects.

In acute cerebrovascular infarction and brain tumors, the lesions that produce field defects may be larger and more disruptive of the function of the entire hemisphere. Conversely, an early atrophic lesion that is highly circumscribed and then removed for the treatment of partial complex seizures might involve functionally deviant tissue and, thereby might not produce a deficit on visually guided stylus maze performances. Specification of extent and recency of involvement is necessary to integrate the disparate results of these studies. With the development of more precise neuroradiographic techniques, such specification should be more readily forthcoming in future research.

The role of the right posterior parietal region in visual-stylus maze performance has been illuminated further by a series of studies of a sizable group of penetrating missile wounds followed 20 years after injury that had been sustained during the Second World War (Newcombe & Russell, 1969; Ratcliff & Newcombe, 1973). While these samples involve static and atrophic lesions, much like those in Milner's series, they differ in terms of age at which they were inflicted and are comprised of penetrating wounds rather than ablations of epileptogenic tissue. However, these studies permit the analyses of processes affected by regional involvement within the hemisphere, as defined by criteria that combine operative reports with lateral and anterioposterior radiographic findings. In the study reported by Newcombe and Russell (1969), a modification of the Mooney Visual Closure Test (1957) and visually guided stylus maze task were utilized. There were hemispheric differences with the right hemisphere group as a whole performing poorly on both tasks, as would be expected. Locus of lesion within the hemisphere was not related to performance on the closure test except for particularly low scores in the right hemisphere group with upper left quadrantic field defects. Presence of a field defect was not related to a deficit on this task in the left hemisphere group. Right hemisphere lesions associated with a hemianopia were related to selectively greater impairment on the maze task, but upper quandrantic field defects did not contribute to impaired maze performances. More severe deficits in closure or maze-learning were related to post-Rolandic lesions, but there was no overlap between those scoring below the twentieth percentile on one task, as compared with the other. Those with particularly severe impairments on the closure task evidenced lesions involving the posterior temporal lobe with relative sparing of the posterior parietal region. Those with severly impaired maze learning had a higher incidence of lesions located in the posterior parietal region and more superiorly. The different pattern of response on these two tests suggests that the site of the lesion was more crucial than was the presence of a visual field defect in determining degree of impairment and that the impairment may have been due to different processes affected by lesions in different portions of the post-Rolandic region of the right cerebral hemisphere. It was concluded that these findings could be best understood to reflect a spatial basis for the maze-learning deficit in right parietal lobe disease, in contrast with a mnestic basis when observed in anterior temporal lobe disease. The posterior temporal lesions that contributed to impairment on closure tasks were similar to the facial recognition deficits described by Milner and reported clinically for patients with lesions in that region (Hécaen, 1962). This study again underscores the need to isolate operationally the processes in multidimensional tasks.

Ratcliff and Newcombe (1973) provided a partial replication of earlier work involving the use of locomotor mazes (Semmes, Weinstein, Ghent & Teuber, 1955, 1960, 1963; Teuber, 1964). These studies reported a deficit in topographical orientation in patients with penetrating missile wounds involving the posterior parietal regions, left or right. Patients with right posterior lesions required a greater number of trials than other posterior groups to reach criterion on the stylus maze task. The bilateral posterior group was equally and severely impaired on the stylus maze and the locomotor maze tasks. However, patients with bilateral anterior lesions performed as well or better than the two (small) unilateral nonposterior groups. Unlike the earlier results, no unilateral group exhibited a deficit in locomotor maze performance. In addition, sizable impairment was observed in a bilateral posterior lesion sample that was added for later analysis. These differing results were attributed to the inclusion of practice trials and the longer postinjury interval in their series of cases rather than to lesion classification, since the left and right posterior lesion groups in the earlier studies performed more poorly than did the unilateral right posterior group in the Ratcliff and Newcombe study. Availability of more exact anatomical criteria, however, might have yielded clearer lateralized deficits. A dissociation between poor performance on the locomotor maze task and the stylus maze task was reflected in somewhat better performances among the bilateral posterior group when compared with the right posterior group on the stylus maze task in the Ratcliff and Newcombe study. This dissociation was reported to be striking in some patients. An a priori analysis of the processes involved in these tasks suggests that the visually guided stylus maze requires a constant orientation but serial processing of choice points and retention of the path, while the locomotor maze produces shifts in orientation from a relatively simple set of markers for otherwise relatively uncomplicated mazes.

SUMMARY AND IMPLICATIONS

This review of the procedural variations that have elicited dissociated deficits in each of the major areas of the association cortex of the right cerebral hemisphere demonstrates the need for a taxonomy of process to guide the design of particular tasks. In addition to the entire range of sensorimotor, perceptual, visuospatial, visuoconstructional, affective, and topographic disturbances associated with right cerebral lesions, there is now evidence of effects of such lesions on the comprehension of language and related symbolic functions (Caramazza, Gordon, Zurif, & DeLuca, 1976; Gardner, Ling, Flam, & Silverman, 1975; Rivers & Love, 1980; Wapner, Hamby, & Gardner, 1981). The participation of the right cerebral hemisphere in language functioning is well established clinically, since early and extensive involvement of the left hemisphere may not prevent language from developing to near normal levels nor necessarily result in definitve aphasic speech in adulthood. In addition, left cerebral hemispherectomy in right-handed adults may result in reestablishment of language function (Smith, 1975). Research reviewed elsewhere in this volume demonstrates some comprehension of language when stimulus input is restricted to the right hemisphere, although the naming function appears to be limited to the left hemisphere (Sperry, Gazzaniga, & Bogen, 1969). Differences in behavioral outcomes between anterior and posterior lesions are readily identified in left cerebral hemisphere involvement, as evidenced by the extensive literature relating to the aphasic syndromes associated with acute and highly circumscribed lesions (Caramazza & Martin, this volume; Geschwind, 1965a, 1965b; Goodglass & Kaplan, 1972). Except for posterior lesions, clinical research has not yielded an analogous typology of deficits or set of syndromes for the right hemisphere. Efforts to develop a taxonomy of symbolic processes subserved by the right hemisphere are underway in the promising studies of Gardner and his associates (Gardner, 1977, 1978; Gardner, Howard, & Perkins, 1974). Qualitative analysis of performances on right hemisphere–related tasks has yielded distinct characterizations of differences between right and left hemisphere lesions (Kaplan, 1980). There is now additional evidence that cognitive and emotional or personality factors are likely to interact in ways that may affect outcomes on verbal tests. For example, Gardner et al. (1975) and Wapner, Hamby, and Gardner (1981) have shown that right hemisphere lesions may affect preferences for jokes and produce inappropriate and unusual reactions to humorous material. Cicone, Wapner, and Gardner (1980) demonstrated impairments in the ability to judge emotion appropriate to a situation, independently of the nature of the material, verbal or nonverbal, whether utilized or applied in making the judgment. Gardner, Silverman, Wapner, and Zurif (1978) elicited difficulties in selecting opposites to materials presented verbally or pictorially, confusing synonymy with antonymy in right hemisphere disease. Similarly, right hemisphere involvement was associated with hesitation to match spoken phrases with graphic patterns of connotative meaning (Gardner & Denes, 1973; Gardner, Silverman, Denes, et al., 1977).

Improved understanding of the functions of the right cerebral hemisphere will depend upon the specification of those symbolic operations, verbal or nonverbal, and the component processes that may be affected differentially by lesions in different portions of the right hemisphere or with involvement of any region of the hemisphere. Given the already rich knowledge of behavioral correlates available in the literature and the prospect for more detailed and precise categorization of the lesion through modern radiographic techniques, clinical investigators have a remarkably strong information base from which to conduct new research. Furthermore, while "extraneous" or "nuisance" factors such as age, sex, etiology, time since symptom onset, chronicity of cerebral disease, individual variation in patterns of cerebral dominance, personality, and premorbid cerebral status need to be controlled as covariates in studies of lateral specialization, they also add to the empirical basis for generating new hypotheses and research questions.

REFERENCES

Annett, M. The distribution of manual asymmetry. *British Journal of Psychology*, 1972, *63*, 343–358.

Annett, M. The binominal distribution of right, mixed, and left-handedness. *Quarterly Journal of Experimental Psychology*, 1967, *19*, 327–333.

Baker, A.B. *An outline of clinical neurology*. Dubuque, Iowa: William C. Brown, 1958.

Bear, D.M., & Fedio, P. Quantitative analysis of interictal behavior in temporal lobe epilepsy. *Archives of Neurology*, 1977, *34*, 454–467.

Benson, D.F., & Barton, M.I. Disturbances in constructional ability. *Cortex*, 1970, *6*, 19–46.

Benton, A. Clinical symptomatology in right and left hemisphere lesions. In V.B. Mountcastle (Ed.), *Interhemispheric relations and cerebral dominance*. Baltimore: Johns Hopkins University Press, 1962.

Benton, A. Visuoperceptive, visuospatial and visuoconstructive disorders. In K.M. Heilman & E. Valenstein (Eds.), *Clinical neuropsychology*. New York: Oxford University Press, 1979.

Benton, A.L. Differential behavioral effects in frontal lobe disease. *Neuropsychologia*, 1968, *6*, 53–60.

Benton, A.L. Aspects of the neuropsychology of aging. Invited address, *Division 40 American Psychological Association*, Los Angeles, August 1981.

Benton, A.L., & Hécaen, H. Stereoscopic vision in patients with unilateral cerebral disease. *Neurology*, 1970, *20*, 1084–1088.

Blumer, D. Temporal lobe epilepsy and its psychiatric significance. In D.F. Benson & D. Blumer (Eds.), *Psychiatric aspects of neurological disease*. New York: Grune & Stratton, 1975.

Blumer, D., & Benson, D.F. Personality changes with frontal and temporal lobe lesions. In D.F. Benson and D. Blumer (Eds.), *Psychiatric aspects of neurological disease*. New York: Grune & Stratton, 1975.

Borkowski, J.G., Benton, A.L., & Spreen, O. Word fluency and brain damage. *Neuropsychologia*, 1967, *5*, 135–140.

Botwinick, J. Intellectual abilities. In J.E. Birren & K.W. Schaie (Eds.), *Handbook of the psychology of aging*. New York: Van Nostrand Reinhold, 1977.

Brain, L. *Diseases of the nervous system*. London: Oxford University Press, 1962.

Branch, C., Milner, B., & Rasmussen, T. Intracarotid sodium amytal for the lateralization of cerebral speech dominance. *Journal of Neurosurgery*, 1964, *21*, 399–465.

Bryden, M. Tachistoscopic recognition, handedness, and cerebral dominance. *Neuropsychologia*, 1965, *3*, 1–8.

Bryden, M. Speech localization in families: A preliminary study using dichotic listening. *Brain and Language*, 1975, *2*, 201–211.

Butters, N., & Barton, M. Effects of parietal lobe damage on the performance of reversible operations in space. *Neuropsychologia*, 1970, *8*, 205–214.

Caramazza, A., Gordon, J., Zurif, E., & DeLuca, D. Right-hemispheric damage and verbal problem solving behavior. *Brain and Language*, 1976, *3*, 41–46.

Carlsson, C.A., von Essen, C., & Lofgren, J. Factors affecting the clinical course of patients with severe head injury. *Journal of Neurosurgery*, 1968, *29*, 242–251.

Carmon, A. Disturbances in tactile sensitivity in patients with cerebral lesions. *Cortex*, 1971, *7*, 83–97.

Carmon, A., & Bechtoldt, H.P. Dominance of the right cerebral hemisphere for stereopsis, *Neuropsychologia*, 1969, *7*, 29–39.

Carmon, A., & Benton, A.L. Tactile perception of direction and number in patients with unilateral cerebral disease. *Neurology*, 1969, *19*, 525–532.

Cattell, R.B. Theory of fluid and crystallized intelligence: An initial experiment. *Journal of Educational Psychology*, 1963, *105*, 105–111.

Cicone, M., Wapner, W., & Gardner, H. Sensitivity to emotional expressions and situations in organic patients. *Cortex*, 1980, *16*, 145–158.

Corkin, S.H. Tactually-guided maze learning in man: Effects of unilateral cortical excisions and bilateral hippocampal lesions. *Neuropsychologia*, 1965, *3*, 339–351.

Corkin, S.H. *Somesthetic function after focal cerebral damage in man*. Unpublished doctoral dissertation, McGill University, 1964.

Costa, L.D., Vaughn, H.G., Jr., Levita, E., & Farber, N. Purdue pegboard as predictor of the presence of the laterality of cerebral lesions. *Journal of Consulting Psychology*, 1963, *27*, 133–137.

Courville, C.B. The structural basis for the common traumatic cerebral syndromes. *Bulletin of Los Angeles Neurological Society*, 1944, *9*, 17.

Courville, C.B., & Ames, E.W. Late residual lesions of the brain consequent to dural hemorrhage. *Bulletin of the Los Angeles Neurological Society*, 1952, *17*, 163.

Craik, F. Age differences in human memory. In J.E. Birren & K.W. Schaie (Eds.), *Handbook of the psychology of aging*. New York: Van Nostrand Reinhold, 1977.

Critchley, M. *The parietal lobes*. London: Edward Arnold, 1953.

Cronbach, L.J. Test "reliability": Its meaning and determination. *Psychometrika*, 1947, *12*, 1–16.

Dahlstrom, W.G., Welsh, G.S., and Dahlstrom, L.E. *An MMPI Handbook. Vol. II: Research Applications*. Minneapolis: University of Minnesota Press, 1975.

Damasio, A. The frontal lobes. In K.M. Heilman & E. Valenstein (Eds.), *Clinical neuropsychology*. New York: Oxford University Press, 1979.

DeRenzi, E. Nonverbal memory and hemispheric side of lesion. *Neuropsychologia*, 1968, *6*, 181–189.

DeRenzi, E., & Nichelli, P. Verbal and nonverbal short term memory impairment following hemispheric damage. *Cortex*, 1975, *11*, 341–353.

DeRenzi, E., Faglioni, P., & Scotti, G. Impairment of memory for position following brain damage. *Cortex*, 1969, *5*, 274–284.

DeRenzi, E., Faglioni, P., & Scotti, G. Judgment of spatial orientation in patients with focal brain damage. *Journal of Neurology, Neurosurgery, and Psychiatry*, 1971, *34*, 489–495.

DeRenzi, E., Faglioni, P., & Villa, P. Topographical amnesia. *Journal of Neurology, Neurosurgery, and Psychiatry*, 1977, *40*, 498–505.

Drewe, E.A. The effect of type and area of brain lesion on Wisconsin Card Sorting Test performance. *Cortex*, 1974, *10*, 159–170.

Drewe, E.A. Go-no go learning after frontal lobe lesions in humans. *Cortex*, 1975, *11*, 8–16.

Durnford, M., & Kimura, D. Right hemisphere specialization for depth perception reflected in visual field differences. *Nature*, 1971, *231*, 394–395.

Fahey, T.J., Irving, M.H., & Miller, P. Severe head injuries: A six year follow-up. *Lancet*, 1967, *2*, 475–479.

Fennell, E., Satz, P., Van den Abell, T. et al. Visuospatial competency, handedness and cerebral dominance. *Brain and Language*, 1978, *5*, 206–214.

Friedman, S.H. *Psychometric effects of frontal and parietal lobe damage*. Unpublished doctoral dissertation, University of Minnesota, 1950.

Gainotti, G. Emotional behavior and hemispheric side of lesion. *Cortex*, 1972, *8*, 41–55.

Gardner, H. Senses, symbols, operations: An organization of artistry. In D. Perkins & B. Leondar (Eds.), *The arts and cognition*. Baltimore: The Johns Hopkins University Press, 1977.

Gardner, H. The development and breakdown of symbolic capacities: A search for general principles. In A. Caramazza & E. Zurif (Eds.), *The acquisition and breakdown of language*. Baltimore: Johns Hopkins University Press, 1978.

Gardner, H., & Denes, G. Connotative judgment by aphasic patients on a pictorial adaption of the semantic differential. *Cortex*, 1973, *9*, 183–196.

Gardner, H., Howard, V., & Perkins, D. Symbol systems: A philosophical, psychological, and educational investigation. In D. Olson (Ed.), *Media and symbols: The forms of expression, communication, and education*. Chicago: University of Chicago Press, 1974.

Gardner, H., Ling, K., Flam, L., & Silverman, J. Comprehension and appreciation of humor in brain-damaged patients. *Brain*, 1975, *98*, 399–412.

Gardner, H., Silverman, J., Denes, G. et al. Sensitivity to musical education denotation and connotation in organic patients. *Cortex*, 1977, *13*, 242–256.

Gardner, H., Silverman, J., Wapner, W., & Zurif, E. The appreciation of antonymic contrasts in aphasia. *Brain and Language*, 1978, *6*, 301–317.

Gasparrini, W., Satz, P., Heilman, K.M., & Coolidge, F. *Hemispheric asymmetries of affective processing as determined by the Minnesota Multiphasic Personality Inventory*. Paper presented at the meeting of the International Neuropsychological Society, Sante Fe, February 1977.

Geschwind, N. Disconnexion syndromes in animals and man. *Brain*, 1965a, *88*, 237–294.

Geschwind, N. Disconnexion syndromes in animals and man. *Brain*, 1965b, *88*, 584–644.

Geschwind, N. Late changes in the nervous system: An overview. In D. Stein, J. Rosen, & N. Butters (Eds.), *Plasticity and recovery of function in the central nervous system*. New York: Academic Press, 1974

Geschwind, N. The clinical setting of aggression in temporal lobe epilepsy. In W.S. Fields & H.W. Sweet (Eds.), *The neurobiology of violence*. St. Louis: Warren H. Green, 1975.

Geschwind, N. Behavioral changes in temporal lobe epilepsy. *Archives of Neurology*, 1977, *34*, 453.

Goldstein, K. The effects of brain damage on the personality. *Psychiatry*, 1952, *15*, 245–260.

Goldstein, K., & Scheerer, M. Abstract and concrete behavior. *Psychological Monographs*, 1941, *53*, (Whole No. 239).

Goldstein, G. & Shelly, C. Does the right hemisphere age more rapidly than the left? *Journal of Clinical Neuropsychology*, 1981, *3*, 65–78.

Goodglass, H., & Kaplan, E. *The assessment of aphasia and related disorders*. Philadelphia: Lea & Febiger, 1972.

Gordon, H. Hemispheric asymmetries in the perception of musical chords. *Cortex*, 1970, *6*, 387–398.

Guerrant, J., Anderson, W.W., Fischer, A. et al. *Personality in epilepsy*. Springfield, Ill.: Charles C. Thomas, 1962.

Halstead, W.C. *Brain and intelligence: A quantitative study of the frontal lobes*. Chicago: University of Chicago Press, 1947.

Heaton, R.P., Baade, L.E., & Johnson, R.L. Neuropsychological test results associated with psychiatric disorders in adults. *Psychological Bulletin*, 1978, *85*, 141–162.

Hebb, D. Distinctive features of learning in the higher animal. In A. Fesard, R.W. Gerard, J. Konorski & J.F. Delafresnaye (Eds.), *Brain mechanisms and learning*. Oxford: Blackwell Scientific Publications, 1961.

Hebb, D.O., & Penfield, W. Human behavior after extensive bilateral removals from the frontal lobes. *Archives of Neurology and Psychiatry*, 1940, *44*, 421–438.

Hécaen, H. Clinical symptomatology in right and left hemispheric lesions. In V.B. Mountcastle (Ed.), *Interhemispheric relations and cerebral dominance*. Baltimore: John Hopkins Press, 1962

Hécaen, H. Mental symptoms associated with tumors of the frontal lobe. In J.M. Warren & K. Akert (Eds.), *The frontal granular cortex and behavior*. New York: McGraw-Hill, 1964.

Heilman, K. Neglect and related disorders. In K.M. Heilman & E. Valenstein (Eds.), *Clinical Neuropsychology*. New York: Oxford University Press, 1979.

Herron, J. *Neuropsychology of left-handedness*. New York: Academic Press, 1980.

Horn, J.L., & Cattell, R.B. Age differences in fluid and crystallized intelligence. *Acta Psychologica*, 1967, *26*, 107–129.

Inglis, J., & Lawson, J.S. Sex differences in the effects of unilateral brain damage on intelligence. *Science*, 1981, *212*, 693–695.

Jarvik, L. Thoughts on the psychobiology of aging. *American Psychologist*, 1975, *30*, 576–583.

Jarvik, L.F., & Falek, A. Intellectual stability and survival in the aged. *Journal of Gerontology*, 1963, *18*, 173–176.

Jones-Gottman, M., & Milner, B. Design fluency: The invention of nonsense drawings after focal cortical lesions. *Neuropsychologia*, 1977, *15*, 653–673.

Joynt, R., & Goldstein, M. Minor cerebral hemisphere. In W.J. Friedlander (Ed.), *Advances in Neurology*, (Vol. 7). New York: Raven Press, 1975.

Kaplan, E. *Process and achievement revisited.* Paper presented at the meeting of the International Neuropsychological Society, San Francisco, 1980.

Kaszniak, A.W., Garron, D.C., Fox, J.H. et al. Cerebral atrophy, EEG slowing, age, education, and cognitive functioning in suspected dementia. *Neurology*, 1979, *29*, 1273–1279.

Kimura, D. Right temporal lobe damage. *Archives of Neurology*, 1963, *8*, 264–271.

Kimura, D. Left-right differences in the perception of melodies. *Quarterly Journal of Experimental Psychology*, 1964, *16*, 355–358.

Kimura, D. Spatial localization in left and right visual fields. *Canadian Journal of Psychology*, 1969, *23*, 445–458.

Kimura, D. The asymmetry of the human brain. *Scientific American*, 1973, *228*, 70–80.

Kinsbourne, M., & Warrington, E. A localizing significance of limited simultaneous form perception. *Brain*, 1963, *86*, 699–702.

Kinsbourne, M. The minor cerebral hemisphere as a source of aphasic speech. *Archives of Neurology*, 1971, *25*, 302–306.

Lansdell, H. Sex differences in hemispheric asymmetries of the human brain. *Nature*, 1964, *203*, 550.

Levin, H., Grossman, R., Rose, J., & Teasdale, G., Long-term neuropsychological outcome of closed head injury. *Journal of Neurosurgery*, 1979, *50*, 412–422.

Levy, J., & Reid, M. Variations in writing posture and cerebral organization. *Science*, 1976, *194*, 337–339

Levy, J., & Reid, M. Variations in cerebral organization as a function of handedness, hand posture in writing and sex. *Journal of Experimental Psychology: General*, 1978, *107*, 119–144.

Luria, A.R. *Higher cortical functions in man*. New York: Basic Books, 1966.

Luria, A.R., & Homskaya, E.D. Disturbances in the regulative role of speech with frontal lobe lesions. In J.M. Warren & K. Akert (Eds.), *The frontal granular cortex and behavior*, New York: McGraw-Hill, 1964.

Luria, A.R., Homskaya, E.D., Blinkov, S.M., & Critchley, M. Impaired selectivity of mental processes associated with a lesion of the frontal lobe. *Neuropsychologia*, 1967, *5*, 105-117.

Matthews, C.G., Shaw, D.J. & Kløve, H. Psychological test performances in neurologic and pseudoneurologic subjects. *Cortex*, 1966, *2*, 244-253.

McGlone, J. Sex differences in human brain asymmetry: A critical review. *The Behavioral and Brain Sciences*, 1980, *3*, 215-263.

McGlone, J., & Kertesz, A. Sex differences in cerebral processes of visuospatial tasks. *Cortex*, 1973, *9*, 313-320.

Meier, M.J. The regional localization hypothesis and personality change associated with focal cerebral lesions and ablations. In J.N. Butcher (Ed.), *MMPI research developments and clinical applications*. New York: McGraw-Hill, 1969, pp. 243-261.

Meier, M.J. Effects of focal cerebral lesions on contralateral visuomotor adaptation to reversal and inversion of visual feedback. *Neuropsychologia*, 1970, *8*, 269-279.

Meier, M.J. *Recovery of neuropsychological functioning after cerebrovascular infarction*. Paper presented at the meeting of the Third International Neuropsychological Society Conference, Chianciano-Terme, Italy, 1980.

Meier, M.J., & French, L.A. Lateralized deficits in complex visual discrimination and bilateral transfer of reminiscence following unilateral temporal lobectomy. *Neuropsychologia*, 1965a, 261-273.

Meier, M.J., & French, L.A. Some personality correlates of unilateral and bilateral EEG abnormalities in psychomotor epileptics. *Journal of Clinical Psychology*, 1965b, *21*, 3-9.

Meier, M.J., & French, L.A. Changes in MMPI scale scores as an index of psychopathology following unilateral temporal lobectomy for epilepsy. *Epilepsia*, 1965c, *6*, 263-273.

Meier, M.J., Ettinger, M.C., & Arthur, L. Recovery of neuropsychological functioning after cerebrovascular infarction. In R. Malatesha & L. Hartlage, (Eds.), *Cognition and neuropsychology*, Sijthoff and Noordhoff: Alphen, The Netherlands, in press.

Meier, M.J. and Okayama, M. Behavior assessment. Stroke (Monograph): U.S. and Japan. Part II. *Geriatrics*, 1969, *24*, 95-110.

Milner, B. *Impairment of visual recognition and recall after right temporal lobectomy in man*. Paper presented at the meeeting of the Psychonomic Society, Chicago, 1960.

Milner, B. Laterality effects in audition. In V.B. Mountcastle (Ed.), *Interhemispheric relations and cerebral dominance*. Baltimore: John Hopkins University Press, 1962.

Milner, B. Some effects of frontal lobectomy in man. In J.M. Warren & K. Akert (Eds.), *The frontal granular cortex and behavior*. New York: McGraw-Hill, 1964.

Milner, B. Visually guided maze learning in man: Effects of bilateral hippocampal, bilateral frontal, and unilateral cerebral lesions. *Neuropsychologia*, 1965, *3*, 317–338.

Milner, B. Brain mechanisms suggested by studies of temporal lobes. In F.L. Darley (Ed.), *Brain mechanisms underlying speech and language*. New York: Grune & Stratton, 1967.

Milner, B. Visual recognition and recall after right temporal lobe excision in man. *Neuropsychologia*, 1968, *6*, 191–209.

Milner, B. Interhemispheric differences in the localization of psychological processes in man. *British Medical Bulletin*, 1971, *27*, 272–277.

Milner, B., & Teuber, H.L. Alteration of perception and memory in man: Reflections on methods. In L. Weiskrantz (Ed.), *Analysis of behavior change*. New York: Harper & Row, 1968.

Mishkin, M. Perseveration of central sets after frontal lesions in monkeys. In J.M. Warren & K. Akert (Eds.), *The frontal granular cortex and behavior*. New York: McGraw-Hill, 1964.

Mooney, C. Age in the development of closure ability in children. *Canadian Journal of Psychology*, 1957, *2*, 219–226.

New, P.F.J., Scott, W.R., Schnur, J.A. et al. Computed tomography with the EMI scanner in the diagnosis of primary and metastatic intracranial neoplasms. *Radiology*, 1975, *114*, 75–87.

Newcombe, F. and Russell, W.R. Dissociated visual perceptual and spatial deficits in focal lesions of the right hemispheres. *Journal of Neurology, Neurosurgery and Psychiatry*, 1969, *32*, 73–81.

Ojemann, G.A., & Whitaker, H. Language localization and variability. *Brain and Language*, 1978, *6*, 239–260.

Oldfield, R.C. The assessment and analysis of handedness: The Edinburgh Inventory. *Neuropsychologia*, 1971, *9*, 97–113.

Ommaya, A., & Gennarelli, T. Cerebral concussion and traumatic unconsciousness. *Brain*, 1974, *97*, 633–654.

Parsons, O.A., & Prigatano, G.P. Methodological considerations in clinical and neuropsychological research. *Journal of Consulting and Clinical Psychology*, 1978, *46*, 608-619.

Paxton, H.L. Jr., & Ambrose, J. The EMI scanner: A brief review of the first 650 patients. *British Journal of Radiology*, 1974, *47*, 530–565.

Penry, J.K. Behavioral correlates of generalized spike-wave discharge in the electroencephalo-gram. In M.A.B. Brazier (Ed.), *Epilepsy: Its phenomenon in man*. New York: Academic Press, 1973.

Peterson, L.R., & Peterson, M.S. Short-term retention of individual verbal items. *Journal of Experimental Psychology*, 1959, *58*, 193–198.

Porteus, S. *The maze test and clinical psychology*. Palo Alto, Calif.: Pacific Books, 1959.

Posner, M. Components of skilled performance. *Science*, 1966, *152*, 1712–1718.

Ratcliff, G., & Newcombe, F. Spatial orientation in man: Effects of left, right, and bilateral posterior cerebral lesions. *Journal of Neurology, Neurosurgery, and Psychiatry*, 1973, *36*, 448–454.

Reitan, R.M. Psychological deficits resulting from cerebral lesions in man. In J.M. Warren & K. Akert (Eds.), *The frontal granular cortex and behavior*. New York: McGraw-Hill, 1964.

Rivers, D., & Love, R. Language performance on visual processing tasks in right hemisphere lesion cases. *Brain and Language*, 1980, *10*, 348–366.

Rizzolati, G., Umiltá, C., & Berlucchi, G. Opposite superiorities of the right and left cerebral hemispheres in discriminative reaction time to physiognomic and alphabetical material. *Brain*, 1971, *94*, 431–442.

Robinson, A.C., Heaton, R.K., Lehman, R.A., & Stilson, D.W. The utility of the Wisconsin Card Sorting Test in defecting and localizing frontal lobe lesions. *Journal of Consulting and Clinical Psychology*, 1980, *48*, 605–614.

Rosvold, H.E., & Mishkin, M. Nonsensory effects of frontal lesions on discrimination learning and performance. In J.F. Delafresnaye (Ed.), *Brain mechanisms and learning*, Oxford: Blackwell, 1961.

Russell, E.W., Neuringer, C. and Goldstein, G. *Assessment of brain damage: A neuropsychological key approach*. New York: Wiley-Interscience, 1970.

Russell, W.R. *The traumatic amnesias*. London: Oxford University Press, 1971.

Russell, W.R., & Smith, A. Post-traumatic amnesia in closed head injury. *Archives of Neurology*, 1961, *5*, 4–17.

Rylander, G. *Personality changes after operations on the frontal lobes*. London: Oxford University Press, 1939.

Satz, P. Left-handedness and brain insult: An explanation. *Neuropsychologia*, 1973, *11*, 115–117.

Satz, P., Achenback, K., Pattishall, E., & Fennell, E. Order of report, ear asymmetry and handedness in dichotic listening. *Cortex*, 1965, *1*, 377–396.

Schaie, K.W. A reinterpretation of age-related changes in cognitive structure and functioning. In L.R. Goulet & P.B. Baltes (Eds.), *Life-span developmental psychology: Research and theory*. New York: Academic Press, 1970.

Schaie, K.W. Quasi-experimental research designs in the psychology of aging. In J.E. Birren & K.W. Schaie (Eds.), *Handbook of the psychology of aging*. New York: Van Nostrand Reinhold, 1977.

Schaie, K.W., & Labouvie-Vief, G. Generational versus ontogenetic components of change in adult cognitive behavior: A fourteen-year cross-sequential study. *Developmental Psychology*, 1974, *10*, 305–320.

Schaie, K.W., & Schaie, J.P. Clinical assessment and aging. In J.E. Birren & K.W. Schaie (Eds.), *Handbook of the psychology of aging*. New York: Van Nostrand Reinhold, 1977.

Seidman, L. Lateralized cerebral dysfunction, personality and cognition in temporal lobe epilepsy (Doctoral dissertation, Boston University, 1980). *Dissertation Abstracts International* 1980, *40*, 5831. (University Microfilms No. 8013298)

Seidman, L., & Mirsky, A. *Hemispheric dysfunction and personality in temporal lobe epilepsy*. Paper presented at the meeting of the International Neuropsychological Society, San Francisco, February 1980.

Semmes, J. Hemispheric specialization: A possible clue to mechanism. *Neuropsychologia*, 1968, *6*, 11–26.

Semmes, J., Weinstein, S., Ghent, L., & Teuber, H.L. Spatial orientation in man after cerebral injury: I. Analysis by locus of lesion. *Journal of Psychology*, 1955, *39*, 227–244.

Semmes, J., Weinstein, S., Ghent, L., & Teuber, H.L. *Somatosensory changes after penetrating brain wounds in man*. Cambridge: Harvard University Press, 1960.

Semmes, J., Weinstein, S., Ghent, L., & Teuber, H.L. Correlates of impaired orientation in personal and extrapersonal space. *Brain*, 1963, *86*, 747–772.

Shallice, T., & Evans, M.E. The involvement of the frontal lobes in cognitive estimation. *Cortex*, 1978, *14*, 294–303.

Shankweiler, D. Effects of temporal lobe damage on perception of dichotically presented melodies. *Journal of Comparative and Physiological Psychology*, 1966, *62*, 115–119.

Smith, A. Speech and other functions after left dominant hemispherectomy. *Journal of Neurology, Neurosurgery, and Psychiatry*, 1966, *29*, 467–471.

Smith, A. Neuropsychological testing in neurological disorders. In W.J. Friedlander (Ed.), *Advances in neurology* (Vol. 7). New York: Raven, 1975.

Smith, A. Principles underlying human brain function in neuropsychological sequelae of different neuropsychological processes. In T.J. Boll & S.B. Filskov (Eds.), *Handbook of clinical neuropsychology*. New York: Wiley, 1981.

Smokler, I.A., & Shevrin, H. Cerebral lateralization and personality style. *Archives of General Psychiatry*, 1979, *36*, 949-954.

Sperry, R.W., Gazzaniga, M.S., & Bogen, J.E. Interhemispheric relationships: The neocortical commisures; syndromes of hemispheric disconnection. In P.J. Viken & G.W. Bruyn (Eds.), *Handbook of clinical neurology*. Amsterdam: North-Holland, 1969.

Stater, E. & Beard, A.W. The schizophrenia-like psychoses of epilepsy. *British Journal of Psychiatry*, 1963, *109*, 95-150.

Strich, S. Shearing of nerve fibers as a cause of brain damage due to head injury: A pathological study of twenty cases. *Lancet*, 1961, *2*, 443-448.

Taylor, A.M., & Warrington, E. Visual discrimination in patients with localized brain lesions. *Cortex*, 1973, *9*, 82-93.

Taylor, D.C. Factors influencing the occurrence of schizophrenia-like psychosis in patients with temporal lobe epilepsy. *Psychological Medicine*, 1975, *5*, 249-254.

Teuber, H.L. The riddle of frontal lobe function in man. In J.M. Warren & K. Akert (Eds.), *The frontal granular cortex and behavior*. New York: McGraw-Hill, 1964.

Thomas, R.S., Hauser, W.A., Strauman, S.E. et al. *Neuropsychological and genetic interactions in epilepsy*. Paper presented at the meeting of the International Neuropsychological Society, San Francisco, February 1980.

Twitchell, T. The restoration of motor function following hemiplegia in man. *Brain*, 1951, *74*, 443-480.

Valenstein, E., & Heilman, K.M. Emotional disorders resulting from lesions of the central nervous system. In K.M. Heilman & E. Valenstein (Eds.), *Clinical neuropsychology*. New York: Oxford University Press, 1979.

Varney, N.R., & Benton, A.C. Tactile perception of direction in relation to handedness and familial handedness. *Neuropsychologia*, 1975, *13*, 449-454.

Victor, M., Adams, R.D., & Collins, G.H. *The Wernicke-Korsakoff syndrome*. Philadelphia: F.A. Davis, 1971.

Wada, J. *Cerebral anatomical asymmetry in infant brains*. Symposium on Sex Differences in Brain Asymmetry presented at the meeting of the International Neuropsychological Society, Toronto, February 1976.

Wapner, W., Hamby, S., & Gardner, H. The role of the right hemisphere in the appreciation of complex linguistic materials. *Brain and Language*, 1981, *14*, 15-33.

Warrington, E.D., & Rabin, P. Perceptual matching in patients with cerebral lesions. *Neuropsychologia*, 1970, *8*, 475-487.

Warrington, E.K., & James, M. An experimental investigation of facial recognition in patients with unilateral lesions. *Cortex*, 1967, *3*, 317–326.

Williams, H. The development of a caudality scale for the MMPI. *Journal of Clinical Psychology*, 1952, *8*, 293–297.

Witelson, S.F., & Pallie, W. Left hemisphere specialization for language in the newborn: Neuroanatomical evidence for asymmetry. *Brain*, 1973, *96*, 641–647.

Zangwill, O.L. *Cerebral dominance and its relation to psychological function*. London: Oliver and Boyd, 1960.

4

Disconnection Syndrome as a Model for Laterality Effects in the Normal Brain

Eran Zaidel

INTRODUCTION: THE HISTORY OF HEMIFIELD TACHISTOSCOPIC STUDIES OF READING

1961 was a turning point for research on hemispheric specialization in humans. In Montreal, Doreen Kimura had just completed a study on laterality effects, correlating the observed ear advantage in dichotic listening with speech dominance determined by unilateral Amytal Sodium to epileptic patients. In Boston, Norman Geschwind and Edith Kaplan were observing the first modern case of a disconnection syndrome due to a natural callosal lesion. And at the California Institute of Technology, Roger Sperry, Michael Gazzaniga, and Joseph Bogen were preparing to study the first complete commissurotomy patient of the California series. The interpretation of Geschwind and Kaplan's case study belonged in the classical clinical neurological tradition of Wernicke, Dejerine, and Liepmann; however, the study was strongly motivated by the animal split-brain studies of Sperry and Meyers on cats and monkeys during the mid-1950s, first at the University of Chicago and later at the California Institute of Technology. Kimura, in turn, combined experimental psychological techniques for stimulus lateralization in the tradition of Donald Hebb's lab at McGill University with the clinical methods of inducing temporary hemispheric anesthesia used by Penfield, Rasmussen, and Milner at the Montreal Neurological Institute. The ensuing years saw a progressive rapproachment between clinical neurology and experimental psychology, ever catalyzed by the human commissurotomy studies, into what is now capable of becoming a systematic and coherent study of hemispheric specialization.

The indispensable catalytic effect of the human disconnection syndrome can be demonstrated by the failure of two earlier sets of hemifield tachistoscopic experiments to gain much scientific attention or following for studies of hemispheric specialization in normal subjects. The first set of studies was carried out by Shepherd Ivory Franz at UCLA in 1933. The second set was performed in Hebb's lab at McGill University beginning in 1952. Although the McGill group was apparently ignorant of Franz's experiments, there were some curious analogies between the two programs. Both arose out of an interest in the question of transfer of visual training across the retina. In addition, both misinterpreted the observed laterality effects because of some confounding effects of ocular scanning directionality in reading. What was missing in both cases was the strong zeitgeist created by the commissurotomy studies in the 1960s.

Shepherd Ivory Franz

When he undertook his hemifield tachistoscopic experiments on hemispheric specialization for linguistic as against nonsense geometric stimuli in normal subjects, Franz was already a veteran neuropsychologist. He had pioneered the method of studying the consequences of cerebral lesions on animals trained preoperatively by observing their effects on a laboratory task. He also taught Karl Lashley how to use the technique during an internship at the McLean Hospital for the Insane in Washington, D.C. In addition, he had conducted cortical mapping studies through brain stimulation in cats and monkeys, he had studied aphasia, and he was especially concerned with functional recovery following cerebral insult. Thus, he was intimately familiar with the doctrine of left hemisphere (LH) specialization for language and particularly for reading in right-handed subjects. More generally, the LH was then widely considered dominant for all higher functions in dextrals, whereas the right hemisphere (RH) was believed dominant, mirror-image fashion, in sinistrals.

Franz's experiments used a gravity tachistoscope, presented bilateral stimuli for 100 msec, and even encouraged fixation by flashing an additional stimulus, a simple geometric design, above fixation. Thus, the experimental paradigm is surprisingly "up-to-date" in design. In the first experiment (Franz & Davis, 1933), Franz split common words, four letters long, into two two-letter halves, presented them bilaterally and horizontally ten degrees of arc apart across the fixation, and required the subjects to report the words or letters that they had seen. He observed a left visual half-field advantage

(LVFA) and interpreted this to signal RH superiority for the task. Franz's experiment reported data from six female subjects. Barbara Gouled-Smith, a graduate student at UCLA, recently replicated and extended this study to both right-handed female and male subjects (Smith, 1981). She found an LVFA for nine out of ten males and for seven out of ten females. Clearly, the task creates a strong bias for left-to-right postexposural attentional scanning of the icon. The left visual field (LVF) letters are reported first and decay the least, resulting in the observed LVFA.

In a second experiment (Franz & Kilduff, 1933), the subject was required to identify, on a multiple-choice card, three nonsense geometric figures eight degrees to the left, right, and above fixation. A consistent right visual half-field advantage (RVFA) was observed! Furthermore, left-handed subjects showed the same pattern as right-handed subjects. Franz interpreted this result as showing LH specialization for "learning to read unfamiliar symbols." This conclusion is in direct contradiction to recent findings (e.g., Gordon & Carmon, 1976; see review in Goldberg & Costa, 1981). However, the result is probably consistent with the recent finding of an RVFA for familiar geometric pattern discrimination and an LVFA for complex geometric figures (Umiltá, Brizzolara, Tabossi, & Fairweather, 1978), since Franz's figures can be verbalized, especially with long, repeated administration, as given by Franz.

This experiment is currently being replicated at UCLA. The original reports are not always explicit concerning the method and procedures used. Consequently, it was necessary to guess at some of the details. It is not clear if Franz's failure to spell out all of the details of his experiment signals a different standard of experimental psychological reporting 50 years ago, if the omitted details were left out because they were presupposed as common practice, or, more likely, that the informal presentation reflects the novelty of the study and the lack of general professional interest in it.

Franz recognized the incompatibility between the results in his reading study and the then current doctrine of unilateral LH dominance for all perceptual, motor, and cognitive functions. Four of his six female subjects showed an LVFA and two showed no visual field advantage (VFA). He did not doubt his results but rather startlingly concluded that we must "alter or give up the conception of cerebral dominance as an anatomical and physiological condition" (Franz, 1933). Thus, Franz abandoned the anatomical interpretation of cerebral dominance and opted for the then radical (but today popular) psychological hypothesis of dynamic control of hemispheric activation as a function of task variables, including attention, set, or gestalt. What was missing in his neuropsychclogical milieu was a concept of complementary RH specialization for specific functions. Milner's work on hemispheric specialization in temporal lobectomy patients may have provided this conceptual background for Kimura, and the disconnection syndrome provided this zeitgeist dramatically for modern neuropsychology in general.

In retrospect, from the vantage point of modern research on hemispheric specialization, it is easy to explain Franz's reading data as artifactual and due to the independent effect of left-to-right reading scanning in English. We now know from more recent hemifield tachistoscopic studies of reading that the VFA can change as a function of degree of separation between the characters about the fixation (see Kimura, 1959). Bilateral words that span the fovea result in an LVFA, and two bilateral words separated far enough around the fixation result in a larger than usual RVFA (Boles, 1979; McKeever & Huling, 1971). However, for Franz there was no experimental base upon which to interpret his findings. Two distinct questions occur. First, why was Franz so willing to abandon the anatomical doctrine of LH dominance on the basis of three experiments? Second, why were his findings and conclusions universally ignored?

The first question is more difficult to answer than the second. I believe he simply did not think his experiments through. He had no body of experimental data to support alternative interpretations and no conceptual model of hemispheric competence to evaluate his conclusions. It is precisely such a model that the work on human disconnection syndrome provided 30 years later. Franz's personality may have been an important contributing factor; he is often remembered as a "nay sayer" and a debunker of myths (A. Benton, personal communication, 1981).

The answer to the second question may be related to the first. Franz's conclusions may have been too radical to gain serious attention; they contradicted some 70 years of clinical neurological tradition. Moreover, they conspicuously lacked a coherent and comprehensive research paradigm (in Kuhn's sense) and were simply not part of the concurrent concern of experimental psychology. However, the question persists — Franz was a well-known psychologist. He was the first chairman of the psychology department at UCLA and was past president of the American Psychological Association (1920). How could he have been ignored? An important part of the answer must be his untimely death in 1933 at the age of 59 soon after the publication of his three papers. Thus, he did not have a chance to validate, refine, and promote his results. Significantly, at that time UCLA did not have a Ph.D. program in psychology, so Franz did not have "converts" who would continue the work and "spread the word" (I. Maltzman, personal communication, 1981).

The McGill Group

Twenty years after Franz, Mishkin and Forgays (1952), working in Hebb's lab at McGill, discovered an RVFA for horizontal English words flashed briefly either to the left or right of central fixation at random locations. These experiments were initiated in the context of studying perceptual learning, not laterality. In connection with his neuropsychological theory (1949), Hebb hypothesized that stimulus equivalence could be established by experience so that increased speed of reading with practice meant a learned extension of the retinal field of perception of letter patterns, that is, it caused selective retinal training. In particular, in English, which is read left to right, the segment immediately following and thus presumably most affected by the reading experience, occurs on the right of the actively read segment in central fixation. One would expect better reading in the RVF than in the LVF for English but the reverse for languages read right to left. Bilingual subjects who were shown English and Yiddish words left and right of fixation, displayed a nonsignificant LVFA for Yiddish together with the usual significant RVFA for English. Alternative interpretations in terms of variations of acuity across the retina, variations in the clarity of patterns, and an attentional bias toward the RVF were thus refuted by the bilingual results, as was a possible interpretation in terms of LH dominance "for vision" (see Bertelson, 1982).

Thus, the hemispheric interpretation was explicitly considered and rejected. In retrospect, Yiddish was a poor choice. This is a hybrid language combining a predominantly High Middle German vocabulary and a Hebrew alphabet and is much more widely spoken than read. Since that time, an RVFA for Hebrew words has been demonstrated (Carmon, Nachon, & Starinsky, 1976). However, it has never been established psychophysically whether or not and to what extent the RVFA in Hebrew is smaller than in English. Determining a baseline in each language is not a trivial problem. The RH would seem to play a more important part in reading Hebrew than English, since Hebrew readers fixate on the right side of an attended word whereas English readers fixate on the left side of an attended word (Pollatsek, Bolozky, Well, & Rayner, 1981).

In any case, hemifield verbal report experiments may be ill suited for tapping RH contribution in any language since they confound reading with speech; lexical decision tasks may be a better choice. The finding that in reading we are attending to about 2 characters before fixation and to about 15 characters following fixation also suggests that, when whole words are flashed unilaterally, equidistant from fixation, postexposural "attentional scanning" to the word in the LVF would require longer "internal eye movements" than to a word in the RVF. This interpretation could explain the usual VFAs without invoking hemispheric specialization, yet it has never been recognized or analyzed. The objection can be partly countered by the observed RVFA for vertically aligned words, but those may not provide good approximations to normal reading.

The McGill experiments were impressively thorough. For example, Mishkin and Forgays found that the RVFA for English words occurred only for eccentricities of 1 degree, 11 minutes to 4 degrees, 46 minutes of arc of the center of stimulus words from fixation. Forgays (1953) found that this RVFA does not begin until the eighth-grade level. Orbach (1952) found a significant LVFA in Yiddish for bilinguals whose first language was Yiddish but a significant RVFA in Yiddish for those whose first language was English. No recent set of experiments is equally systematic and yet the authors reached the wrong conclusions, namely that the RVFA was due to factors other than hemispheric specialization for reading!

Heron (1957), continuing the work in Hebb's lab, presented rows of letters either on one side of the fixation or simultaneously on both sides. He obtained an RVFA for unilateral presentations (maximal at eccentricities of five or six degrees of arc and minimal when subjects were informed on which side the stimuli would occur) and an LVFA for bilateral presentations. The LVFA virtually replicates Franz's data and extends it from split words to nonsense character strings. Both are likely due to a left-to-right scanning habit in English, an explanation that presupposes the concept of a fading trace or iconic image. Heron interpreted all his findings in terms of attentional biases due to reading habits, although the applicability of this interpretation to unilateral presentations seems less clear. In this case, in particular, it is difficult to disentangle the "reading scanning habits" and the "perceptual learning" hypotheses. Heron also rejected the hemispheric interpretation. This shows the powerful binding power of scientific paradigms and prevailing zeitgeists on the conduct of experiments and the interpretation of data: one does not find that for which one is not looking, and there is a tendency to assimilate new data into an old conceptual framework.

However, the hemispheric interpretation must not have been far from the collective unconscious of the McGill group. Kimura was Heron's student; she did her master's thesis on hemifield tachistoscopic recognition of letters as a function of separation across the fixation and followed his suggestion in adapting the Broadbent dichotic listening method to studying hemispheric specialization for auditory stimuli. The persistent concern with hemispheric specialization at McGill must have been partly the influence of Brenda Milner's work at the Montreal Neurological Institute and perhaps partly the influence of Sperry's animal work.

Fortunately, the work on the human disconnection syndrome came soon enough afterward to revive and reevaluate the old experiments and to support the hemispheric interpretation of new ones. Again at McGill, Orbach (1967) examined the combined effects of handedness and direction of reading using bilingual English-Hebrew subjects and concluded that both LH specialization and reading scanning habits were effective, with handedness attenuating the specialization but not the scanning effect. He thus reached a multifactor account of laterality effects in normal subjects that is shared by most workers in the field today (see Bertelson, 1982).

THE CONCEPTUAL STATUS OF THE DISCONNECTION SYNDROME

Methodological Problems with the Clinical-Neurological Approach

To date, the main source of data on hemispheric specialization remains clinical-neurological data from patients with cognitive deficits subsequent to hemispheric lesions. In the past 100 years, the logic of the clinical research paradigm has been the same: observe the behaviors of selected individual patients and correlate those behaviors with clinical anatomical findings. Until recently, the methods for observing and analyzing behavior did not change conceptually. Lately, the rapproachment among clinical neurology, experimental psychology, and linguistics has yielded new and more sophisticated experimental protocols. The shift is most noticeable in the theoretical linguistic influence on aphasia research and in the effects of the information-processing brand of cognitive psychology on studies of hemispheric specialization (see Caramazza & Martin, this volume). Standardized clinical tests are being replaced by laboratory tasks that systematically vary the experimental parameters and seek to determine the stage-of-processing locus of observed deficits. However, in contrast with the rather recent change in behavioral assessement, the clinical-neurological approach has consistently emphasized the development of ever new methods of anatomical localization of lesions and functions: sensory-motor deficits, postmortem anatomical examination, EEG, cerebral angiography, pneumoencephalography, isotope scan, CAT scan, PET scan, ERP, and magnetoencepholography.

Suppose now that one wants to compare the functional specialization of the two cerebral hemispheres. The method of comparing individual case studies with localized left and right lesions is inadequate since it is impossible to match exactly the size, type, location, and etiology of the lesions. This sampling problem can be resolved by statistical studies of large populations of patients with unilateral lesions. That was the approach taken, for example, by

DeRenzi in Italy. Unfortunately, population averages lose some of the most dramatic patterns of cognitive deficits associated with unique individual patients. Moreover, in all cases of studying the diseased brain, one infers behavioral-anatomical relations indirectly from deficit. This may be logically invalid. The fact that a lesion in location x results in a disorder in function y does not mean that x "controls" y in the normal brain, much less that x is the "center" for y. Suppose that the RH has a more diffuse functional representation than the LH (see Semmes, 1968). Then comparable homologous lesions in the two sides will result in relatively severe deficits of discrete functions in the LH but milder and more numerous functional deficits in the RH (Nebes, 1974). In any case, it is never clear whether the behavioral pattern of the lesioned brain reflects functional compensation by the remaining tissue on the diseased side, takeover by healthy tissue on the contralateral side, and/or pathological inhibition of the healthy by the diseased tissue.

Negative Inference from Deficit Versus Positive Competence

Most of these methodological problems can be solved by studying hemispheric specialization in the split brain. Here, with appropriate techniques, one can compare the positive competence of the two hemispheres on tasks of interest. Since the two hemispheres of the same patient are automatically matched for sex, age, education, and so forth, they constitute mutual controls. Thus, a systematic comparison of patterns of hemispheric specialization in the disconnected hemispheres and in the hemisphere-lesioned brain provides the convergent evidence that neither approach by itself could produce. In principle, the comparison allows one to separate the pathological effect of the diseased brain from residual competence in undamaged tissue. This distinction is not merely theoretical. Extensive studies of commissurotomy patients have made it clear that the disconnected hemispheres are remarkably free of some of the more severe cognitive deficits subsequent to localized lesions, such as global aphasia following left cerebral insult and visuospatial agnosia, prosopagnosia, or unilateral neglect of the left half of space following right cerebral insult. The disconnected RH is not globally aphasic, and the disconnected LH is not prosopagnosic.

Relative Versus Exclusive Specialization

From their beginning, disconnection studies emphasized the view of each cerebral hemisphere as an independent cognitive system with its own perceptions, cognitions, memories, language, cognitive style, and even personality. This leads to the view that hemispheric specialization encompasses a wide range of behaviors throughout the sequence of information-processing stages from sensory registration to motor response. That view may be labeled as the "complete range" conceptualization of hemispheric specialization. Further, many tasks can be performed by both hemispheres, although not necessarily with equal competence and usually using different strategies. This pattern supports a "relative specialization" model of hemispheric functions, in contrast with the "exclusive specialization" model often suggested by classical clinical-neurological syndromes. Studies of patients who have had temporal lobectomy for epilepsy are perhaps unique among clinical-neurological preparations in generally supporting a relative specialization pattern. Temporal lobe excisions often result in mild cognitive deficits, and the observed left-right differences, although statistically significant, are commonly small and not reliable in individual patients (see Milner, 1978).

A natural and productive research question to result from the interface between hemispheric specialization and cognitive psychology has been the search for the information-processing locus of hemispheric specialization. Moscovitch (1979) argues that hemispheric differences first occur at relatively late stages of processing and that they will thereafter be evident at all subsequent stages (transitivity). The "complete range" conceptualization inspired by the disconnection syndrome argues, on the contrary, that laterality effects can occur at any stage. The "relative specialization" model suggested by the same data implies that hemispheric differences in performance strategies applied to any stage of processing need not result in differences in performance that may be detected with the standard latency and accuracy measures. Thus, a failure of a laterality effect to emerge in a given task may simply reflect a failure of the task to tap the differential strategies used by the two hemispheres. Furthermore, there are examples with the commissurotomy patients in which a presumed earlier stage of processing (reading qua matching of printed words with pictures of their references) yields a strong LH superiority, whereas an apparently subsequent stage (lexical decision for the same words) does not (see below.) Conversely, the failure of transitivity in laterality may be taken as evidence against a particular sequential or stage model of processing a given task. This is an example of the most important contribution of the disconnection syndrome to laterality research with normal subjects; it provides a powerful heuristic source of intuitions, hypotheses, and limit-case data.

Operational Meaning of "Degree of Hemispheric Specialization"

There is a much more important theoretical contribution of the disconnection syndrome to studies of hemispheric specialization in normals. The split-brain operationalized the concept of "degree of hemispheric specialization" by demonstrating conditions of independent processing of the same task by each hemisphere. The demonstration is so dramatic, general, and convincing that anyone who has worked with these patients for any length of time quickly begins to use expressions such as "the RH was very good at that task," or "the LH became really upset when the RH was correct." Strictly and logically, such linguistic usage is not quite justified. The disconnected hemispheres share a variety of midline structures, and one cannot exclude the possibility that the RH, for instance, uses some LH mechanisms not available to linguistic awareness on the left when the former processes stimuli presented exclusively in the left sensory field. The crucial experiment is to take the LH temporarily and completely out during RH processing. Unilateral Amytal anesthesia has several methodological shortcomings, but undoubtedly in the next 50 years there will be an arsenal of neurochemical and neuroelectric techniques for creating very well localized, both anatomically and functionally reversible, benign lesions.

Thus, the disconnection syndrome makes it well defined and coherent to use expressions such as, "hemisphere x scored y on test z." From this, it is easy to go on and operationalize the concept, "hemisphere x performed better than hemisphere y by amount z." In other words, the split-brain provides a criterial experiment for the concept of relative hemispheric specialization in the normal brain (see Harshman, 1980.) Once the concepts of "complete range" and "relative specialization" are accepted, the next theoretical task is to explicate the concept of interhemispheric interaction. If the two hemispheres represent two independent processors, how do they communicate to create apparently unified behavior? The split-brain cannot answer this question, of course, except indirectly in relation to subcallosal transfer and ipsilateral sensory-motor control. However, through negative contrast, the split-brain draws immediate attention to the concept of "callosal connectivity" as a factor independent from relative hemispheric specialization in interhemispheric dynamics.

Hemispheric Specialization Versus Callosal Connectivity

The twin concepts of relative hemispheric specialization and callosal connectivity, in turn, provide a conceptual basis for interpreting behavioral laterality effects in normal subjects. It is possible to interpret laterality experiments with normals as simulations of callosal section in the intact brain, using latency and accuracy performance measures (see Filbey & Gazzaniga, 1969). The rationale for such an interpretation is provided by regarding the corpus callosum as a channel of communication with a finite capacity, a measurable transition time, and a definite loss of information or stimulus quality during transit. The second set of assumptions underlying the interpretation of laterality effects in the normal brain is that of predominantly contralateral sensory-motor representation.

Consider a hemifield tachistoscopic task for which exclusive specialization had been demonstrated in the lesioned brain and in the disconnected hemispheres. If patterns observed in the disconnection syndrome are generalizable to the normal brain, one would expect a massive laterality effect in the split-brain but a consistent, modest, and reliable effect in the intact brain. Suppose the stimulus is flashed to the unspecialized hemisphere in the normal brain; it will have to shuttle across the corpus callosum at a measurable cost in time and accuracy. If, however, the stimulus is flashed directly to the specialized hemisphere, it will be processed immediately, that is faster and more accurately. In the split-brain, if the stimulus is flashed to the specialized hemisphere, it will also be processed immediately. But when it is flashed to the unspecialized hemisphere, it will not be processed accurately at all, yielding a massive laterality effect. I shall refer to this interpretation as the "callosal relay model."

Consider next a hemifield tachistoscopic task for which relative specialization has been demonstrated in the disconnected hemispheres. There are two possible interpretations for an observed laterality effect with the same task in normal subjects. The first assumes that the stimulus will shuttle to the relatively specialized hemisphere when projected to the other side. Again, this is the callosal relay model. With the second interpretation, however, the hemisphere that receives the stimulus first will also process it, for better or worse, without recourse to callosal transfer. With this view, the laterality effect in the normal brain is due to the difference in relative competence for the task between the two hemispheres. I shall refer to this interpretation as the "direct access model." The direct access model emphasizes relative hemispheric specialization, whereas the callosal relay model focuses on callosal connectivity. It is theoretically possible that all complex tasks involve interhemispheric interactions so that no real task will fit either model. The next section will develop some behavioral criteria for the two models, and the subsequent section will present "existence proofs," showing that cognitive tasks fitting each model do exist.

MODELS OF LATERALITY EFFECTS IN THE NORMAL BRAIN

Direct Access and Callosal Relay Models

A common procedure for studying hemispheric specialization in the normal brain is to restrict sensory input and motor response each to one hemisphere, and then to measure latency or accuracy in all possible pairings. In the case of visual or somesthetic input, predominantly contralateral innervation guarantees that LVF or left-hand information will go first to the RH. In the case of auditory input, this can only be assumed when two acoustically similar but not identical stimuli reach both ears simultaneously (dichotic listening.) For motor responses, it is usually assumed that manual behavior is contralaterally controlled and that speech originates from the LH. Of course, these assumptions "beg the question" when the object of the study is to determine the extent of RH speech or, for example, of ipsilateral motor control of the right hand by the RH. It will be shown below that the assumption of contralateral manual control or of its consequences in terms of callosal transfer may fail if the response is too simple a function of the stimulus, as in binary choices.

As already mentioned, studies of patients with hemispheric damage tend to highlight severe linguistic deficits leading to "exclusive specialization" views, where one hemisphere alone is said to control the linguistic ability in question. With this view, if linguistic information within the domain of this ability is introduced to the "wrong" hemisphere, it will have to shuttle across the corpus callosum to the proper processing centers, at some cost in latency and accuracy. This leads to the "callosal relay" interpretation of laterality effects in normal subjects. Split-brain studies, however, suggest that each hemisphere has a wide language-processing repertoire, capable of handling many tasks. This "relative specialization" view, in turn, leads to "direct access" models of some linguistic laterality effects in normals, where each hemisphere is said to process its own sensory input, although with unequal competence.

A direct access model predicts the same small laterality effects in normal and split-brains, whereas a callosal relay model predicts much larger laterality effects in the split-brain than in the normal brain. A comparison of the laterality effects for a given task in the split-brain and normal brain can then serve as a decision procedure to determine whether the task is of the direct access or callosal relay variety. This is one example of the importance of converging clinical and experimental studies.

There is now evidence that both types of tasks do exist. For example, dichotic listening to nonsense stop–consonant vowel (CV) syllables requires callosal relay to the LH, whereas lexical decision tasks, certain versions of dot localization tasks (Bryden, 1976; Gordon & Zaidel, unpublished data, 1982), and matching-to-sample of nonsense shapes of intermediate complexity (Hellige & Cox, 1976; Letai, 1981) seem to be processed in either hemisphere. The distinction between callosal relay and direct access tasks is theoretically crucial because it separates laterality effects due to hemispheric specialization per se from those due to degrees of callosal connectivity, which presupposes hemispheric specialization. The two factors may contribute independently and unequally to individual differences in laterality effects, including those due to sex and handedness. A general research program would then call for development of a battery of direct access (for each hemisphere), callosal relay (in each direction), and probably also some "bilateral-interaction" tasks, and for administration of them to subject populations of interest. Experimental variables that affect callosal connectivity alone should result in laterality differences on the callosal relay but not the direct access task. Variables affecting hemispheric competence, however, should result in laterality differences exclusively for the direct access tasks.

The first step toward such a research program is to catalog a variety of direct access and callosal relay tasks, both left and right hemispheric, verbal and visuospatial, and visual as well as auditory. As noted above, a comparison of laterality effects between the split-brain and the normal brain provides a decision procedure for distinguishing direct access from callosal relay tasks. However, this requires a special subject population that is neither generally available nor necessarily always representative of the normal brain. Two main alternative decision procedures have occasionally been used.

The first relies on the facts of contralateral sensory-motor innervation and requires pairing of both stimulus VFs with both response hands or with another lateralized motor channel. If the LH is specialized for processing the task (or its dominant components), LVF stimulus presentation requires right-left cross callosal relay of the visual information prior to processing, and left-hand motor response requires left to right cross callosal relay of the motor command following central processing. A direct access model predicts a shorter reaction time with LVF–left hand pairing than with LVF–right hand pairing, whereas the converse is predicted by a callosal relay model. This is called the "contralateral advantage" test. Springer (1971) introduced related concepts, and Moscovitch (1973) discussed an early version of these considerations in a pioneering paper.

The second procedure involves a task with a variable central processing load but fixed or indistinguishable lateralized sensory-motor components. Suppose the LH is specialized for the task — introducing several increasing processing loads to the inferior RH would result in a parallel curve with a higher intercept than obtained for the LH, if callosal relay obtains, but also a curve with a higher slope, reflecting accumulating RH disadvantage, if direct access holds (Figure 4.1). Any experiment demonstrating different effects in the LVF than in the RVF suggests independent RH processing, but this second decision procedure ("processing dissociation") is independent of the first ("contralateral advantage") criterion. The processing dissociation criterion can be tested in data that do not involve manual responses, whereas the contralateral advantage test applies only to lateralized motor, usually manual or verbal, responses. Only when both are satisfied can one be secure in inferring RH competence. When the second but not the first criterion is satisfied, the experiment may involve interhemispheric interaction.

Different performance styles with input to the two visual half-fields, for example, different error types, may be regarded as examples of the process dissociation criterion, suggesting a direct access model. But what about the occurrence of more false-positive errors in the inferior field during a stimulus discrimination or binary identification task? This could suggest a callosal relay since stimulus degradation due to callosal transfer should make the decision harder. If the decision criteria remain unchanged (or are relaxed), loss of features should result in acceptance of stimuli that are incorrect when complete. The argument assumes that callosal transfer results in loss of features rather than in feature distortion (see Figure 4.1).

One important class of application of the processing dissociation criterion involves correlations of performance level in the two lateralized conditions, as a function of complexity of test items. The callosal relay model predicts a high positive correlation, whereas the direct access model, together with the

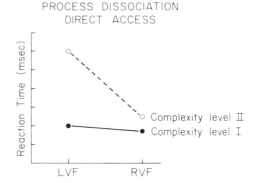

Figure 4-1. *Schematic representation of the processing dissociation criterion for direct access in a behavioral laterality experiment.*

assumption of differential hemispheric strategies, predicts a low, or a high negative, correlation. A variation of this application is the correlation across individuals of performance in central vision with performance in each lateralized condition and with the laterality effect (difference between the two lateralized conditions) (Ladavas & Umiltá, 1982). In particular, a positive correlation between performance in central vision and each hemifield, together with no correlation between performance in central vision and laterality effect, would suggest exclusive specialization and callosal relay.

Behavioral Criteria for Model Fitting

Manual Response

These considerations can be made more explicit. They presuppose an additive information-processing model where sensory relay, central processing, and motor response are identifiable, independent, and temporally sequential stages of an information-processing sequence. Consider a paradigmatic hemifield tachistoscopic experiment with manual reaction time as the dependent variable. Let $V_L(V_R)$ represent the transmission time of the sensory stimuli from the LVF (RVF) to the occipital cortex (area 17) of the RH (LH). There is no anatomical reason to suppose that $V_L \neq V_R$ for identical stimuli. Although there may be slight differences between decussating (crossed) and nondecussating projections such that (the crossed projection) V_L from the LVF to the RH through the left eye is in some sense "stronger" than either (the uncrossed) V_R through the left eye or (the uncrossed) V_L through the right eye, one can ignore these differences in binocular presentations, assuming no effect of eye dominance. For direct access scenarios, let $P_R(P_L)$ represent the central processing time for the stimulus in the RH (LH), and let $M_L(M_R)$ represent the latency from the initiation of a motor response in the RH (LH) to the conclusion of the appropriate button press with the left hand (right hand). Manual dominance suggests that, for right-handers, $M_L > M_R$, but these differences are usually negligible. For callosal relay scenarios, also let $CV_{RL}(CV_{LR})$ represent the delay in response due to cross-callosal transfer of the visual information from the RH to the LH (from the LH to the RH), and let CM_{LR} represent cross-callosal transmission of the motor command from the processing LH to the motor cortex of the RH controlling the responding left hand. This model presupposes that contralateral motor control predominates over possible ipsilateral connections, so that left-hand responses are always controlled by the motor cortex of the RH, and so forth (Figure 4-2).

Direct access models assume that the hemisphere that receives the visual input is the one that will process the information. If the hand ipsilateral to

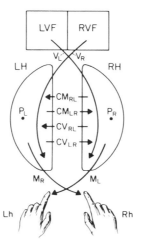

	DIRECT ACCESS	
Input VF	Output hand	Response time
L	L	$V_L + P_R \qquad\qquad + M_L$
L	R	$V_L + P_R + CM_{RL} + M_R$
R	L	$V_R + P_L + CM_{LR} + M_L$
R	R	$V_R + P_L \qquad\qquad + M_R$
Simplified,		
L	L	$V + P_R \qquad\quad + M$
L	R	$V + P_R + CM + M$
R	L	$V + P_L + CM + M$
R	R	$V + P_L \qquad\quad + M$

	CALLOSAL RELAY	
Input VF	Output hand	Response time
L	L	$V_L + CV_{RL} + P_L + CM_{LR} + M_L$
L	R	$V_L + CV_{RL} + P_L \qquad\qquad + M_R$
R	L	$V_R \qquad\quad + P_L + CM_{LR} + M_L$
R	R	$V_R \qquad\quad + P_L \qquad\qquad + M_R$
Simplified,		
L	L	$V + CV + P + CM + M$
L	R	$V + CV + P \qquad\quad + M$
R	L	$V \qquad\quad + P + CM + M$
R	R	$V \qquad\quad + P \qquad\quad + M$

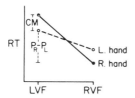 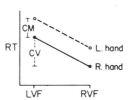

Figure 4-2. *Direct access and callosal relay analyses of a tachisto-scopic laterality experiment in which hemifield presentations are paired with unimanual responses. V_L = transmission time of sensory stimuli from the LVF to the occipital cortex of the right hemisphere (RH); P_R = central processing time for the stimulus in the RH; M_L = latency from the initiation of a motor response in the RH to its conclusion by the left hand; CV_{RL} = delay in response due to cross callosal transfer of the visual information from the RH to the LH; CM_{LR} = cross-callosal transmission of the motor command from the processing LH to the motor cortex of the RH controlling the responding left hand; and so forth.*

110

that hemisphere must respond, the motor command must first travel to the motor cortex of the other hemisphere through the corpus callosum. Thus, the reaction times shown in Figure 4-2 are predicted for the various lateralized stimulus-response combinations. We can assume that $M_L = M_R$ and that $CM_{LR} = CM_{RL}$ to obtain the simplified model shown. Assuming $P_L < P_R$ (i.e., LH specialization) and $(P_R - P_L) > CM$, we obtain the graph on the left that shows that a necessary, although not sufficient, condition for direct access is a visual field times response-hand interaction in an analysis of variance experimental design. In this model, hemispheric specialization is indicated by a main visual half-field effect (here an RVF advantage). However, a direct access model may hold without a VF effect, and then one can conclude that both hemispheres are equally competent for the task. On the other hand, the absence of a laterality effect cannot by itself be taken as evidence of direct access; it may simply represent a negative result reflecting the insensitivity of the experiment.

In contrast to direct access, callosal relay assumes that the specialized hemisphere (here the LH) always processes the input and that stimulus presentation to the LVF simply results in callosal transfer of at least some data from the RH to the LH. This model is also sketched in Figure 4-2 and leads to the predictions detailed on the right. The simplifications, $V_L = V_R = V$, $CM_{LR} = CM_{RL} = CM$, and $M_L = M_R = M$, lead to the predictions and the graph shown on the right. The model is characterized by parallel lines and thus by a main response-hand effect and an absence of visual half-field times response-hand interaction. Overriding this must be a main visual half-field laterality effect (here an RVF advantage). Consequently, the lower line in the right-sided graph must represent responses by the hand contralateral to the specialized hemisphere (here, the right hand). Conversely, conditions for refuting the callosal relay model include a main hand effect without a main visual hemifield effect, or a main hand effect opposite to the hemifield effect.

Verbal Report

The classical basis for interpreting laterality effects in normal subjects has been the use of verbal responses together with the assumption, supported equally by clinical neurology and until recently by split-brain data, that speech is controlled exclusively by the LH, at least in most right-handed adult males. Consider a classical hemifield tachistoscopic experiment requiring verbal responses. As can be seen in Figure 4-3, the assumption of LH specialization simply yields an RVFA for both the relay and direct access models, and the two cannot be distinguished from each other by the experimental data Thus, such data cannot speak to the issue of RH participation in reading. The alternative is to use this approach in conjunction with the processing dissociation test. Such results have been reported but are clearly less stringent than the criteria possible for the manual response paradigm.

It should be noted that laterality effects in complex tasks involving verbal responses, such as reading, may be due to the verbal response selection component rather than to the reading per se. Many experiments in the literature fail to make this elementary distinction. In principle, the solution is to compare the laterality effects in an identical task that omits the verbal response, such as lexical decision. However, there is generally no way to ensure that the new task really represents the initial stages of the older one, short of a detailed information-processing analysis of both tasks. Furthermore, the proposed solution presupposes a sequence of independent additive stages that can be separated at any link. On the contrary, it is possible that different components of the task interact with each other in complex ways. This may well vary from task to task. If one is fortunate, the task will satisfy the chronometric criteria for independent stages of processing outlined in Sternberg's well-known paper (1969). Alternately, we may select tasks that are known to satisfy those assumptions and that have some inherent interest in other contexts.

Interhemispheric Transfer Time

Different callosal relay delays occur in different tasks. Simple motor reaction time experiments yield callosal transmission time estimates of 4 msec and have the clearest anatomical interpretation (Bashore, 1981; Poffenberger, 1912; Rizzolatti, 1979). Here the estimate is plausibly due to the presence of an extra synapse, assuming that the largest callosal fibers are responsible for the behavioral response. In contrast, estimates of callosal transmission time obtained from choice reaction time experiments are on the order of 30 msec. Although this estimate is also consistent with callosal transmission through many small myelinated and unmyelinated fibers, the estimate is probably a reflection of psychological (i.e., dynamic) as well as fixed or prestructured anatomical effects. As Rizzolatti (1979) points out, in choice reaction time experiments, a transfer of information cannot occur at the level of the primary visual cortical areas, where hemispheric differences in analyzing stimuli are unlikely, because these areas are not, as far as is known, connected with each other across the callosum except along the vertical meridian. Thus, transfer time may well be a function of the complexity of the stimuli. This is especially true if transfer occurs past some level of psychological processing by the receiving hemisphere in the callosal relay situation. In that case, some "translation" is necessary with some latency cost. At the present time, there is no anatomical basis for such variations in callosal connectivity as a function of

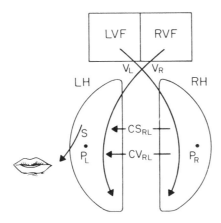

DIRECT ACCESS

Input VF	Response time
L	$V_L + P_R + CS_{RL} +$ Speech
R	$V_R + P_L \qquad + S$

Simplified,

L	$V + P_R + CS_{RL} + S$
R	$V + P_L \qquad + S$

CALLOSAL RELAY

Input VF	Response time
L	$V_L + CV_{RL} + P_L + S$
R	$V_R + \qquad + P_L + S$

Simplified,

L	$V + CV \quad + P_L + S$
R	$V \qquad + P_L + S$

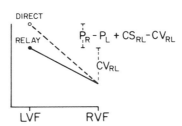

Figure 4-3. *Analyses of a laterality experiment with verbal report.* S = *latency for initiating a speech response;* CS_{RL} = *cross-callosal transmission time from right hemisphere (RH) to LH of the information to be converted into a speech response; others are as in Figure 4-2.*

psychological variables. One way to search for underlying anatomical models would focus, for example, on modality-specific callosal effects, for which some specificity of callosal connections is already established.

Model Fitting

A quick difference between the direct access and callosal relay models is provided by conditions 1 and 2 (Figure 4-2). Thus, for direct access, LVF-left hand pairing results in faster reaction time than LVF-right hand pairing, whereas the converse is true for callosal relay (the "contralateral advantage" test). Conditions 3 and 4 are identical for both models. Both models are underdetermined by the data. Direct access yields four equations with eight unknowns, or four equations with five unknowns in the simplified model. Callosal relay, in turn, yields four equations with seven unknowns, or simplified, four equations with five unknowns. However further constraints, such as $P_L < P_R$ or requiring nonzero positive solutions, limit the degrees of freedom and can often determine whether or not a model fits the results of a specific experiment. The presence or absence of a visual half-field by response-hand interaction or a main hand effect are two useful tests of the fit of direct or callosal relay access to an experiment, respectively, but a more precise model fitting is possible by estimating the hypothetical variables (V, P, CV, CM, M) and testing whether variations in values obtained for the same variable fall within the statistical limits of noise.

It is rare to find a laterality experiment that provides the data necessary for model fitting and that shows a consistent fit. I have reviewed hemifield reading experiments that involved manual responses, that included data for both hands, and that appeared in one of the journals, *Cortex*, *Neuropsychologia*, or *Brain and Language* between 1970 and 1980. In addition, I looked at certain experiments that directly addressed the issue of right hemisphere reading. Only 1 of the 14 experiments that included all the requisite data yielded a consistent model fit (Day, 1977, expt. I). Here a lexical-decision task of abstract words showed a main RVFA and a main right-hand advantage and thus demonstrated a callosal relay model with LH specialization.

A much quoted experiment by Klatzky and Atkinson (1971) illustrates the frustrations of a systematic attempt at model fitting. The first task required the subjects to determine whether the name of a lateralized picture started with a letter belonging to a memorized set, and a second task inquired whether a lateralized letter itself belonged in the memory set. The results showed a (probably insignificant) LVF advantage for the letter task, a (significant?) RVF advantage for the picture task, and a significant VF times task interaction. Furthermore, reaction times as a function of increasing memory set showed parallel lines for the two VFs, suggesting a callosal relay model. Thus, the failure of the processing dissociation criterion for model fitting supports a relay model. Unfortunately, the reaction time data for each task do not include analyses of variance with visual half-field or with hand; thus, the tests outlined above could not be applied. But what, as appears likely at least for the letter task data, if it did not support the callosal relay interpretation, that is, did not reveal significant main VF and hand effects?

Actual model fittings usually show that $CM_{LR} \neq CM_{RL}$, $M_L, \neq M_R$, and $CV_{LR} \neq CV_{RL}$. Furthermore, widely different estimates of these variables are obtained from different experiments. Experiments with split-brain patients suggest that there is a very weak noncallosal visual projection from the LVF to the LH but a significant motor control of the LH over the left hand, which, in turn, is stronger than RH control of the right hand. It follows that the cross-callosal visual transfer hypothesized above, CV, is obligatory, whereas the cross-callosal motor transfer, CM, is perhaps optional.

As can be expected, the callosal relay model applies much more frequently than does direct access, since substantial hemispheric specialization on a task can naturaly result in complete hemispheric control on the task under brief, taxing experimental conditions, even if the inferior hemisphere is competent in isolation and participates in related natural processes. Direct access and callosal relay may be thought of as representing limit cases of a theoretical continuum, where the two hemispheres interact to greater or lesser extents during task performance. It is not clear as yet how to formalize the concept of "degree of interaction" in terms of some hypothetical variables that could then be estimated from empirical data.

Ipsilateral Motor Control

Both the direct access and callosal relay models assume exclusively contralateral sensory-motor connections, that is, that LVF stimulation must reach the visual cortex of the RH first and that left-hand (Lh) control must be from the motor cortex of the RH. Actually, research with commissurotomy patients shows that the two assumptions are not equally plausible. Brief left hemifield presentations consistently fail to be verbalized correctly by split-brain patients, and even prolonged ocular scanning with one hemifield can, at best, yield very gross visual information of the kind provided by the second, extrageniculostriate visual system. On the other hand, there is evidence for good ipsilateral efferent manual control by both hemispheres, even in choice reaction time tasks. Such ipsilateral control may be stronger in the LH over the Lh; but it can occur spontaneously with either hemisphere under conditions of conflict, as one of them assumes control because of its specialization for the type of information to be processed.

To the extent that these observations are generalizable to the normal brain, the differences between right-hand and left-hand responses to stimuli in the same VF may reflect the contralateral-ipsilateral advantage rather than callosal transfer time. This may explain why estimates of cross-callosal motor transfer are often not symmetric, that is, why often $CM_{LR} \neq CM_{RL}$. Let

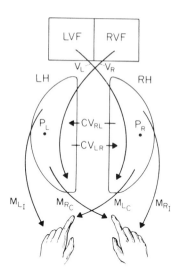

DIRECT ACCESS		
Input VF	Output hand	Response time
L	L	$V_L + P_R + M_{L_C}$
L	R	$V_L + P_R + M_{R_I}$
R	L	$V_R + P_L + M_{L_I}$
R	R	$V_R + P_L + M_{R_C}$

CALLOSAL RELAY		
Input VF	Output hand	Response time
L	L	$V_L + CV_{RL} + P_L + M_{L_I}$
L	R	$V_L + CV_{RL} + P_L + M_{R_C}$
R	L	$V_R \quad\quad + P_L + M_{L_I}$
R	R	$V_R \quad\quad + P_L + M_{R_C}$

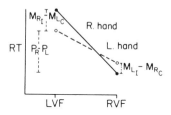

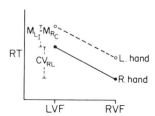

Figure 4-4. *Analyses of a laterality experiment, pairing hemifield presentations with manual responses but assuming ipsilateral motor control.* M_{L_I} = *latency of executing a motor response of the left hand in the LH using ipsilateral control;* M_{R_C} = *latency of executing a motor response of the right hand in the LH using the usual contralateral control; and so forth.*

M_{L_I} represent the time necessary to activate the left hand *i*psilaterally from the LH, and let M_{L_C} represent the time necessary to activate the left hand *c*ontralaterally from the RH in a given response paradigm (Figure 4-4). For a fixed manual response paradigm, one may still assume that at least M_{R_C} and M_{L_C} are fairly constant. The problem is to know when exclusively contralateral motor control obtains and when ipsilateral manual control is possible. If ipsilateral control obtains consistently, then the result is the model equations in Figure 4-4, and with the simplifications $V_L = V_R$ and $M_{L_I} M_{R_I}$, the result is the graphs in Figure 4-4. Both models yield four equations with five unknowns, and the relay model yields four equations with six unknowns. The split-brain preparation could provide estimates of manual ipsilateral and contralateral response times for either hand in a given response paradigm, assuming that these estimates are not subject to large interindividual differences, that they are not sensitive to processing demands of the main task, and that they do not reflect postoperative neural readjustments in the patients.

An early split-brain paper by K.U. Smith on one of Von Wagenen's and Akelaitis's patients claims that section of the corpus callosum did not change the crossed minus uncrossed response time differential [(LVF-Rh + RVF-Lh) - (LVF-Lh + RVF-Rh)] in a simple motor reaction time task (see Swanson, Ledlow, & Kinsbourne, 1978). This suggests that crossed field-hand combinations (LVF-Rh or RVF-Lh) reflect ipsilateral motor control (by the RH or LH, respectively) rather than callosal transfer of motor commands. However, Smith's study failed to show any effect of the surgery, and the Akelaitis-Von Wagenen series generally is notable for its failure to demonstrate any disconnection effects. Therefore, one can question the Smith data and await results from more recent patients.

Just such results were obtained recently in a lateralized lexical-decision and facilitation task carried out with both commissurotomy and normal subjects (Radant, 1981; Temple, 1981; E. Zaidel, 1982b). The split-brain patients received briefly lateralized target-letter strings in various facilitation conditions and were asked to press a button when the target was a word. Each facilitation condition was administered in three blocks. In the first, the patient was asked to respond with the hand ipsilateral to the target VF; in the second, the patient responded with the right hand throughout; and in the third, the patient pressed with the left hand only. Unmatched t-test comparisons of left- and right-hand response latencies to the same stimulus combinations were carried out and generally failed to show significant differences!

One may suspect that manual responses employing distal movements are more likely to be contralaterally represented. Yet precisely such responses were used in the lateralized lexical-decision task that failed to show the contralateral advantage in the disconnected hemispheres. The commissurotomy patients actually show asymmetrical ipsilateral control, both proximal and distal (D.

Zaidel & Sperry, 1977; E. Zaidel, 1978b), but all these patterns may reflect postsurgical readjustments that are not representative of the normal brain.

If the absence of an advantage of contralateral over ipsilateral manual control in the split-brain for the lexical-decision task is representative of the normal brain, one can no longer use the effect of response hand on degree of observed laterality as a criterion for either direct access or callosal relay. This is what Temple found when she administered one form of the lexical-decision task to normal subjects (Temple, 1981). In her experiment, response hand actually changed the balance of hemispheric processing on the task in complex ways. This is not universally true; some studies using counterbalanced response hands do result in the laterality effects expected from contralateral innervation and some do not (see discussion in Swanson et al. 1978). In particular, since Poffenberger (1912), parametric analyses of simple manual reaction time to lateralized unpatterned visual stimuli routinely disclose a hemifield by response-hand interaction, supporting direct access and providing consistent estimates of interhemispheric transfer times (about 3 msec). These estimates do not appear to vary as a function of handedness or sex and are not sensitive to spatial compatibility effects (see review in Bashore, 1981). By minimizing both cognitive and response demands, a reasonably pure measure of input and output operations can be derived (Bashore, 1981). The simple tasks can be executed relatively quickly and with smaller variance so that the brief interhemispheric transfer time can be measured reliably.

Within certain small limits, there is an apparent inverse relation between RT and interhemispheric transfer time. Thus, slower RTs due to eccentric stimuli or crossed hands tend to produce shorter estimates of callosal transfer. As tasks demand increase in complexity, for example, when stimulus detection or response decisions are required, longer and more variable RTs, as well as longer estimates of callosal transfer time, are obtained. Thus, estimates of interhemispheric transfer time that derive from two-choice RT experiments are generally longer than those from simple RT and stimulus detection studies and are also much more sensitive to spatial compatibility effects. Practice is said to reduce the S-R compatibility effect for the dominant hand in the crossed and uncrossed response conditions, whereas this effect persists in the nondominant hand (Brebner, 1973, cited in Bashore, 1981). This suggests that spatial compatibility is a consequence of hemispheric specialization rather than the general cause of laterality effects or a factor independent of hemispheric specialization.

Bashore (1981) speculates that fast callosal transfer in simple RT tasks is mediated by large-diameter, myelinated axons that account for 10% of callosal fibers, whereas slower callosal transfer in choice RT tasks is mediated by the 60% of smaller and slower fibers. The question occurs as to whether the spatial distribution of different types of fibers in the corpus callosum can be associated with differences in type and modality of the conveyed information.

Complex RT tasks rarely yield a VF by response-hand interaction (but see expt. 2 in Moscovitch, Scullion, & Christie, 1976). The reason for this becomes clear when one considers that response hand should not affect the total reaction time much when the difference involves the callosal transfer of a mere binary choice (e.g., go or no-go, yes or no). This is especially true since hand activation occurs at the last stage of processing and is more susceptible to noise. The solution may be to use tasks that require more complex manual (e.g., identification) responses as a function of stimulus parameters and are therefore more likely to show the expected hand effects. Until a general rationale for predicting the effect of hand use on observed laterality is available, each experimental task needs to be evaluated on a case-by-case basis. Again, the split-brain provides a useful baseline in specific cases.

Anatomical Considerations

The foregoing analysis suggests that the absence of a laterality effect in a hemifield tachistoscopic experiment does not imply a lack of hemispheric specialization on the task. If there is no main visual half-field (VF) effect but there is a significant visual half-field by response hand (VFxh) interaction, the direct access model holds without hemispheric specialization, and one can infer hemispheric equipotentiality for the task. Since the callosal relay model does not allow an absence of a main VF effect, the failure of such a VF advantage to occur where one should reasonably be expected (together with an absence of VFxh interaction, i.e., no direct access), suggests that the task requires complex parallel interhemispheric interactions. Unfortunately, as mentioned above, there is not yet a model to account for such interactions, even though most laterality tasks probably fall within this category.

As tasks increase in complexity, they would seem less likely to fit either the direct access or callosal relay model and should be more likely to invoke interhemispheric interactions and to involve considerably longer response times than either callosal relay or especially direct access tasks. Paradoxically, this is not always the case. Dahlia W. Zaidel has recently administered a hemifield tachistoscopic test of category membership with pictorial examplars to normal subjects and has found a significant interaction between visual half-field and degree of typicality of category instances (1981). Furthermore, she obtained a massive and highly significant overall LVFA of about 400 msec. This complex task that taps long-term semantic memory and requires rather long RTs (mean 1400 msec for positive responses by male subjects) still satisfies the processing dissociation criterion of direct access. Perhaps the direct access and callosal relay models are not as extreme as they appear and do fit directly a variety of complex tasks, variously consistent with the "complete range" and "exclusive specialization" views of hemispheric functions, respectively.

A major challenge to laterality research with normal subjects is the need to articulate increasingly explicit anatomical rationales for new behavioral effects; thus far, this has been rare. Kimura and Durnford (1974) offer two intriguing hypotheses about the dependence of visual laterality effects on anatomical asymmetries. First, they note that visual laterality effects are only likely to occur in tasks that activate cortical areas receiving early or direct visual input. As the visual information is subjected to consecutive stages of processing and more abstract representation several synapses away from the primary visual cortex, it is also subjected to increasingly extraneous influences at each synaptic stage. Consequently, the hemisphere of input will be less and less a determinant of the final response.

Thus, they argue, although hemispheric specialization may occur in late stages of information processing, one is not very likely to detect it by comparing the results of restricting the visual input to one visual half-field or the other. This means that the hemifield tachistoscopic paradigm is biased in favor of perceptual (i.e., early) as opposed to cognitive (late) laterality effects for visual information. It is interesting that Kimura and Durnford's logical argument is in contrast with the empirical claim of Moscovitch (1979), who argues (incorrectly, I believe) that laterality effects occur during relatively later rather than early stages of information processing.

The second hypothesis of Kimura and Durnford argues that anatomical facts may have serious methodological consequences; they may mask an authentic underlying hemispheric specialization or may even signal an opposite effect misleadingly. Suppose that LH specialization for language resulted in a "crowding" effect for visual functions, so that the visual areas that are responsible for form perception in the posterior LH are smaller and hence closer in transmission time to the primary visual areas than is the corresponding connection in the RH. This may result in an RVF (LH) advantage for certain form perception tasks, even though the RH is actually specialized for them. On the surface, this hypothesis errs in assuming that small differences in transmission due to synaptic length can counteract differences in processing due to hemispheric specialization; the former is on the order of milliseconds, while the latter is on the order of tens of milliseconds. Still, the difference in callosal transfer between simple motor reaction time tasks (3 to 5 msec) and choice reaction time tasks (20 to 50 msec) suggests that the same synaptic pathway may result in widely divergent transmission times as a function of the complexity of the transferred information or of the translation required.

Another interesting example of an anatomically inspired interpretation of laterality effects in normal subjects comes from Berlucchi, Heron, Hyman et al.

(1971). Consider simple reaction times to lateralized visual stimuli and the difference between reactions with the ipsilateral and contralateral hand. The authors suggest that, if this difference changes as a function of degree of eccentricity of the visual stimuli, interhemispheric transfer occurs at the level of the visual, rather than, for instance, the motor cortex. This is presumably because only the cortical areas related to the vertical meridian of the visual field give origin to and receive commissural fibers. More eccentric stimuli that do not have direct commissural connectons would then require longer cross-callosal transfer time and result in a bigger difference between crossed and uncrossed visual field-hand responses (the former require visual callosal transfer, the latter do not). An eccentricity effect would imply a callosal relay model. Failure of the eccentricity effect to occur would remain ambiguous. It could be due to exclusively motor transfer, thus supporting a direct access model, or it could reflect more anterior callosal transfer of more processed or abstract visual information, which is consistent with a callosal relay model. The data of Berlucchi et al. did not show an eccentricity effect (on the difference between crossed and uncrossed responses) and did show a VFxh interaction, which fits with a direct access model.

What experimental conditions will give evidence of RH language competence in the normal brain? Usually, this will consist of an experiment that fits the direct access model. In principle, it is also possible to find a callosal relay condition with RH specialization, but this must be rare.

Problems of Measurement and Inference

These problems are discussed in more detail in E. Zaidel (1979a). As mentioned, few visual laterality experiments include or permit a systematic model fitting. Where inferences about models are possible, studies of reading involving phonological recoding seem to suggest exclusive LH specialization and callosal relay. However, lexical decision of concrete, imageable words seems to allow direct access. When the data of a laterality reading experiment do not fit either the direct access or callosal relay models, there is no rationale for interpreting the experiment, and in the absence of further information, it should remain undecided. This would apply to many, perhaps most, experiments in the literature, but even where one of the models applies, serious methodological difficulties remain.

One problem is that the applicability of one or the other models is conventionally determined by main effects in an analysis of variance research design. Yet such a design, in effect, uses difference and ratio measures as indexes of hemispheric specialization, and these indexes are notoriously unreliable (Harshman, 1980.) A better approach than using LVF and RVF as two levels of an independent experimental variable would be to compute a laterality index (such as $f = (Rc\text{-}Lc)/(Rc+Lc)$ if $Rc+Lc<100\%$ and $f = (Rc\text{-}Lc)/(Re\text{-}Le)$ if $Rc+Lc>100\%$, where Rc = percentage of correct RH (LVF or left hand) responses, Re = percentage of incorrect RH responses, etc.) (Marshall, Caplan, & Holmes, 1975) for each individual in each experimental condition and to use this as a dependent variable.

The choice of a laterality index is related to the issue of possible interaction between perfomance level and degree of laterality. Laterality indexes that are theoretically independent of performance level may be desirable in some situations, such as developmental studies. However, many models of laterality effects in the normal brain, such as that the RH is selectively involved in processing novel stimuli leading to quick but errorful responses, yield specific predictions about the relation of the laterality index to overall accuracy (E. Zaidel, 1979a).

Another problem is that both the reliability and validity of most laterality tests in normals are disturbingly low. There is at present no compelling rationale either for choosing a laterality index or for regarding experimental laterality effects and the underlying hemispheric specialization as continuous and correlated variables in the general population. That is, one cannot infer relative degrees of hemispheric specialization from degrees of laterality effects. Furthermore, given conservative estimates from clinical data about the relationship of handedness and language dominance, it has been argued that inferences of the existence of RH language from LVF superiority are very unlikely to be correct (Satz, 1977). However, different language tasks may tap differentially specialized functions for which relevant clinical estimates are not available; thus, tasks need to be assessed on a case-by-case basis. Unfortunately, most of the tasks studied in the laboratory are quite artificial and of limited relevance to normal function. This is especially true for reading vertically aligned words or for words split in the peripheries of the left and right visual half-fields.

EXISTENCE "PROOFS" FOR THE CALLOSAL RELAY AND DIRECT ACCESS MODELS

It now appears quite likely that direct access and callosal relay tasks exist that are left hemisphere and right hemisphere specialized, verbal and nonverbal, auditory and visual. However, there is nothing logically necessary about this. The more complex a task is, the more likely it is to involve interhemispheric interaction and thus not to qualify as either direct access or callosal relay. Even if no real task of interest fit the models, they could still have theoretical value in explicating the microstructure of cross-callosal communication during strategic points in the information-processing sequence. As a matter of fact, a variety of tasks seems to exist instantiating both models. Both models will be illustrated with linguistic tasks — one auditory, the other visual. This will provide an opportunity to discuss dichotic listening and hemifield tachistoscopy, with special reference to the contribution of the commissurotomy syndrome.

Callosal Relay: Dichotic Listening to Nonsense Syllables

Three Assumptions

Following a suggestion of Woody Heron, Kimura adapted Broadbent's dichotic listening technique to the study of hemispheric specialization for auditory stimuli in normal subjects. Instead of analyzing the technique parametrically, Kimura established its validity by comparing the observed ear advantage as an index of contralateral hemispheric dominance for speech with speech dominance determined by Amytal Sodium injection. Kimura's dichotic tape consisted of three pairs of digits that the subject had to repeat. This tape allowed for strong attentional biases, and the interpretation of the right ear advantage (REA) as evidence for left hemisphere dominance for language is not as straightforward as with other dichotic stimuli. Fortunately, the observed REA was robust enough to withstand the possible effects of attention, memory, and other complicating factors.

Kimura also observed that left temporal lobectomy erased the REA and reduced performance in both ears to chance. Right temporal lobectomy, however, resulted in an increased REA, due to reduced left ear scores. There, the laterality effects reflected an additive combination of hemispheric specialization and lesion effects. This acted to magnify the laterality effect and to demonstrate its relation to hemispheric specialization.

Consider a dichotic tape with linguistic stimuli. More accurate perception of right ear stimuli is commonly considered as evidence of LH specialization for language. Three independent assumptions are made in this interpretation. First, it is assumed that the LH is specialized for processing the input signal (Kimura, 1961a). Second, it is supposed that the ipsilateral signal from the left ear to the LH is suppressed, perhaps at a subcortical level (Kimura, 1967). Berlin (1977) suggests that ipsilateral suppression occurs at the medial geniculate bodies. Third, stimuli presented to the left ear will first reach the RH, then cross the corpus callosum to be processed in the LH. This left ear signal then competes or interferes with, but does not dominate, the direct contralateral right ear signal, resulting in the observed REA (Sparks & Geschwind, 1968).

Although most experiments interpret the observed ear advantage as evidence for hemispheric specialization in the perception of the auditory stimuli, many of the studies include other task components, such as verbal responses or memory requirements that could be separately responsible for the laterality effect. Similarly, the assumption of ipsilateral suppression is usually made without any direct evidence. Although some partial, early supporting animal models exist (e.g., Rosenzweig, 1951), there is no definite information on the mechanism or anatomical locus of ipsilateral suppression. In particular, until recently, it has not been generally known whether ipsilateral suppression occurs subcortically and whether it shows cortical influences.

The split-brain offers a unique opportunity for testing the three assumptions. Milner, Taylor, and Sperry (1967) verified the suppression of the left ear signal by showing that commissurotomy patients could verbally report very few digits reaching the left ear during dichotic presentation of Kimura's tape. However, Sparks and Geschwind (1968) found weaker suppression and increasing left ear intrusions with practice in another commissurotomy patient. Furthermore, the verbal report used in both studies precluded RH responses so that RH competence was never tapped.

In 1974 I presented a paper at the UCLA conference on Human Brain Function, verifying the three hypotheses on a task with natural tokens of the dichotic stop consonant–vowel nonsense syllables, ba, da, ga, pa, ta, and ka, prepared at Haskins Laboratory in New Haven (E. Zaidel, 1976). The stop-consonant syllables were chosen because they are highly coded phonetically. The LH is said to be specialized for phonetic analysis, whereas both hemispheres may be able to do acoustic analysis (Studdert-Kennedy & Shankweiler, 1970). Perception of the dichotic pairs was assessed separately by verbal report and by lateralized visual probes. In the visual probe condition, each dichotic pair was followed immediately by a triplet of letters (from the set B,D,G,P,T,K, corresponding to the six dichotic syllables) representing the left ear syllable, the right ear syllable, and a syllable differing from both in one or two phonetic features (voicing and place of articulation). The subjects were required to point to the letter representing the sound they were most sure of having heard in either ear. These tests were administered to normal subjects, hemispherectomy patients, and commissurotomy patients.

The results showed a small but reliable REA in normal subjects in verbal report and in either visual half-field with visual probes (Figure 4-5). Commissurotomy patients showed a massive REA but not as complete as a case of right hemispherectomy. Monotic presentation resulted in good and equal verbal report (LH) from either ear. The RH could not perceive either ear in both the dichotic and monotic condition. Thus, all three assumptions

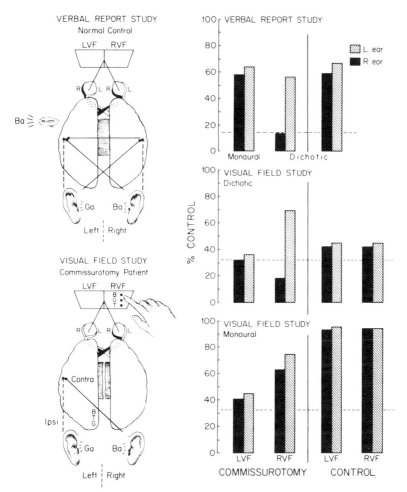

Figure 4-5. *Results of dichotic listening to nonsense CV syllables using verbal responses or lateralized visual probes (E. Zaidel, 1976). L. ear = left ear score, RVF = right hemifield, and so forth.*

were verified. In particular, given the verification of exclusive LH specialization and of ipsilateral left ear suppression, the large difference between the REA in normals and in split-brain patients verified the assumption of callosal interference and demonstrated that this is a callosal relay task. Furthermore, there was some evidence for different amounts of left ear suppression, depending upon the task and phonetic feature differences between the two ears, suggesting that ipsilateral suppression was affected by cortical processes, particularly by hemispheric specialization itself.

Modulation of Hemispheric Specialization and Ipsilateral Suppression

A more recent study in collaboration with B. Kashdan has extended the lateralized probe technique in several important ways. The meaningfulness of the CV syllables was manipulated, only one lateralized probe followed each dichotic pair, the delay between the auditory pair and the probe was varied, and ear attention was manipulated. The question was whether and how the common variables of meaningfulness and attention separately affected hemispheric specialization and ipsilateral suppression in contributing to a possible difference in overall laterality effect (REA). First, the verification of the three assumptions and the instantiation of the callosal relay model will be illustrated again, using data from this study. It will also be shown that the experimental modulations of specialization and suppression, although real, are relatively small in relation to status of this as a callosal relay task. The range of modulation of ipsilateral suppression is of secondary relevance to the demonstration of the existence of a callosal relay task, but it is very important in showing that small task differences can result in changes in ipsilateral suppression. The latter, therefore, needs to be assessed on a case-by-case basis until its mechanism is better understood.

A dichotic tape with pairs of syllables from the set, Bee, Dee, Gee, Pee, Tee, and Kee, was produced at Haskins Labs from natural tokens. These syllables are phonetically similar to the usual CV, Ba, Da, Ga, Pa, Ta, and Ka, but each can refer to a letter (e.g., B) or an object (e.g., the insect bee). Each dichotic pair was followed by a picture flashed briefly and randomly either to the left or to the right of a central fixation dot. The subject then pointed with the hand ipsilateral to the stimulated half-field to the words "yes" or "no" in order to indicate whether the picture did or did not match the sound heard in either ear. In the "letter" condition the flash consisted of an uppercase letter (B, ..., K) and in the "picture" condition the flash contained a simple line drawing (a bee, a girl named Dee, a boy named Guy, a pea pod, a tea cup, and a key). This cross-modal lateralized task allowed each disconnected hemisphere to respond separately. Monotic and binaural control conditions were also administered.

In addition, the delay between the dichotic pair and the lateralized flash was varied from zero through one-fourth, one-half to one second. Attention instruction varied between attending to both ears in the usual manner, attending to one ear for the whole test, or attending to the random ear receiving a brief beep 1 sec before the dichotic pair.

Subjects consisted of four patients with complete sections and two patients with partial section of the neocortical commissures, as well as 40 college undergraduates.

Six Commissurotomy Patients

Callosal section was performed to alleviate intractable epilepsy. Complete section included the corpus callosum, anterior commissure, and hippocampal commissure. Partial section left the splenium intact. The partially sectioned patients showed no visual, auditory, or tactile disconnection effects. The case histories are summarized in Table 4-1. For further details see Bogen and Vogel (1975) and Gordon, Bogen, and Sperry (1971). The patients were first tested in the zero delay and no attention conditions. Right visual half-field (RVF) (LH) performance in commissurotomy patients showed a large REA that was variable with performance level and higher for consonants than for picture probes. LVF (RH) score was consistently above chance in only one patient (L.B.), and occasionally in another (N.G.). Thus, LH specialization for the task was verified.

An analysis of variance was performed on the five patients' data with visual half-field (L, R), ear (L, R), and probe type (consonant, picture) as independent within-subject variables and with d′, a bias-free measure of sensitivity, as a dependent variable. d′ was generated from the accuracy data for each subject in all conditions by pairing the probability of hits with the probability of false alarms. The ANOVA disclosed a significant REA, confirming hemispheric specialization and a significant field × ear interaction (Figure 4-6). d′ for the left ear in the LVF was significantly above zero, but d′ for the right ear in the LVF was not. Similarly, d′ for the left ear in the RVF was essentially zero, confirming ipsilateral suppression. No significant effects or interactions due to probe type occurred.

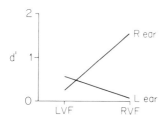

Figure 4-6. *Dichotic listening to nonsense CV syllables by five commissurotomy patients using lateralized visual probes. d′ is the signal detection sensitivity index. L ear = left ear; RVF = right hemifield, and so forth.*

Effects of Probe Type on Hemispheric Competence in Patients L.B. and N.G. Separate ANOVAs on the zero delay condition were performed for patients L.B. and N.G. because they were the only ones showing some, albeit minimal,

TABLE 4-1.
Summary of Case Histories

Patient	Sex	Reason for surgery	Surgery	Age at surgery	Years postop. at testing (1975)	Age at onset of symptoms	IQ history[a]		Predomin. extra callosal damage
							Preop.	Postop.	
N.G.	F	Intractable epilepsy	Complete cerebral commissurotomy: Single-stage midline section of anterior commissure, corpus callosum (and presumably psalterium), massa intermedia and right fornix. Surgical approach by retraction of the right hemisphere	30	12	18	Wechsler–Bellvue 76 (79,74) at age 30	WAIS 77 (83,71) at age 35	RH(BI)
L.B.	M	Intractable epilepsy	As above but massa intermedia was not visualized	13	10	3 : 6[b]	WISC 113 (119,108) at age 13	WAIS 106 (110,100) at age 16	RH
R.Y.	M	Intractable epilepsy	As above. (Normal cerebral development until 13)	43	9	17		WAIS 90 (99,79) at age 45	RH
N.W.	F	Intractable epilepsy	As above. Massa intermedia divided. Partial damage to left fornix	36	9	8	WAIS 93 (97,89) at age 36 at age 13	WAIS 93 (97,89) at age 38 age 16 : 8	RH
A.A.	M	Intractable epilepsy	As above. Difficult operation	14	10	5 : 6		WAIS 78 (77,82) age 17 : 8	LH(BI)

| D.M. | M | Intractable epilepsy; Seizures; To close attributed head injury at age 11 | Surgery involved the anterior commissure, the anterior 5 cm of the corpus callosum, and presumably the hippocampal commissure. Massa intermedia was absent. Especially smooth postoperative course and rapid recovery | 23 | 7 | 11 | WAIS 76 (70,87) at age 23 | WAIS 94 (108,76) at age 24 | BI |
| N.F. | F | Intractable epilepsy | Surgery as above. Callosal section seen to include all the genu and body and the anterior part of the splenium. Right-sided unilateral convulsion on 7th postoperative day and transient aphasia and hemiplegia | 27 | 6 | 14 | WAIS 101 at age 27 | | BI |

[a] WISC and WAIS scores are expressed: full-scale IQ (verbal IQ, performance IQ).

[b] Age x : y = x yr and y months old.

RH competence. Both patients showed a (nonsignificant) trend for a VF x probe interaction (Figure 4-7).

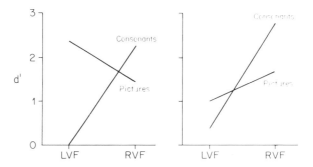

Figure 4-7. *Dichotic listening to nonsense CV syllables. Interaction of type (letter vs. picture) with hemifield of visual probe for patients L.B. (right) and N.G. (left).*

The RE score in the RVF (LH) is unchanged whether the signal is dichotic or monotic, that is, regardless of whether there is a competing signal in the LE. This also verifies the ipsilateral suppression of the LE in the LH. Further, with monotic presentations in the LH of one channel to only one ear, the LE signal is reported somewhat less accurately than is the RE. Thus, the ipsilateral LE → LH channel is somewhat weaker than the crossed RE → LH channel, even without dichotic competition. This laterality effect disappeared, and somewhat lower scores for either ear were obtained with binaural presentations of the same signals to both ears. Therefore, the ipsilateral signals would seem to have some functional significance even when they simply duplicate the contralateral ones.

A similar subtle asymmetry was observed in initial training, with one hand pointing to the picture of the stimulus among six exposed in free vision. Here monotic LE signals yielded slightly higher initial error rates with right-hand pointing; RE signals first showed more errors with left-hand pointing; and binaural signals showed more initial left-hand errors, thus demonstrating LH control. However, either hand pointing to one of the six choice pictures in free vision in the dichotic condition shows the same massive REA; thus, hand pointing is not a reliable index of contralateral hemispheric control.

Effects of Delay on Hemispheric Competence in Patients N.G. and L.B. The effects of stimulus meaningfulness, ear attention, and delay between dichotic pair and visual probe was only investigated in the two patients who showed some RH competence, L.B. and N.G.. ANOVA of the delay data, where trials were partitioned into delay (0.5 or 1 sec) and no-delay conditions, revealed (the usual significant VF, ear, ear × VF effects and) a significant VF × ear × delay interaction (Figure 4-8). While delay had no effect on the LH, it affected the RH in complex ways, both interacting with probe type and showing an effect of the length of the delay.

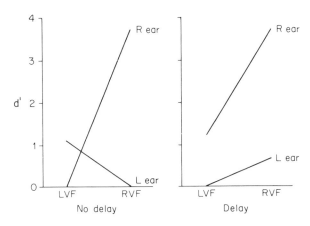

Figure 4-8. *Effect of delay on hemispheric perception of dichotic signals by commissurotomy patient L.B. L ear = left ear score; RVF = right hemifield probes, and so forth.*

Effect of Delay in Patient L.B. Patient L.B. illustrates this pattern best in Figures 4-9 and 4-10. Here percentage accuracy scores for each ear are represented in an accuracy space with the x-axis representing the left ear, and the y-axis representing the right ear. Let a laterality index be defined by $f = (Lc-Rc)/(Lc+Rc)$ if $Lc + Rc < 100\%$ and $f = (Lc-Rc)/(Le+Re)$ if $Lc + Rc > 100\%$, where Lc = percentage correct left ear responses, Re = percentage erroneous right ear responses, and so forth (Marshall et al., 1975). Then line mn denotes a uniform 50% accuracy line and traverses the whole range of f, from –1 to +1, with equal distances representing equal values of f. Lines parallel to mn represent points of equal accuracy. The lines connecting o and p and intersecting mn denote points of equal laterality value.

L.B.'s LH showed a massive REA at all delays and equally for letter and picture probes. By contrast, at zero delay the RH showed a significant LEA for pictures but a nonsignificant REA for letters. A simple mathematical model suggested RH response control for the pictures but LH cross-cuing and control (with poor ipsilateral visual transfer LVF → LH) for the pictures. Thus, the degree of LE suppression in the RH for the same auditory dichotic pairs varied as a function of stimulus meaningfulness (letter vs. picture).

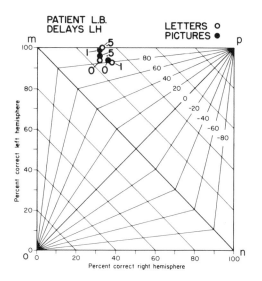

Figure 4-9. *Effect of delays on dichotic listening in the left hemisphere of patient L.B. See text for details. Dots denote picture probes; circles denote letter probes.*

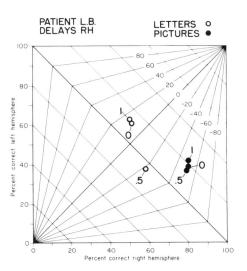

Figure 4-10. *Effect of delays on dichotic listening in the right hemisphere of patient L.B. See Figure 4-9.*

When the visual probes followed the auditory dichotic pair by 0.5 seconds, the RH controlled performance to produce an LEA for both pictures and letters. The LEA was larger for pictures. At 1-sec delay the RH showed a massive LEA for pictures but a reversal to a nonsignificant REA, signaling LH cross-cuing and control, for letters. Thus, the hypothesis of uniform subcortical ipsilateral suppression in dichotic listening is not supported by this data. Rather, ipsilateral suppression is seen to depend upon a variety of cognitive variables and particularly on hemispheric specialization. Whether the lability of ipsilateral suppression is associated with poor competence in either hemisphere or only in the RH remains to be found.

Effects of Attention on Hemispheric Competence in Patient L.B. The effects of attention are even more complex. In L.B., instructions to attend to one ear throughout the test had the effect of reducing the laterality effect in the hemisphere contralateral to the unattended ear without affecting the laterality effect in the hemisphere contralateral to the attended ear. In other words, in each hemisphere attention to the contralateral ear had little influence on the laterality effect, whereas attention to the ipsilateral ear resulted in a substantial change. This change was especially strong and unpredictable in the RH (Figure 4-11). The attention set can affect both the contralateral and ipsilateral ear signals in the "unattended hemisphere." In contrast with delay, attention affected both hemispheres and resulted in substantial changes in laterality effects, especially in the blocked (set) condition.

However, when attention was signaled by random beeps to one ear before the dichotic pairs, LE beeps decreased the laterality effect in both hemispheres but primarily in the LH, whereas RE beeps increased the laterality effect in the RH without affecting that in the LH (Figure 4-11). It seemed that the affect of attention here was mediated by the LH, either to decrease its REA or to decrease its interference with the LEA in the RH.

Normal Subjects

Thirty-six of forty (90%) right-handed normal subjects showed an REA on the dichotic listening test with picture probes. Similar laterality effects were observed in the LVF and in the RVF. Letter probes yielded a slightly larger REA, especially in the RVF. Set attention had no effect on the REA in either visual field (Figure 4-12). Thus, the test seems unusually valid and reliable.

Analysis of variance of the accuracy data (visual field × ear × probe) for the normal subjects revealed a significant REA. Analysis of variance of the latency data showed that letters were recognized significantly faster than pictures and that LVF probes were recognized significantly faster than RVF probes.

Thus, it would seem that accuracy data emphasized the LH advantage in processing the auditory stimuli, whereas latency data emphasized RH superiority in processing the visual probes, even though those have linguistic associations.

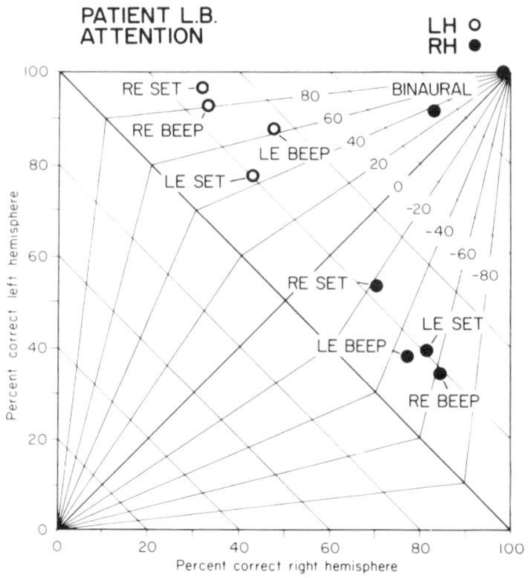

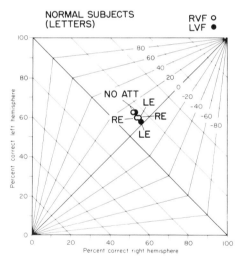

Figure 4-11. *Effect of attention on dichotic listening in the LH and RH of patient L.B. RE set = attention to the right ear for a whole set of trials; LE beep = attention to the left ear indicated by a random beep to the ear prior to the dichotic pair.*

Figure 4-12. *Effect of attention on dichotic listening to nonsense CV syllables by normal subjects using lateralized letter probes. LE = attention to the left ear for a whole set of trials; NO ATT = listening to both ears; dots denote LVF probes: circles denote RVF probes.*

In a second validation study (Kashdan, 1979) with 16 normal right-handed subjects, an ANOVA with d′ as the dependent variable disclosed a significant REA but no effect of probe or VF. In a third validation study

(Kashdan, 1979), letter and picture probes were introduced as between-subject variables with identical results. A fourth study (Kashdan, 1979) manipulated attention in blocks and found a decrease in the REA that showed only a trend (p > .09).

The failure of the REA in normal subjects to be affected by probe type, that is, stimulus meaningfulness, parallels the pattern observed in the disconnected LH but not in the RH. This confirms again exclusive LH specialization and callosal relay to the LH on this task. The effects of attention were seen to be mixed. It can counteract ipsilateral suppression while reducing the contralateral signal. Attention seems to have a much larger effect on the disconnected LH than on the intact LH, suggesting that its effect on ipsilateral suppression can be partly mitigated by the commissures.

Overall, the results in split-brain patients, although complex, warrant optimism about obtaining valid and reliable indexes of hemispheric specialization in normal subjects by manipulating stimulus and task variables.

The Paradoxes of Callosal Relay

Serious conceptual problems persist with the third assumption above (callosal competition) and the callosal relay model for dichotic listening to nonsense syllables. First, it is not known which part of the neocortical commissures transmit the cross-callosal left ear signal to the LH. Anatomical considerations point to the middle third of the corpus callosum (Hamilton, 1982) but the clinical data are conflicting. Some studies do and some do not show auditory disconnection with middle callosal section (e.g., Geffen, Walsh, Simpson, & Jeeves, 1980). Some useful data in this regard can come from cases of paradoxical left ear extinction for our dichotic listening test, where an LH lesion results in reduced left ear scores. Such cases are usually interpreted as auditory disconnection syndromes, and the responsible lesions may invade projections from the corpus callosum rather than callosal fibers directly (Damasio & Damasio, 1979).

The second paradox is the failure of some plausible consequences of callosal relay to be supported by seemingly relevant experiments. Thus, callosal relay is said to result in measurable temporal delay and signal degradation. Yet temporally advancing the stimulus to the inferior ear does not decrease the observed perceptual asymmetry (Berlin & McNeil, 1976). Similar failures were observed in visual tests with bilateral hemifield presentation (McKeever & Huling, 1971). Correspondingly, increasing the intensity of the left ear signal in a consonant-vowel dichotic listening test does not erase the right ear advantage (Studdert-Kennedy & Shankweiler, 1970). The intensity manipulation also failed to erase the REA in the commissurotomy patients (Cullen, 1975; Efron, Yund, & Bogen, 1977).

The reasons for these counterintuitive results have not been explored. It is not clear, for example, whether the temporal offset in the lag manipulation should be in the range of 5 msec (callosal transfer of a motor command in a simple RT task), in the range of 50 msec (callosal transfer in a choice RT task), or other. The lag condition may introduce an independent backward masking effect that dominates the change in ear advantage (Bertelson, personal communication, 1982).

Direct Access: Lexical Decision and Semantic Facilitation

Next will be described a lexical decision task with concrete, imageable targets and pronounceable nonwords, which can be performed by both disconnected hemispheres. I will argue that the decision task fits the direct access model. The behavioral criteria cited in evidence consist of the observation of a relatively small and comparable VFA in the split-brain and in the normal brain and of a pattern of results with normal subjects satisfying the processing-dissociation criterion for direct access in semantic facilitation. Thus, although the disconnected RH is seen to be inferior to the normal RH in semantic facilitation, the two are similar in competence for lexical decision per se.

The Split-brain

The same six patients were used for this study as for the dichotic listening study (Table 4-1).

Stimuli and Procedures

The lexical decision lists were developed by Allen Radant at UCLA and included 128 pairs of prime and target-letter strings (Radant, 1981). The primes and half of the targets were all highly imageable, concrete, and frequent words. The other half of the targets were orthographically regular nonwords. Half of the word targets were highly associated with their primes and half were not. An equal number of associated target word pairs (eight), unassociated target word pairs (eight), and target nonword pairs (sixteen) was assigned to each of four presentation conditions: 1. prime in the LVF and target in the LVF (LL), 2. prime in the RVF and target in the LVF (RL), 3. prime in the left and target in the right (LR), and 4. prime in the right and target in the right (RR). The subjects had to press a left button with the left hand if an LVF target was a word and press a right button with the right hand if an RVF target was a word. No response was required for nonword targets. Thus, LL and RR represented within-hemisphere conditions, while LR and RL represented across-hemisphere conditions.

Tasks

Three tests were used.

1. *Visual priming*. This is the task described above where the prime was flashed for 100 msec to one visual half-field and the target was flashed for 100 msec either to the same or to the opposite visual half-field, following an interstimulus interval of 500 msec.

2. *Auditory priming*. In this version the primes were spoken aloud rather than flashed, followed about 250 msec later by 100-msec targets.

3. *Targets alone*. In this simpler version, no primes were presented. Targets were simply flashed for 100 msec.

Tasks were administered in that order in one-month intervals.

Results and Discussion

Targets Alone. Lexical decision of lateralized targets alone without primes disclosed bilateral competence. All patients except one (N.G.) could lexically decide targets in both VFs. Most patients showed more accurate LH decision, but, of those patients whose accuracy was above chance bilaterally, most were equally fast with both hemispheres. This test also provided a control for the auditory and visual facilitation tests by showing that there was no systematic bias in the targets assigned to the unassociated (A–) and associated (A+) prime conditions.

Partial commissurotomy patient, N.F., showed a pattern of latency and accuracy that was entirely consistent with that of the complete commissurotomy patients. Like most of them, she could decide RVF targets significantly more accurately than LVF targets, and her latency data also did not show hemispheric differences. If anything, her responses to LVF targets were slightly faster than responses to RVF targets. Thus, her performance pattern supports the hypothesis of direct access for lexical decision.

Visual Primes. Lexical decision of lateralized targets with lateralized primes showed bilateral competence in three patients (L.B., N.G., and N.F.) and bilateral incompetence in one patient (R.Y.). There was a generally insignificant trend for more accurate LH decisions but no consistent hemispheric difference in latency. It is noteworthy, again, that only N.F., with partial commissurotomy, showed RH superiority in latency.

Only one patient (L.B.) showed significant facilitation, that is, shorter RTs in the A+ than in the A– condition, and then only in the LH.

The standard administration of the test called for the subject to respond with the hand ipsilateral to the stimulated visual half-field. The test was later repeated twice: once with right-hand responses to stimuli in either VF and then with left-hand responses. From the assumption of contralateral motor innervation, one would expect responses to LVF targets to show an RT decrease or no change from the "both hands" to the "left hand–only" condition. The latter prediction is due to the optimization of RH responses and minimization of LH interference when blocked left hand–only responses were used. The predictions were supported neither by the accuracy nor by the latency data. Thus, neither (four) complete nor (two) partial commissurotomy patients supported the putative advantage of contralateral over ipsilateral manual responses in this choice RT task. It follows that a main effect of response hand or significant interaction of response hand by target VF cannot serve as behavioral criteria for callosal relay and direct access, respectively, in this task!

Auditory Primes. Lexical decision of lateralized targets with free auditory primes showed bilateral competence and no consistent hemispheric superiority in accuracy. Latency data showed significant but mixed hemispheric superiorities. Furthermore, auditory facilitation was about equally likely to occur in either hemisphere.

The data are summarized in Table 4-2. Together, the results show that both disconnected hemispheres could perform lexical decision and show some form of semantic facilitation. There was either no hemispheric, or occasionally LH, superiority. Thus, the pattern is consistent with a direct access model.

Normal Subjects

The visual facilitation test used with the commissurotomy patients was originally designed and administered to normal subjects by Allen Radant for an honors undergraduate psychology thesis at UCLA (Radant, 1981). These experiments were continued and extended by Christine Temple and myself. Radant's original experiment randomly assigned words matched for frequency, concreteness, and imageability to four different lists of primes and targets: LL (prime in *L*VF, target in *L*VF), RL (prime in *R*VF, target in *L*VF), LR, and RR. In particular, in each condition, different sublists were assigned to the unassociated (A–) and associated (A+) conditions. In addition, in the experiment described below, prime and target lists were counterbalanced between left and right hemifields. A go/no-go paradigm was used requiring speeded right-hand presses to word targets. All subjects saw the lateralized

TABLE 4-2.
Summary of Lexical Decision and Semantic Facilitation Data with Commissurotomy Patients

	Targets alone	Visual primes	Auditory primes
Lexical decision	BI 4/5 RH 5/5 LH	BI 3/4 RH 3/4 LH	BI 4/5 RH 4/5 LH
Semantic facilitation	—	LH?	BI 4/5 RH 4/5 LH
Hemispheric specialization	LH	Mixed	Mixed

BI = bilaterial competence, LH = left hemisphere, RH = right hemisphere.
3/4 RH = 3 out of 4 right hemispheres, etc.

prime for 100 msec, and after an ISI of 500 msec, they saw the lateralized target for 50 msec.

An ANOVA of RTs to target words with sex as a between-subject factor and association (A-, A+), prime VF, and target VF as within-subject factors showed main effects of association (associated targets were faster than unassociated targets) and target VF (RVF targets were decided faster than LVF targets) and a significant interaction of prime VF by target VF (Figure 4-13). The same interaction occurred for associated and for unassociated primes.

In principle, the prime × target interaction is consistent with both the callosal relay and direct access models, if one assumes a second effective factor, independent of facilitation. However, the control experiment in which only targets with no primes were presented provides evidence that is more suggestive of direct access in lexical decision. In each of the four conditions (LL, LR, RL, RR) the difference between the "targets only" and "primes plus targets" conditions may represent some combination of inhibition and priming of the target by the unassociated prime and facilitation of the target by the associated prime. Figure 4-14 plots the difference in RT between the "targets only" and "primes plus targets" in the A- and A+ conditions, as a function of processing hemisphere (LL = RH, RR = LH). The figure illustrates a classic processing dissociation, indicating direct access. It means that there is no inhibition and little facilitation in the normal LH, but strong inhibition and even greater facilitation in the normal RH.

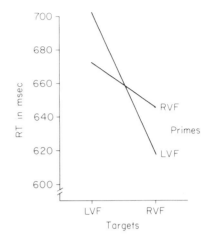

Figure 4-13. *Replication of Radant's experiment. Interaction of prime visual half-field and target visual half-field.*

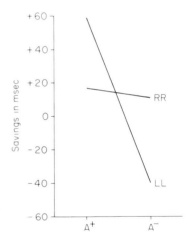

Figure 4-14. *Lexical decision by normal subjects. Difference between primes plus targets and targets only: interaction between hemifield of prime/target and association of prime.*

CONCLUSION: GENERALIZABILITY OF DISCONNECTION SYNDROME

The disconnection syndrome, although based initially on a relatively small group of subjects, served as an important catalyst, both conceptual and empirical, for the study of hemispheric specialization in humans. Conceptually, the disconnected brain serves as a criterial experiment for the concepts, "degree of hemispheric competence" and "degree of relative hemispheric specialization." Empirically, the disconnection syndrome complements inferences from deficit following hemispheric lesions by providing evidence of positive competence. The comparison supports some of the lessons of clinical neurology, such as LH specialization for speech; it qualifies others, such as LH specialization for language in general including, for example, auditory comprehension; and it does not support yet others, such as exclusive RH specialization for constructional praxis. The disconnected hemispheres are generally free of some of the most dramatic deficits consequent to hemispheric damage. Thus, posterior RH lesions can result in devastating contralateral neglect and denial syndromes, and yet the disconnected LH shows no evidence of neglect (Zaidel, Zaidel & Sperry, 1981). It follows that left-sided neglect is a consequence of pathological influence by an RH lesion, rather than of residual LH competence.

The disconnection syndrome, in turn, yielded models for interpreting laterality effects in the normal brain. By focusing upon the twin factors of hemispheric competence and callosal connectivity, the split-brain suggests the two models of direct access and callosal relay, respectively. In principle, the split-brain can index the contribution of hemispheric competence alone to a laterality task, and the comparison with the normal brain can then index the role of callosal transfer. Most complex cognitive tasks may well call for complex interhemispheric interactions. Even for those, the direct access and callosal relay models are useful, since they account for the two independent components of hemispheric competence and callosal transfer in the interactions. I have demonstrated above not only that both models actually exist but that they represent surprisingly complex cognitive operations. The two models, then, represent the limit cases of a continuum of models for laterality effects in the normal brain.

Comparisons with the disconnection syndrome presuppose that the commissurotomy patients represent normal hemispheric organization. Do these patients represent abnormal hemispheric organization due to early brain pathology caused by epileptogenic lesions? Do they show patterns of ipsilateral sensory-motor control and noncallosal interhemispheric interaction, due to postsurgical compensatory adjustment? These questions cannot be answered in the abstract; they raise empirical issues. In general, whether a brain-damaged patient shows compensatory readjustment in hemispheric control of higher cognitive functions or not depends upon the nature, extent, and etiology of that patient's extracallosal damage. Severe, early LH lesions in the language areas can result in a language shift to the RH, but this is certainly not the case with most epileptics. It is simply a matter of the neurological history of the particular patients that were selected for surgery.

There is no evidence of abnormal language organization in the disconnected hemispheres of the California series. There is, however, considerable interindividual variability. The patients vary widely in etiology and localizing symptoms, yet they exhibit the same general pattern of hemispheric specialization. With the linguistic tasks described above, all the commissurotomy patients showed exclusive LH specialization for the perception of dichotic nonsense CV syllables, all showed bilateral competence for lexical decision and auditory facilitation, and none appeared to have speech in the disconnected RH.

Is lexical decision indicative of functional reading? A recent argument that nonfoveal facilitation does not occur in normal reading (Inhoff, 1982) is based upon artificial tasks that seem to be poor approximations to natural reading. Marcel and Patterson (1978) showed peripheral facilitation in both VFs of normal subjects. Conversely, Cohen and Freeman (1978) showed phonological effects (defacilitation due to nonword homophones of real words) in the RVF but not in the LVF of normal subjects, supporting the conclusion drawn from the disconnected RH that RH lexical reading does not involve intermediate phonological representation (Zaidel & Peters, 1981). In our experiment, the same targets used in the lexical decision task were subsequently used for a reading task in which patients L.B. and N.G. were required to point to a multiple-choice array of pictures exposed in free vision, in response to the lateralized target. Hemispheric performance estimates for both hemispheres were generally higher for the reading than for the lexical decision task (E. Zaidel, 1982b). Furthermore, the tachistoscopic assessment of reading competence in these patients actually underestimated the hemispheric reading vocabularies, as assessed with a custom-made contact lens technique! It would seem, therefore, that lexical decision provides a conservative estimate of RH competence for reading.

Similar conclusions follow from comparing lexical decision and semantic facilitation in the disconnected and intact RHs. The disconnected RH did not show evidence and the intact RH did show evidence of semantic facilitation from lateralized printed words, yet both showed lexical decision. Hence, the disconnected RH seems to underestimate the contribution of the normal RH to reading.

How does the evidence on RH language in commissurotomy patients compare with clinical neurological data? The pattern observed in the disconnected RH resembles that observed in adults with dominant hemispherectomy for late lesions (Burklund, 1972) and in temporal lobe epileptics whose RH is temporarily anesthetized by sodium amobarbital (Rasmussen & Milner, 1977). Conversely, the "exotic" pattern of the disconnected RH (no speech, good auditory comprehension, intermediate reading, good lexical and poor sentential analysis, good semantics and poor phonology, etc.) contrasts sharply with language in the RH following left hemispherectomy for infantile hemiplegia, for which early damage leads to rather complete and uniform language representation in the intact RH.

More recently, there has been a resurgence of interest in RH language in aphasics. Many case studies are now available, providing evidence of RH takeover of various language functions in aphasia (e.g., Cummings, Benson, Walsh, & Levine, 1979; Heilman, Rothi, Campanella, & Wolfson, 1979). The syndrome of deep dyslexia, in particular, lends itself to an interpretation in terms of RH support of semantic lexical access during reading (Coltheart, Patterson, & Marshall, 1980; E. Zaidel, 1982a). Furthermore, right brain damage in right-handed adults has now been shown to selectively impair diverse communication functions, ranging from the appreciation of humor, proverbs, and metaphor (Gardner, Hamby, Wapner, et al., 1979; Gardner, Ling, Flamm, & Silverman, 1975) to thematics of discourse (Ulatowska, personal communication, 1982) and the control of prosody and intonation (Ross, 1981). Finally, there is growing awareness of special linguistic roles for the RH during the initial stages of acquiring reading (Silverberg, Gordon, Pollack, & Bentin, 1980), at least in some children (Bakker & Moerland, 1981), or in supporting a second language (Vaid & Genessee, 1980).

The results with the lexical decision, semantic facilitation, and dichotic listening tasks extend to the six available commissurotomy patients of the Bogen-Vogel series and to some conclusions reached on the basis of more extensive contact lens studies with patients, N.G. and L.B. These latter two were chosen to be fitted with contact lenses because they were relatively free of extracallosal damage in comparison with other patients in the series and because they differed in sex, IQs, and clinical history. Yet the RHs of these two patients, as well as that of a patient with dominant hemispherectomy at age ten (for a tumor showing first symptoms at age eight), all showed similar receptive language profiles (e.g., E. Zaidel, 1979b). In fact, L.B. and N.G. are suspected of having predominant RH rather than LH extracallosal damage. This would lead to the conjecture that their RHs underestimate the linguistic competence of an intact RH.

In general, predominant laterality of extracallosal damage in these patients (Table 4-1) does not predict laterality effect in either visual or auditory tasks, although it does seem to predict somatosensory deficits and compensatory readjustments in ipsilateral manual efferent and afferent control (E. Zaidel, 1978a, 1978b). Even so, it is easy to demonstrate consistent tactile hemispheric specialization effects in these patients (e.g., Milner & Taylor, 1972). However, I have tested these patients recently with several "reputedly RH" visuospatial tests (such as Street's Gestalt Completion, Benton's Line Orientation, The Mooney Faces) and have failed to find the expected RH superiority. We need to establish the limits of this apparent failure and its dependency upon subtle task demands (such as response mode) before considering the more radical interpretation that some RH language development in the disconnected RHs occurred "at the expense of" more traditional RH functions.

The disconnection syndrome has been especially important in focusing attention upon RH functions and upon nonverbal experimental paradigms that tap these functions. Testing the linguistic capacity of the disconnected RH has particularly drawn my own attention to issues of partial competence—its characterization and assessment—and of variability in RH performance. Observed RH superiority can often be reversed by small changes in the conditions of the task, and the LH is more likely to interfere with the RH and to assume control over ipsilateral pathways and behavior in free vision than the other way around (E. Zaidel, 1978a). Tasks for which the disconnected RH has only partial competence often show highly erratic behavior, characterized by frequent failures, occasional successes, and considerable variability, but the short-term variability is masked by long-term stability of RH performance. Quite frequently, overall chance performance by the RH on some task contains nonrandom sequences of alternatively correct and incorrect responses. The source of such long sequences is not clear as yet, but they may signal attentional shifts to and away from RH control, perhaps due to LH interference. Reviewing laterality effects in hemifield tachistoscopic studies in normal subjects, Bertelson (1982) reached similar conclusions. The observed LVFAs for "RH stimuli" (e.g., dot localization and identification or matching of nonsense shapes) are generally smaller than the LVFAs found for words or letters, and they often prove more difficult to replicate.

One theoretical significance of RH functions is related to the concept of masked or hidden competence. A standard interpretation of language competence in the disconnected RH is in terms of ability that is not accessible to verbal description and that is masked under certain conditions of testing and pathology. In that sense, RH functions in the disconnected brain can serve as a paradigm case for the recent illustration of masked competence, as in blind sight (Weiskranz, Warrington, Sanders, & Marshall, 1974), in release from agraphia with the aid of prosthesis for the dominant, hemiplegic hand (J. Brown, 1982), and in the "hidden observer" under hypnosis (Hilgard, 1977).

The promise of the distinction between direct access and callosal relay models lies in their explication of individual differences in hemispheric organization. The question for future research is whether or to what extent individual differences (e.g., sex, handedness, extreme cognitive profiles, or idiosyncratic information-processing strategies) correspond to selective differences in right or left hemispheric competencies, as against differences in functional callosal connectivity for complex information. In particular, how do these differences vary as a function of modality, material, attention, hemispheric priming, and overloading?

ACKNOWLEDGMENTS

Thanks to John Maslow and Elizabeth Maslow for assistance and to Joseph Bogen, Avraham Schweiger, and Joe Hellige for helpful suggestions. This work was supported by NSF grant BNS 79–29177 and NIMH RSDA MH 000179 to the author, and by NIMH grant MH 03372 to R.W. Sperry.

REFERENCES

Bakker, D.J. and R. Moerland (1981) Are there brain-tied sex differences in reading? In A. Ansara, N. Geschwind, A. Galaburda, M. Albert and N. Gartell (Eds.) *Sex Differences in Dyslexia*. Townson, Md., The Orton Society, 109–117.

Bashore, T.R. (1981) Vocal and manual reaction time estimates of interhemispheric transmission time. *Psychological Bulletin*, *89*, 352–368.

Berlin, C.I. (1977) Hemispheric asymmetry in auditory tasks. In S. Harnad, R.W. Dody, L. Goldstein, J. Jaynes, & G. Krauthamer (Eds.), *Lateralization in the Nervous System*. New York: Academic Press, pp. 303–308.

Berlin, C. & M.R. McNeil (1976) Dichotic listening. In N.J. Lass (Ed.), *Contemporary Issues in Experimental Phonetics*. New York: Academic Press, pp. 327–391.

Berlucchi, G., W. Heron, R. Hyman et al. (1971) Simple reaction times of ipsilateral and contralateral hand to lateralized visual stimuli. *Brain*, *94*, 419–430.

Bertelson, P. (1982) Lateral differences in normal man and lateralization of brain function. *International Journal of Psychology*, *17*, 173–210.

Bogen, J.E. & P.J. Vogel (1975) Neurologic status in the long term following complete cerebral commissurotomy. In F. Michel and B. Schott (Eds.), *Les Syndromes de Disconnexion Calleuse Chez l'Homme*. Lyon: Hôpital Neurologique, pp. 227–251.

Boles, D.B. (1979) The bilateral effect: Mechanisms for the advantage of bilateral over unilateral stimulus presentation in the production of visual field asymmetry. Unpublished doctoral dissertation, Department of Psychology, University of Oregon.

Bryden, P. (1976) Response bias and hemispheric differences in dot localization. *Perception and Psychophysics*, *19*, 23–28.

Burklund, C.W. (1972) Cerebral hemisphere function in the human: Fact versus tradition. In W. Lynn Smith (Ed.) *Drugs, Development, and Cerebral Function*. Springfield, Ill.: Charles C. Thomas.

Carmon, A., T. Nachshon, & R. Starinsky (1976) Developmental aspects of visual hemifield differences in perception of verbal material. *Brain and Language*, *3*, 463–469.

Cohen, G. & R. Freeman (1978) Individual differences in reading strategies in relation to handedness and cerebral asymmetry. In J. Reguin (Ed.), *Attention and Performance VII*. Hillsdale, N.J.: Lawrence Erlbaum, pp. 411–426.

Coltheart, M., K. Patterson, & J.C. Marshall (Eds.) (1980) *Deep Dyslexia*. London: Routledge & Kegan Paul, pp. 326–380.

Cullen, J.K., Jr. (1975) Tests of a model for speech information flow (doctoral dissertation, Louisiana State University). *Dissertations Abstracts International*, *36*, 1167A (University Microfilms No. 75-19, 262)

Cummings, J.L., D.F. Benson, M.J. Walsh, & H.L. Levine (1979) Left-to-right transfer of language dominance: A case study. *Neurology*, *29*, 1547–1549.

Damasio, H. and A. Damasio (1979) Paradoxical ear extinction in dichotic listening: possible anatomic significance. *Neurology*, *29*, 644–653.

Day, J. (1977) Right hemisphere language processing in normal right handers. *Journal of Experimental Psychology* [Human Perception], *3*, 518–528.

Efron, R., E.W. Yund, & J.E. Bogen (1977) Perception of dichotic chords by normal and commissurotomized human subjects. *Cortex*, *13*, 137–149.

Filbey, R.A. & M.S. Gazzaniga (1969) Splitting the normal brain with reaction time. *Psychonomic Science*, *17*, 335–336.

Forgays, D.G. (1953) The development of differential word recognition. *Journal of Experimental Psychology*, *45* 165–168.

Franz, S.I. (1933) The inadequacy of the concept of unilateral cerebral dominance in learning. *Journal of Experimental Psychology*, *16*, 873–875.

Franz, S.I. & E.F. Davis (1933) Simultaneous reading with both cerebral hemisheres. *Studies in Cerebral Function, IV*. Publications of the University of California at Los Angeles in Education, Philosophy, and Psychology, *1*, 99–106.

Franz, S.I. & S. Kilduff (1933) Cerebral dominance as shown by segmental visual learning. *Studies in Cerebral Function, II*. Publications of the University of California at Los Angeles in Education, Philosophy, and Psychology, *1*, 79–90.

Gardner, H., S. Hamby, W. Wapner et al. (1979) The role of the right hemisphere in the organization of linguistic materials. Paper presented at the seventeenth annual meeting of the Academy of Aphasia, San Diego.

Gardner, H., P.K. Ling, L. Flamm, & J. Silverman (1975) Comprehension and appreciation of humorous material following brain damage. *Brain*, *98*, 349–412.

Geffen, G., W. Walsh, D. Simpson, & M. Jeeves (1980) Comparison of the effects of transcortical and transcallosal removal of intraventricular tumors. *Brain, 103*, 773–778.

Goldberg, E. & L.D. Costa (1981) Hemispheric differences in the acquisition and use of descriptive systems. *Brain and Language, 14*, 144–173.

Gordon, H.W., J.E. Bogen & R.W. Sperry (1971) Absence of disconnection syndrome in two patients with partial section of the neocommissures. *Brain, 94*, 327–336.

Gordon, H.W. & A. Carmon (1976) Transfer of dominance in speed of verbal response to visually presented stimuli from right to left hemisphere. *Perceptual and Motor Skills, 42*, 1091–1100.

Hamilton, C.R. (1982) Mechanisms of interocular equivalence. In D.J. Engle, M.A. Goodale, & R. Mansfield (Eds.), *Analysis of Visual Behavior*. Cambridge: MIT Press.

Harshman, R. (1980) The meaning and measurement of differences in degree of lateralization. Paper presented in the symposium on Methodological and Statistical Issues in Neuropsychological Research, chaired by S.A. Berenbaum. Eighth Annual Meeting, INS, San Francisco, January 29–February 2.

Hebb, D.O. (1949) *The Organization of Behavior*. New York: Wiley.

Heilman, K.M., L. Rothi, D. Campanella, & S. Wolfson (1979) Wernicke's and global aphasia without alexia. *Archives of Neurology, 36*, 129–133.

Hellige, J.B. & P.J. Cox (1976) Effects of concurrent verbal memory on recognition of stimuli from the left and right fields. *Journal of Experimental Psychology* [Human Perception], *2*, 210–221.

Heron, W. (1957) Perception as a function of retinal locus and attention. *American Journal of Psychology, 70*, 38–48.

Hilgard, E.R. (1977) *Divided Consciousness*. New York: Wiley.

Inhoff, A.W. (1982) Parafoveal word perception: A further case against semantic preprocessing. *Journal of Experimental Psychology* [Human Perception], *8*, 137–145.

Kashdan, E. (1979) Speech perception and cerebral asymmetry. Honors undergraduate thesis, Department of Psychology, Dartmouth College.

Kimura, D. (1959) The effect of letter position on recognition. *Canadian Journal of Psychology, 13*, 1–10.

Kimura, D. (1961a) Cerebral dominance and the perception of verbal stimuli. *Canadian Journal of Psychology, 15*, 166–171.

Kimura, D. (1961b) Some effects of temporal-lobe damage on auditory perception. *Canadian Journal of Psychology, 15*, 156–165.

Kimura, D. (1967) Functional asymmetry of the brain in dichotic listening. *Cortex, 3*, 166–178.

Kimura, D. & M. Durnford (1974) Normal studies on the function of the right hemisphere in vision. In S.J. Dimond & J.G. Beaumont (Eds.), *Hemisphere Function in the Human Brain*. London: Elek Science, pp. 25–47.

Klatzky, R.I. & R.C. Atkinson (1971) Specialization of the cerebral hemispheres in scanning for information in short-term memory. *Perception and Psychophysics*, *10*, 335–338.

Ladavas, E. & C. Umiltá (1982) Do laterality measures relate to speed of response in central vision? Unpublished manuscript.

Letai, A.D. (1981) Performance on lateralized visual and auditory single and dual tasks. Department of Psychology, UCLA.

Marcel, A.J. & K.E. Patterson (1978) Word recognition and production: Reciprocity in clinical and normal studies. In J. Reguin (Ed.), *Attention and Performance VII*. Hillsdale N.J.: Lawrence Erlbaum, pp. 209–226.

Marshall, J.C., D. Caplan, & J.M. Holmes (1975) The measure of laterality. *Neuropsychologia*, *13*, 315–322.

McKeever, W.F. & M.D. Huling (1971) A note on Filby and Gazzaniga's "Splitting the brain with reaction time." *Psychonomic Science*, *22*, 222.

Milner, B. (1978) Clues to the cerebral organization of memory. In P.A. Buser & A. Rougeul-Buser (Eds.), *Cerebral Correlates of Conscious Experience*. Amsterdam: North-Holland, pp. 139–153.

Milner, B. & L. Taylor (1972) Right-hemisphere superiority in tactile pattern-recognition after cerebral commissurotomy: Evidence for nonverbal memory. *Neuropsychologia*, *10*, 1–15.

Milner, B., I. Taylor, & R.W. Sperry (1967) Lateralized suppression of dichotically presented digits after commissural section in man. *Science*, *161*, 184–185.

Mishkin, M. & D.G. Forgays (1952) Word recognition as a function of retinal locus. *Journal of Experimental Psychology*, *43*, 43–48.

Moscovitch, M. (1973) Language and the cerebral hemispheres: Reaction time studies and their implications for models of cerebral dominance. In P. Plimer, T. Alloway, & L. Krames (Eds.), *Communication and Affect: Language and Thought*. New York: Academic Press, pp. 89–126.

Moscovitch, M. (1979) Information processing and the cerebral hemispheres. In M.S. Gazzaniga (Ed.), *Neuropsychology, Handbook of Behavioral Neurobiology*. (Vol. 2). New York: Plenum Press, pp. 379–446.

Moscovitch, M., D. Scullion, & D. Christie (1976) Early vs. late stages of processing and their relation to functional hemispheric asymmetries in face recognition. *Journal of Experimental Psychology* [*Human Perception*], *2*, 401–416.

Nebes, R.B. (1974) Hemispheric specialization in commissurotomized man. *Psychological Bulletin*, *81*, 1–14.

Orbach, J. (1952) Retinal locus as a factor in the recognition of visually perceived words. *American Journal of Psychology*, *65*, 555–562.

Orbach, J. (1967) Differential recognition of Hebrew and English words in left and right visual fields as a function of cerebral dominance and reading habits. *Neuropsychologia*, *5*, 127–134.

Poffenberger, A.T. (1912) Reaction time to retinal stimulation with special reference to time lost in conduction through nerve centers. *Archives of Psychology*, *23*, 17–25.

Pollatsek, A., S. Bolozky, A.D. Well, & K. Rayner (1981) Asymmetries in the perceptual span for Israeli readers. *Brain and Language*, *14*, 174–180.

Radant, A. (1981) Facilitation in a lexical decision task: Effects of visual field, sex, handedness and anxiety. Honors undergraduate thesis, Department of Psychology, UCLA.

Rasmussen, T. & B. Milner (1977) The role of early left-brain injury in determining lateralization of cerebral speech functions. In S.J. Dimond & D.A. Blizard (Eds.), *Evolution and Lateralization of the Brain. Annals of NY Academy of Science*, *299*, 355–369.

Rizzolatti, G. (1979) Interfield differences in reaction times to lateralized visual stimuli in normal subjects. In I.S. Russell, M.W. Van Hoff, & G. Berlucchi (Eds.), *Structure and Function of Cerebral Commissures*. Baltimore: University Park Press, pp. 390–399.

Rosenzweig, M.R. (1951) Representation of the two ears at the auditory cortex. *American Journal of Psychology*, 167, 147–158.

Ross, E.D. (1981) The aprosodias: Functional-anatomical organization of the affective components of language in the right hemisphere. *Archives of Neurology*, 1981, *38*, 561–569.

Satz, P. (1977) Laterality tests: An inferential problem. *Cortex*, *13*, 208–212.

Semmes, J. (1968) Hemispheric specialization: A possible clue to mechanism. *Neuropsychologia*, *6*, 11–26.

Silverberg, R., H. Gordon, S. Pollack, S. Bentin (1980) Shift of visual field preference for Hebrew words in native speakers learning to read. *Brain and Language*, *11*, 99–105.

Smith, B.G. (1981) Visual laterality effects for words. Unpublished manuscript, Department of Psychology, University of California, Los Angeles.

Sparks, R. & N. Geschwind (1968) Dichotic listening in man after section of neocortical commissures. *Cortex*, *4*, 3–16.

Springer, S.P. (1971) Ear asymmetry in a dichotic detection task. *Perception and Psychophysics*, *10*, 239–241.

Sternberg, S. (1969) The discovery of processing stages: Extensions of Donder's method. In W.J. Koster (Ed.), *Acta Psychologica 30, Attention and Performance II*. Amsterdam: North-Holland, pp. 276–315.

Studdert-Kennedy, M. & D. Shankweiler (1970) Hemispheric specialization for speech perception. *Journal of Acoustical Society of America*, *48*, 579–594.

Swanson, J., A. Ledlow, & M. Kinsbourne (1978) Lateral asymmetries revealed by simple reaction time. In M. Kinsbourne (Ed.), *Asymmetrical Function of the Brain*. New York: Cambridge University Press, pp. 274–292.

Temple, C.M. (1981) Lateralized lexical decision involving facilitation. Unpublished manuscript, Department of Psychology, University of California at Los Angeles.

Ulatowska, H. (1982) Personal communication.

Umiltá, C., D. Brizzolara, P. Tabossi, & H. Fairweather (1978) Factors affecting face recognition in the cerebral hemispheres: Familiarity and naming. In J. Reguin (Ed.), *Attention and Performance VII*. Hillsdale, N.J.: Laurence Erlbaum.

Vaid, J. & F. Genessee (1980) Neuropsychological approaches to bilingualism. *Canadian Journal of Psychology*, *34*, 417–445.

Weiskranz, L., E.K. Warrington, M.D. Sanders, & J. Marshall (1974) Visual capacity in the hemianopic field following a restricted occipital ablation. *Brain*, *97*, 709–728.

Zaidel, D.W. (1982) Long-term memory and hemispheric specialization: Semantic organization for pictures (doctoral dissertation, University of California at Los Angeles). *Dissertation Abstracts International*, *42* (University Microfilms No. 82–06,093)

Zaidel, D. & R.W. Sperry (1977) Some long term motor effects of cerebral commissurotomy in man. *Neuropsychologia*, *15*, 193–204.

Zaidel, E. (1976) Language, dichotic listening and the disconnected hemispheres. In D.O. Walter, L. Rogers, & J.M. Finzi-Fried (Eds.), *Conference on Human Brain Function*. Brain Information Service, BRI Publications Office, UCLA, pp. 103–110.

Zaidel, E. (1978a) Concepts of cerebral dominance in the split brain. In P.A. Buser & A. Rougeul-Buser (Eds.), *Cerebral Correlates of Conscious Experience*. Amsterdam: Elsevier, pp. 263–284.

Zaidel, E. (1978b) Long-term asterognosis and sensory integration across the midline following brain bisection in man. Manuscript.

Zaidel, E. (1979a) On measuring hemispheric specialization in man. In B. Rybak (Ed.), *Advanced Technobiology*. Alphen aan den Rijn: Sijthoff & Noordhoff, pp. 365–403.

Zaidel, E. (1979b) The split and half brains as models of congenital language disability. In C.L. Ludlow & M.E. Doran-Quine (Eds.), *The Neurological Bases of Language Disorders in Children*:

Methods and Directions for Research (NINCDS Monograph No. 22). Washington, D.C.: U.S. Government Printing Office, pp. 55–89.

Zaidel, E. (1982a) Reading in the disconnected right hemisphere: An aphasiological perspective. In Y. Zotterman (Ed.), *Dyslexia: Neuronal, Cognitive and Linguistic Aspects*. Oxford: Pergamon, pp. 67–91.

Zaidel, E. (1982b) Lexical decision and semantic facilitation in the split brain. Unpublished manuscript, Department of Psychology, UCLA.

Zaidel, E. & Peters, A.M. (1981) Phonological encoding and ideographic reading by the disconnected right hemisphere: Two case studies. *Brain and Language*, *14*, 205–234.

Zaidel, E., Zaidel, D.W., & Sperry, R.W. (1981) Left and right intelligence: Case studies of Raven's progressive matrices following brain bisection and hemidecortication. *Cortex*, *17*, 167–186.

5

Competence versus Performance after Callosal Section: Looks Can Be Deceiving

John J. Sidtis
Michael S. Gazzaniga

The classic approach to relating sensory, perceptual, and cognitive functions to specific brain areas has been to characterize the behavioral deficits that accompany damage to the areas in question. Functional significance is thereby established by inference: areas in which damage causes profound or relatively permanent deficits are generally assumed to subserve a more important role in the impaired function than are areas in which damage causes a less severe or more transient loss. Although this approach is not foolproof (for example, general regulatory areas may be assigned the same functional importance as areas that perform specific operations) the analysis of cognitive deficits following focal brain damage has provided the foundations for neurological and neuropsychological understanding of the functions of the left and right cerebral hemispheres.

An unusual complement to the classical approach to the study of lateralized cerebral function became available with the advent of the neurosurgical procedure of callosal section for the control of otherwise intractable epilepsy. Certainly, the classic approach has been and continues to be used in studying the human split-brain syndrome. The analysis of deficits in interhemispheric transfer and integration after surgical lesions to this tract has established the role of the corpus callosum in interhemispheric communication. The commissurotomy population also provides a situation in which the functions of each hemisphere can be studied directly, without recourse to defectology. In this approach, the comparison between the performance obtained from each callosally disconnected hemisphere allows subjects to serve as their own controls, since callosal section does not result in focal damage of either hemisphere. The interpretation of the results of such interactions must take into account each patient's neurological history as well as the epileptic focus. In commissurotomized patients with two relatively intact cerebral hemispheres, the absence of any gross neurological deficits due to disconnection is striking.

It is the apparently normal behavior of commissurotomy patients that led to the first of several paradoxical findings in the history of split-brain research, namely, the early claims that surgical section of the corpus callosum produced no behavioral changes. As is now known, the first look at the split-brain subject was deceiving. In this chapter, several areas will be discussed in which the performance of commissurotomy patients provides the strongest impetus to reconsider the traditional ways in which lateralized cognitive functions are conceptualized.

NORMAL BEHAVIOR WITHOUT A CORPUS CALLOSUM

In the face of nearly a century of clinical-neurological observations and descriptions that strongly demonstrated that the left and right hemispheres mediated very different mental functions, A.J. Akelaitis purported to show that surgical section of the corpus callosum, the major interconnection between the cerebral hemispheres, had very little effect on behavior. In a series of studies that included 26 patients with either a partial or complete section of the corpus callosum, Akelaitis and his colleagues concluded that the callosum had no significant role in functions such as vision, gnosis, praxis, or language (e.g., Akelaitis, 1941, 1944; Akelaitis, Risteen, Herren & Van Wagenen, 1942; Smith & Akelaitis, 1942).

The role of the callosum in interhemispheric information transfer began to be understood with the animal work of Myers and Sperry (1953). By sectioning the optic chiasm in cats, information could be lateralized to one of the hemispheres by using a monocular training procedure. Myers and Sperry demonstrated that, whereas monocularly trained animals could perform the learned discrimination with either the trained or the untrained eye when the callosum was intact, the training was not bilaterally available when the callosum was sectioned. Subsequent work confirmed the importance of the callosum in the transfer of visual information between the hemispheres (e.g., Myers, 1956, 1962). It was in this context that a new series of human commissurotomy studies was initiated.

When Akelaitis's approach was repeated on this new series of patients, operated on by Bogen and Vogel, the results were similar to those reported by Akelaitis in the 1940s. However, when the methodology was modified so that information was lateralized to a single hemisphere, when visual guidance of motor acts was eliminated where inappropriate, and when the opportunities for cross-cuing were restricted, the human split-brain syndrome became apparent. Contrary to the conclusions drawn by Akelaitis, the corpus callosum was shown to play a major role in the interhemispheric transfer of sensory information, as well as in ipsilateral cortical control of distal motor activities (e.g., Gazzaniga, 1970; Gazzaniga, Bogen, & Sperry, 1962, 1965, 1967).

The study of commissurotomized patients and of patients with callosal lesions of vascular and neoplastic etiologies has revealed some of the important functional properties of the corpus callosum. The posterior part of the callosum provides a sensory window through which information about a hemisphere's ipsilateral sensory field is transferred. The splenium, which is at the most posterior extent of the callosum, is responsible for the interhemispheric transfer of visual information (e.g., Gazzaniga & Freedman, 1973; Maspes, 1948; Sugishita, Iwata, Toyokura, et al., 1978; Trescher & Ford, 1937). Anterior to the splenium but within the posterior half are the areas responsible for the transfer of audition, touch, and motor control (e.g., Sidtis, Volpe, Holtzman, et al., 1981a; Springer & Gazzaniga, 1975; Volpe, Sidtis, Holtzman, et al., 1982). The patient who has undergone surgical section of the posterior half of the callosum, then, looks like the completely commissurotomized patient in many respects. Table 5-1 presents performance on naming stimuli presented to the left and right sensory fields prior to and following section of the posterior callosum.

Unlike the patient with a complete callosal section, however, the patient with the posterior callosal section may not verbally deny right hemisphere stimulation. In one such patient, J.W., the left hemisphere language system could not name right hemisphere stimuli because of the absence of sensory transfer, yet he did express a sense of knowing what the stimulus was. The interhemispherically transferred information that provided this sense of knowing enabled the patient's left hemisphere language system to interact with the examiner in a game of "20 questions" regarding the right hemisphere stimuli. By using this strategy, J.W. could name right hemisphere stimuli at levels significantly better than chance. During a ten-week interoperative period when only the anterior portion of the callosum was intact, the patient learned to describe his sense of right hemisphere stimuli in a form much like that of a mental image. His descriptions were rarely that of the stimulus itself, but were typically of a context or episode related to the stimulus. For example, the word *stove* elicited a description of his aunt's kitchen; the word *onion* elicited a description of a family garden. Following completion of his callosal section, the

TABLE 5-1.

Naming Accuracy (percentage correct) on Stimuli Presented to the Left and Right Sensory Fields Prior to and Following Surgical Section of the Posterior Half of the Corpus Callosum

Modality	Left sensory field		Right sensory field	
	Callosum intact	Posterior callosum sectioned	Callosum intact	Posterior callosum sectioned
Vision				
Pictures	93	28[a]	93	91
Words	63	13[b]	92	96
Tactile				
Objects	100	20[b]	100	90
Audition				
C-V syllables	67	23[b]	77	100

[a]Reflected patient's use of 20-question interaction (see text).

[b]Not significantly better than chance.

patient could no longer access this information for verbal description. In fact, like the classic split-brain patient, he verbally denied right hemisphere stimulation. The kinds of responses produced at each surgical stage are depicted in Figure 5-1. The observations of cognitive transfer in J.W. suggest that the anterior callosum was providing the left hemisphere with mnestic information activated by the right hemisphere. The left hemisphere then had to search the memory to retrieve the original referent.

The corpus callosum, then, provides interhemispheric communication at several levels. It plays an important role in supplying visual, auditory, and somatosensory information from the ipsilateral sensory fields, and it also mediates ipsilateral motor control of the distal extremities. This tract also provides higher-order information, transferring the results of cognitive processing in each hemisphere.

Although, in retrospect, there may be a temptation to summarily dismiss the work of Akelaitis, his reports make an important point about the human split-brain syndrome. When two intact cerebral hemispheres are separated, there is little discernible loss of function at a gross behavioral level, except the capacity to cross-integrate information from the left and right sensory fields. Even the cross-integration deficits are not obvious in unconstrained behavioral situations, as is evident from Akelaitis's extensive negative results and from

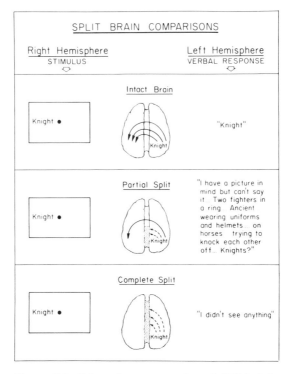

Figure 5-1. *Schematic representation of J.W.'s left-visual-field naming ability with the corpus callosum intact, with the posterior portion of the callosum sectioned, and with the entire callosum sectioned (after Sidtis et al., 1981a).*

simply observing commissurotomy patients' behaviors in normal situations. The comparative subtlety of the split-brain syndrome compared with other neurological syndromes emphasizes the enormous behavioral plasticity available to two intact hemispheres. To compensate for the absence of neural interhemispheric communication, split-brain patients attempt to ensure that communication by using any available information. Much of this information can be provided by behavioral means, such as eye movements, visual guidance of motor acts, and auditory cross-cuing. Moreover, since there is no apparent loss of specific cognitive function in either hemisphere, the subject has not one, but two brain systems contributing to the behavioral compensation for disconnection, without having to additionally compensate for cognitive gaps in mental function. The grossly normal performance of commissurotomy patients, then, is not evidence of the competence of subcortical commissures in the normal interhemispheric integration of cortical sensory and motor activity. Rather, such performance demonstrates the competence of intact cognitive systems in using neural, perceptual, and behavioral information to integrate left and right hemisphere functions in the absence of the corpus callosum.

TWO KINDS OF VISUAL FUNCTION

The ability of split-brain patients to use behavioral cross-cuing strategies to compensate for callosal disconnection can account for some but not all aspects of their behavior. In general, each hemisphere receives direct sensory input largely from the contralateral sensory hemifield, with the ipsilateral hemifield supplied by the callosal window. Through the geniculostriatal projections, for example, occipital areas in each hemisphere receive information about the contralateral visual field, while the splenium of the corpus callosum supplies the ipsilateral visual fields. When the posterior portion of the callosum is cut, each hemisphere can subserve visual identification and recognition only for its contralateral hemifield, and the ability to integrate visual information from the two hemifields is lost (e.g., Sidtis et al., 1981a). In spite of this, visual-motor function in both the partial-posterior and complete commissurotomy patient is intact for a wide range of activities for which one might expect at least some dysfunction: running, throwing, catching a ball, swimming, and even riding a bicycle. Such goal-directed behaviors, which require integration of information across the visual midline, are somewhat paradoxical in light of the striking disconnection phenomena one can demonstrate in the laboratory.

Based upon the visual disconnection observed when commissurotomy subjects are required to identify stimuli, one might expect one or both of the following situations to occur during the execution of goal-directed visual-motor acts. If both hemispheres vied for the control of motor acts, one would observe a constant state of competition, likely to be marked by hesitancy, abrupt starts and stops, and misdirected movement. However, if a single hemisphere dominated the control of such acts, one might expect to observe some form of hemispatial neglect or inattention. Whereas both situations can be elicited under certain laboratory conditions, neither is common under normal conditions.

One possible explanation for this discrepancy is that the processes underlying visual identification and those underlying the control of visual attention are dissociable, both behaviorally and neurophysiologically. Whereas the processes underlying identification in each hemisphere have access only to information from the contralateral visual field after commissurotomy, the process underlying the control of attention in either or both hemispheres may retain bilateral access to visual information. The possible dissociation of the control of visual attention from explicit identification after commissurotomy was examined in a study that incorporated a spatial priming paradigm (Holtzman, Sidtis, Volpe et al., 1981).

The question in these studies was straightforward: although it was well known that visual information used for stimulus identification could not be integrated across the midline after commissurotomy, could the control of visual attention use information accessed from a source not restricted to a single hemifield? To examine the question of whether information used in the control of visual attention had a bilateral representation after commissurotomy, Holtzman et al. used a spatial priming paradigm, in which subjects had to judge whether a digit briefly presented at various spatial positions in one of the visual fields was odd or even. The spatial location of the digit was constrained to a cell in one of two three-by-three cell matrixes that were presented continuously, four degrees of visual angle to the left and right of fixation. Each presentation of a digit was preceded by a cue (the letter x); a valid cue would appear in the same cell as the digit, an invalid cue would appear in a different cell, and a neutral cue would appear at the fixation point between the two grids. These contingencies occurred under both within- and between-visual field conditions. In the between-field condition, the valid cue appeared in the cell homologous to the one in which the digit would appear in the opposite visual field. Likewise, the invalid cue in the between-field condition appeared in a cell other than the one in which the digit would appear, in the opposite visual field. The neutral cue was the same in both within- and between-field conditions. Figure 5-2, B, depicts a typical within-field valid trial, in which a cue appears in the right visual field, followed by the number 3 in the same spatial position in the same field. In Figure 5-2, C, a between-field trial, the number 3 appears in a homologous location in the opposite visual field. In both cases, the patient would respond appropriately by pressing the odd key.

The performance of normal subjects has been shown to benefit when an antecedent cue provides valid information about the spatial location of a subsequent target (e.g., Posner, Snyder, & Davidson, 1980; Shulman, Remmington, & McClean, 1979). As expected, the performance of two commissurotomy patients, P.S. and J.W., also showed such a benefit in the within-field condition. The critical data, however, are in the between-field condition, where performance was quite similar to that observed in the within-field condition. These results are presented in Figure 5-3. One can see that, in both the within- and between-field conditions, there was a significant effect of cue type: performance was best when the cue was valid and worst when the

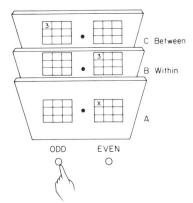

Figure 5-2. *Typical within-field (b) and between-field (c) trials in the spatial priming study.*

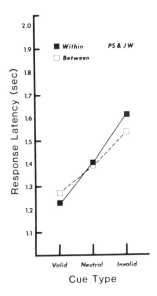

Figure 5-3. *Response latency as a function of spatial cue type. Data are presented separately for the within-field condition and the between-field condition. Each data point represents the average of two observers, with each given equal weight (after Holtzman et al., 1981).*

cue was invalid. Not only was spatial location information accessible within a visual field but also across fields.

A second experiment was carried out to determine whether or not spatial location information was bilaterally accessible for explicit interfield comparisons. As in the first experiment, three-by-three grids were presented continuously to the left and right of central fixation. In this study, however, the digit was replaced by the letter x, and the subject had to make a "same" response if the antecedent cue and the subsequent target appeared in the same or homologous cells or make a "different" response if the two stimuli appeared in different cells. Both patients showed good performance in the within-field conditions, but performance in the between-field condition was at or near chance. The spatial information that was bilaterally accessible for the control of attention was not accessible for explicit interfield comparisons.

The results of these two studies strongly suggest the operation of two dissociable cognitive components in visual information processing—one subserving identification and the other subserving the control of visual attention. Whereas the former is mediated by the primary geniculostriate pathways, which cortically represent the contralateral visual hemifield, and by the splenium of the corpus callosum, the latter probably reflects information processing in the parietal lobe, which appears to maintain access to both visual fields after callosal disconnection. It is probably the selective loss of one or the other of these two visual functions that is responsible for the clinical reports of blind-sight after occipital lesions (e.g., Perenin & Jeannerod, 1975; Weiskrantz, Warrington, Sanders, & Marshall, 1974), and of hemi-attentional deficits after parietal lesions (e.g., Friedland & Weinstein, 1977).

It should be emphasized, however, that the integration of visual information for attentional control is observed in the context of the classic split-brain syndrome. Although a cue appearing in the left visual field may either facilitate or interfere with the classification of a subsequent target, information appearing in this field cannot be accessed by the language systems in the left hemisphere. Commissurotomy patients cannot report left-visual field cues or targets and typically deny any experience after stimulation of that field. Thus, some of the information processing that contributes to the control of attention operates outside the sphere of verbal awareness.

Whereas the apparently normal performance of the commissurotomy patient under a wide range of conditions led Akelaitis to overestimate his subjects' competence in interhemispheric integration, there are other conditions for which the commissurotomy patient's poor performance under some conditions may lead to an underestimate or an inaccurate characterization of a hemisphere's competence. Two areas for which such conditions exist will be considered: the so-called visuospatial functions of the right hemisphere and the language functions of the right hemisphere.

VISUOSPATIAL VERSUS MANIPULOSPATIAL FUNCTION

In contrast with the role of the left hemisphere in language, the functional characteristics of the right hemisphere have been poorly understood. The descriptions of the cognitive strength of this side of the brain have emphasized its relative superiority over the left hemisphere for functions such as construction (Patterson & Zangwill, 1944; Piercy & Smyth, 1962), manipulation and spatial appreciation (e.g., DeRenzi, Faglioni, & Scotti, 1970; Weisenburg & McBride, 1935), synthesis (Denny-Brown & Banker, 1954), and holistic processing (Levy-Agresti & Sperry, 1968). Although none of the functional descriptions of the right hemisphere approached the detail provided by aphasiology for the left hemisphere, most of them shared an emphasis on visual and spatial abilities (see Meier & Thompson, this volume).

The so-called visuospatial dominance of the right hemisphere was also observed in early commissurotomy patients (Bogen & Gazzaniga, 1965). Prior to callosal section, both W.J. and N.G. could copy three-dimentional drawings better with their right hands than with their left hands. However, after surgery, better performance was produced by their left hands; for both patients, right-handed attempts at copying a cube produced drawings that failed to convey depth. A right hemisphere advantage was also observed on the block design subtest of the Wechsler Adult Intelligence Scale. Whereas the left hand of W.J. was able to accurately reproduce each of the seven designs tested, the right hand accurately reproduced two.

The right hemisphere advantage for visuospatial processing was reexamined in a patient, P.S., from the Wilson series (LeDoux, Wilson, & Gazzaniga, 1977). LeDoux et al. noted that, although many of the descriptions of right hemisphere function emphasized visual and spatial characteristics, most of the observations on which such descriptions were based were made in situations in which manual manipulation was required in the response. If, in fact, the right hemisphere's advantage was based upon a visual-perceptual superiority, they reasoned, it should be observed even when a manipulative response was not required.

Like W.J. and N.G., after complete callosal section, P.S. could only convey depth in the copy of a cube produced by his left hand, although prior to surgery this could be accomplished with either hand. Similarly, he accurately completed five out of six block designs with his left hand but only three out of six with his right hand. Two other tests of spatial processing were also used, and similar results were obtained. In the wire figures test (Milner & Taylor, 1972), a series of nonsense shapes fashioned out of wire were tactually presented, and after each figure was palpated, the subject was asked to manually select the figure from a set of four alternatives. P.S.'s left hand was errorless on this task, but his right hand performed at chance. A fragmented figures test was also administered (Nebes, 1972). In this test, the patient tactually explored three geometric shapes and was required to select the shape that corresponded to a visually presented "unfolded" version of the shape. Again, the right hand performed at chance, while the left hand's accuracy ranged between 75 and 90%.

When these tests were readministered without requiring a manual manipulative response, the previously observed right hemisphere advantage was eliminated or reduced. When the patterns from the block design test were visually lateralized to either hemisphere and the patient had to point to the correct design, the previously observed right hemisphere advantage was eliminated. Similarly, when the wire figure designs were presented visually, neither hemisphere erred, and when the fragmented figures task was presented in this fashion, left hemisphere performance improved to 85%, while the right hemisphere remained at 100%.

One of the important points of these results was, that for many of the spatial tests of right hemisphere function, the manipulative aspects of the response were more important than the demands of simply discriminating the test patterns visually. This is not to say that, under some circumstances, right hemisphere visual-perceptual advantages do not occur (e.g., Gazzaniga & Smylie, in press; Moscovitch & Klein, 1980), but rather that the right hemisphere's apparant advantage in spatial processes may be most salient when some form of pattern manipulation is required, either mentally or in terms of a manual response.

LANGUAGE FUNCTIONS OF THE RIGHT HEMISPHERE

Among the growing group of commissurotomy patients, at least 40 of whom have been studied, there are only five established cases of right hemisphere language in left hemisphere–dominant individuals. These few subjects have generated intense interest, since they provide a means by which a right hemisphere language system can be studied directly and with some degree of independence from the left hemisphere system. Inferring right hemisphere linguistic ability from the performance of such patients is even less straightforward than in the case of spatial tasks, however, since there is as yet only a crude understanding of the composition of right hemisphere language in cases of bilateral representation.

One of the most important points that can be made about the subgroup of commissurotomy patients with right hemisphere language is that the intersubject variability, in its extent, exceeds that observed for their left hemisphere language (Sidtis, Volpe, Rayport et al., 1981b). Whereas, in the least linguistically proficient right hemispheres, such capacity consists of little more than the ability to comprehend common words, the most linguistically proficient right hemispheres can gain access to the speech system. For the patients with only right hemisphere receptive language function, there has been a general agreement as to what this system can understand. Right hemisphere comprehension has been shown to be strongest for nouns (Gazzaniga & Hillyard, 1971), and although it has been suggested that the comprehension of verbs is similar to that found for nouns when word frequency is taken into account (Zaidel, 1976a), there is a marked deficiency for the execution of verbal commands by the nonexpressive right hemisphere (Gazzaniga & Hillyard, 1971; Sidtis et al., 1981b; Volpe et al., 1982). Further, there is little or no capacity for syntactic processing in the nonexpressive right hemisphere (Gazzaniga & Hillyard, 1971; Zaidel, 1977). In contrast, the two patients with expressive right hemisphere language not only comprehend but can also follow verbal commands, produce fluent writing, and generate speech from the right as well as the left hemispheres (Gazzaniga, Volpe, Smylie et al., 1979; Sidtis et al., 1981b). While different patients can perform different linguistic tasks with their right hemispheres, one function common to all such patients is the ability to comprehend the meaning of words. One may well ask what sort of linguistic competence this ability represents.

One way to begin to address this question is to examine the kinds of semantic relationships that the right hemisphere can recognize. Semantic judgments of visually presented words were obtained from two patients whose right hemisphere language capacities reflected the range of function found in the commissurotomy population. Patient J.W., from Wilson's surgical series, had a right hemisphere language capacity similar to that found in patients L.B. and N.G. in the earlier Bogen and Vogel surgical series (Gazzaniga & Sperry, 1967). These are the patients with some right hemisphere comprehension but no expression (see Zaidel, this volume). At the other end of the range, V.P., a patient in Rayport's surgical series, had both receptive and expressive abilities comparable to those of patient P.S. (also from Wilson's series). In both of these patients, the right hemisphere could follow commands, write using the left hand, and produce some speech (Sidtis et al., 1981b; Gazzaniga et al., 1979).

In order to test each hemisphere's performance in making various semantic judgments, a series of high-frequency words (rated A and AA on the Thorndike-Lorge word count) were briefly presented on a video monitor lateralized to the left or right of a center fixation point. Following the presentation of each word, the subject was presented with a response card in free vision, on which four words were printed. The subject was asked to select the word that best fit a specified semantic relationship, using the hand ipsilateral to the visual field in which the stimulus word was presented. Five tests were constructed to assess the recognition of the following semantic relationships: synonym (e.g., boat-ship), antonym (e.g., day-night), function e.g., clock-time), superordinate category membership (e.g., lake-water), and subordinate category membership (e.g., tree-oak).

The left and right hemisphere results obtained from J.W. and V.P. are presented in Table 5-2. Across all five tests, the left hemisphere accuracy of these two patients was nearly identical and, in both cases, consistently higher than right hemisphere accuracy. J.W.'s right hemisphere performance was consistently lower than that observed for V.P., suggesting that the intersubject differences found in right hemisphere expression were also present in word comprehension, albeit to a lesser extent. Also of note was the consistency of right hemisphere performance across semantic judgments: for V.P., accuracy on four of the five judgements was within 4 percentage points, while for J.W., accuracy on four of the five judgements was within 10 percentage points. For both subjects, the remaining test, on which right hemisphere performance was lowest, was also the test on which the left hemisphere produced the poorest performance. Thus, while the left hemisphere was consistently more accurate than the right hemisphere, there was no indication that a qualitative difference existed in the kinds of semantic judgments that each hemisphere made.

TABLE 5-2.

Left and Right Hemisphere Accuracy Scores (percentage correct) on Five Tests of Semantic Relationships Obtained from Two Subjects Who Have Undergone Complete Section of the Corpus Callosum

Semantic relationship	V.P.		J.W.	
	Hemisphere			
	Left	Right	Left	Right
Synonym	96.0	80.0	87.0	43.5
Antonym	92.3	70.8	100.0	62.5
Function	100.0	84.0	100.0	66.7
Superordinate	96.0	80.0	96.0	68.0
Subordinate	95.8	80.8	100.0	72.0
Mean	96.0	79.2	96.7	62.8

Note: Each percentage is based on at least 23 trials.
Source: After Sidtis et al., 1981b.

The question of right hemisphere linguistic ability can be pursued further by determining the level at which the right hemisphere's disadvantage in recognizing semantic relationships occurs. Apart from a general difficulty in responding to verbal material (e.g., Sidtis et al., 1981b), the relatively poorer performance of the right hemisphere, compared with that of the left hemisphere on semantic judgments, may reflect left/right differences at either or both of two levels of function. The semantic system that is accessed by the right hemisphere may be uniformly less extensive than that accessed by the left hemisphere. Alternatively, the processes involved in reading and auditory comprehension that provide the right hemisphere with access to the semantic system may be less efficient than those available to the left hemisphere. A recent study of semantic activation after commissurotomy strongly suggests that the limiting factor in right hemisphere comprehension is not the extent of semantic representation available to it.

The previously described interhemispheric cognitive interaction that was observed after partial posterior-callosal section suggested a very close correspondence between the episodic and semantic memory representations activated by each hemisphere. Had there been qualitative differences in either the form or the substance of the memory representations accessed by each hemisphere, the observed cognitive interactions would have been unlikely. Although after complete callosal section, overt interhemispheric interaction no longer occurred, the possibility remained that the close correspondence between the semantic information available to the left and right hemispheres reflected each hemisphere's access to a functionally common semantic system. This possibility was examined by using the phenomenon known as semantic priming.

For normal subjects, processing the meaning of a word can have a significant effect on judgments made on subsequent words. Semantic relatedness, for example, can significantly facilitate word/nonword judgments (e.g., Meyer & Schvaneveldt, 1976; Schvaneveldt & McDonald, 1981) and semantic category judgments (e.g., Durso & Johnson, 1979) made on the second item of a related word pair. This facilitation, or so-called priming effect, is interpreted as reflecting both the organization of the semantic system and the process by which this system is activated. This effect was used to examine two questions for the commissurotomy patient with left and right hemisphere language: do both hemispheres benefit from processing a semantically related antecedent word, and is the benefit available to a hemisphere when the semantically related antecedent was processed by the other hemisphere? Whereas the first question addresses left/right differences in semantic activation, the second question addresses the independence of semantic processing in each hemisphere.

In one study, a commissurotomy patient, J.W., was presented with a series of high-frequency nouns that were flashed to the left or right of a central fixation point on a video screen. After each word was presented, the patient was asked to classify it as referring to something artificial or natural, by manually pressing one of two keys. Four conditions were tested in each hemisphere. Target words were preceded by either an unrelated word in the same category (e.g., ship-gate) or a related word in the same category (e.g., ship-boat), and the preceding word appeared in either the same visual field as the target (the within-hemisphere condition) or in the visual field opposite that in which the target appeared (the between-hemisphere condition). These contingencies are depicted in Figure 5-4.

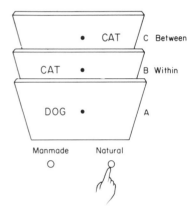

Figure 5-4. *Typical within-field (b) and between-field (c) semantically related trials in the study of semantic priming.*

Some of the results of this study are presented in Table 5-3 (Sidtis, Holtzman & Gazzaniga, 1981). As in the previously described study of semantic processing, left hemisphere performance (86%) was significantly better than right hemisphere performance (69%) across conditions (chi-square(1) = 10.899; $p < 0.01$). Across hemispheres, there was a significant facilitation due to semantic relatedness, seen in both within-field accuracy (chi-square(1) = 10.790; $p < 0.01$) and between-field accuracy (chi-square(1) = 7.752; $p < 0.01$). A significant effect due to semantic relatedness was also found in latency of response $(F(1) = 11.028; p < 0.001)$. There was no significant difference between the within- and between-field conditions on either measure. For the present discussion, the important results are the presence of an interhemispheric facilitation effect and the absence of a difference in the within- and between-field conditions.

These data suggest that, after complete section of the corpus callosum, right and left hemisphere language systems maintain access to a functionally common semantic system. The language systems in each hemisphere, then, are not completely independent functional units, since they extract information from the same semantic store. This raises another paradox, however, because

TABLE 5-3.

Accuracy (percentage correct) and Latency (msec) of Semantic Categorization
Judgments When the Preceding Word Was Either Semantically Related or
Unrelated and Presented to Either the Same Hemisphere as the Subsequent
Word or to the Opposite Hemisphere

Condition	Left hemisphere		Right hemisphere	
	Related	Unrelated	Related	Unrelated
	Percentage correct			
Within hemisphere	92.6	79.5	82.1	60.9
Between hemisphere	92.0	82.9	88.5	58.3
	Latency (SEM)			
Within hemisphere	1390 (64)	1469 (65)	1142 (62)	1493 (66)
Between hemisphere	1427 (76)	1604 (68)	1385 (77)	1723 (79)

Note: The standard errors of the means (SEM) for the latencies are presented in
parentheses.

in spite of this interhemispheric semantic interaction, neither hemisphere in
this patient can verbally name words presented to the right hemisphere. Like
the interfield interaction in the control of visual attention, the semantic
interaction occurs in the context of the classic split-brain syndrome: whereas
semantic activation by one hemisphere can facilitate a subsequent judgment
made by the other hemisphere, the activation alone does not provide the subject
with sufficient information for explicit naming. Although the extent to which
semantic activation alone can be used by an unstimulated hemisphere has yet
to be fully determined, it does appear that, when provided with some context,
such information is more useful to the left than to the right hemisphere (Sidtis,
Holtzman, & Gazzaniga, 1981).

The bilaterality of language in these patients does not strictly imply the
existence of two completely independent systems, even in the comprehension
process. At least for high-frequency nouns, each hemisphere appears to have
access to the same semantic information, although this common access provides
neither a means of cross-cuing nor an avenue of paracallosal transfer
(Gazzaniga, Sidtis, Volpe et al., 1982).

The limitations in right hemisphere word comprehension would appear to
occur largely in the processes through which the semantic system is accessed.
At least for the patients in whom there is only right hemisphere comprehension, there has been little consensus about how such access is gained. Based
upon such patients' inability to recognize rhyming relationships with their
right hemispheres (Levy & Trevarthen, 1977), some reports have suggested

that language comprehension is mediated by qualitatively different processes in each hemisphere. According to such claims, the right hemisphere analyzes spoken language through some unspecified "acoustic-gestalt" process and written language through ideographic interpretation. Phonetic analysis is believed not to play a role in either hypothetical process, since the capacity for such process is supposed to be restricted to the left hemisphere (Levy & Trevarthen, 1977; Zaidel, 1976a). An examination of the range of right hemisphere linguistic capacities, however, suggests that, at least in some patients, the right hemisphere is indeed capable of phonetic processing.

One of the ways in which phonetic discrimination was assessed was by the use of dichotically presented consonant-vowel syllables. The test consisted of pairs of natural-speech syllables selected from among the following six: ba, da, ga, pa, ta, ka. Each member of a dichotic pair was aligned on a single channel of audio tape, using the pulse-code modulation system at the Haskins Laboratories, so that when played stereophonically, competing syllables had a simultaneous onset. Under the standard testing conditions, each dichotic pair was followed by a right-hand written response in which the subject was asked to report both items. In the discrimination form of the test, each pair was followed by a binaurally presented probe item, which matched the right ear stimulus 25% of the time, the left ear stimulus 25% of the time, and neither stimulus 50% of the time. After the probe item, the subject was asked to make a manual "yes" response if the probe matched the sound in either ear or a manual "no" response if it did not. As with this case, when there is sufficient stimulus competition, the dichotic technique functionally lateralizes stimuli to the hemisphere contralateral to the stimulated ear (Sidtis, 1978; Springer, Sidtis, Wilson, & Gazzaniga, 1978).

The results obtained from V.P., J.W., and a group of ten normal subjects on the standard form of the dichotic speech test are presented in Table 5-4. The left ear scores for both commissurotomy subjects were below those found in normal subjects, while their right ear scores were above the normal performance level. For J.W., preoperative testing was also performed, and both left (67%) and right (77%) ear accuracies were with the normal range. These results demonstrate the classic effects of callosal section on the auditory system; stimuli lateralized to the right hemisphere are not transferred to the responding left hemisphere and, hence, are not reported by the subject. The stimuli lateralized to the left hemisphere, however, are processed without interference from the competing information normally transferred through the callosum (Milner, Taylor, & Sperry, 1968; Sidtis, 1978; Sparks & Geschwind, 1968; Springer & Gazzaniga, 1975; Springer et al., 1978).

Although the standard form of the dichotic speech test assesses auditory disconnection, it does not provide a test of right hemisphere capacity, since a right hand response is used. Therefore, the standard test was readministered,

TABLE 5-4.
Accuracy (percentage correct) of
Identification of Consonant-Vowel
Syllables Lateralized to the Left and Right
Hemispheres in Two Commissurotomy
Patients and Ten Normal Subjects

Patient	Hemisphere	
	Left	Right
V.P.	100.0	8.0
J.W.	100.0	23.0
Normal subjects (N = 10)	78.0	65.0

Source: After Sidtis et al., 1981b.

using the left hand to provide a written response. When this was attempted out of vision so that the language-dominant left hemisphere could not visually guide the left hand by exerting ipsilateral control, V.P. performed at chance on both right (20%) and left (17%) ear stimuli, while J.W. refused to respond, claiming that he could not move his left hand.

In order to evaluate phonetic discrimination in the right hemisphere, independent of the capacity for linguistic expression, the discrimination form of the dichotic speech test was also administered to both patients. The results obtained for both left and right hand responses are presented in Figure 5-5. When the right hand was used to respond, the pattern was identical to that found with the standard test requiring a written response. For V.P., however, this pattern was reversed when the left hand was used to respond. Performance on left ear (right hemisphere) speech sounds rose to a nearly perfect level, while right ear (left hemisphere) performance fell to chance. No such reversal was observed for J.W.

Phonetic processing was also examined, using a visual rhyming test. High-frequency nouns were briefly presented to the left or right of a central fixation point on a video monitor. After each word was presented, the subject was asked to choose a word that rhymed with the stimulus (e.g., leg-egg, note-boat) from among four alternatives presented on a response card. Subjects used the hand homotopic to the visual field in which the stimulus word occurred. As with the auditory tests, V.P. and J.W. differed in their right hemisphere performance on the rhymes test. Whereas the left hemispheres of both subjects performed at 100% accuracy, J.W.'s right hemisphere performance (25%) was not significantly different than chance. Conversely, V.P.'s right hemisphere performance was well above chance, at 75% correct.

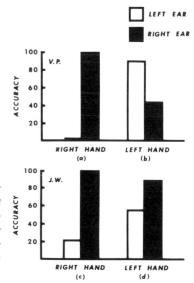

Figure 5-5. *Accuracy of discrimination (percentage correct) of consonant-vowel syllables as a function of ear of presentation and hand of response. CV syllables presented to the right ear are lateralized to the left hemisphere, while those presented to the left ear are lateralized to the right hemisphere.*

For both J.W. and V.P., the standard dichotic speech test demonstrated both the absence of interhemispheric auditory transfer and the ability of the left, but not the right, hemisphere to provide a written transcription following a dichotic trial. Although these results appeared to show that only the left hemispheres of both subjects were capable of phonetic processing, this picture was altered in V.P., when the task was changed to discrimination rather than identification and a nonlinguistic response was allowed. When each hemisphere's contralateral hand responses were compared under these conditions, V.P.'s right hemisphere performance was nearly as accurate as that of her left hemisphere. In contrast, J.W.'s right hemisphere showed no evidence of phonological processing on either the standard or the discrimination form of the dichotic speech test.

The presence of right hemisphere phonological capacity in V.P. and its apparent absence in J.W. was also demonstrated on the visual rhymes test. Although either hemisphere in V.P. could use phonological rules to generate rhyme, only the left hemisphere in J.W. could perform this task. Thus, the marked difference between these two patients in right hemisphere expressive capacity is also present in phonological processing, a function that plays a role in both auditory and visual comprehension.

At least for the commissurotomy patients with the most right hemisphere language, the capacity for phonological processing is present. For the commissurotomy patients with less extensive right hemisphere language, caution should be exercised in interpreting that system's phonological deficit. Phonological rules may be absent, or they may be present in a weak or incomplete fashion in the limited right hemisphere language system. In either case, the available data are beginning to identify the extent to which some linguistic functions can be bilaterally represented but, as of now, do not provide sufficient evidence that the left and right hemispheres subserve qualitatively different language systems.

As the language functions represented in some callosally disconnected right hemispheres have come under study, several things have become clear. There is significant intersubject variability in the representation of expressive and some receptive functions. Further, there is a paradoxical independence between the language functions in each hemisphere. Although both access a functionally common semantic system, the interhemispheric interactions that occur as a consequence of shared access are subtle and do not provide enough information for either explicit naming or even an awareness that any interaction is occurring. Finally, one of the receptive language functions that appears to limit the right hemisphere's capacity for comprehension is phonological processing, although it is inaccurate to say that such capacity is always restricted to the language-dominant hemisphere. Thus, it is reasonable to conclude that, at least in the commissurotomy population, there is no specific entity that could be reasonably termed right hemisphere language. In some of these patients, there is a bilateral representation of a greater number of language functions than in others, and for those functions that are represented bilaterally, there is considerable intersubject variability in the extent of their right hemisphere representation.

CONCLUSIONS

Although the preceding discussion has dealt with studies of cortical function in commissurotomy patients, a number of points can be made that are of general importance to the study of brain and cognition.

First, while it is obvious that cognitive systems process information from both internal and external sources, this fact takes on added importance when attempts are made to attribute cognitive function to specific areas of the brain. Even in the most general case of cortical localization, that is, ascribing particular functions to one hemisphere or the other, the corpus callosum is a significant source of information at cognitive as well as sensory levels of processing. The role of the callosum should not be understated, especially in studies of normal subjects. Whereas most stimulus lateralization procedures appear to provide the experimenter with a preferred channel of information flow into a hemisphere, caution should be exercised in the interpretation of lateral differences obtained with such techniques, since extensive interhemispheric communication exists in the normal, intact brain. Similarly, the extensive and sometimes sophisticated behavioral strategies employed by commissurotomy patients to ensure some degree of interhemispheric communication further suggest that lateralized cognitive systems actively use callosal information: when it is surgically removed, behavioral compensation is actively pursued.

The second point also pertains to sources of information for lateralized cognitive systems. The studies of visual attention and semantic activation after commissurotomy indicate that not every source of information available to a cognitive system is also necessarily available to consciousness, at least at the level of verbal report. However, the subtlety of these effects should not obscure their significance. For both spatial-location and semantic information, each hemisphere had access to common data, although such information was not interhemispherically transferred through the callosum. Some kinds of information, then, may also be available at other levels of the nervous system, albeit in a limited form, and restricted to specific operations in a cognitive system. The independence of cognitive function in either hemisphere is, therefore, limited not only by the degree to which callosal transfer is necessary but also by the degree to which such functions rely upon other common sources of information.

Finally, a point can be made about lateralized cognitive function and left/right differences. As was demonstrated in the examples of spatial processing and right hemisphere linguistic function, some of the general descriptions of these functions belie the extent of ignorance regarding their fundamental characteristics. Neither the spatial characteristics of right hemisphere perceptual and motor function nor the linguistic characteristics of right hemisphere word comprehension, when it exists, are understood. Caution is urged both in broadly characterizing lateralized functions and in invoking the presumed existence of poorly understood functions to account for either normal or pathological behaviors.

The study of split-brain subjects has provided a great deal of information about the functions of the left and right hemispheres. More generally, though, it has also provided a view of the relationships existing between the brain and cognition, which is different from that available from normals and other neurological populations. Through this view, a new picture of subtle interhemispheric interaction is beginning to emerge.

ACKNOWLEDGMENTS

This work was supported by USPHS Grant Number NS15053-02, the Alfred P. Sloan Foundation, and the McKnight Foundation. We wish to thank Dr. Jeffrey D. Holtzman for his comments on this paper. Please address all correspondence to Dr. John J. Sidtis.

REFERENCES

Akelaitis, A.J. (1941) Studies on the corpus callosum. II. Higher visual functions in each homonymous field following complete section of three corpus callosum. *Archives of Neurology and Psychiatry, 45*: 788–796.

Akelaitis, A.J. (1944) A study of gnosis, praxis and language following section of the corpus callosum and anterior commissure. *Journal of Neurosurgery, 1*: 94–102.

Akelaitis, A.J., Risteen, W.A., Herren, R.Y., & Van Wagenen, W.P. (1942) Studies on the corpus callosum. III. A contribution to the study of dyspraxia in epileptics following partial and complete section of the corpus callosum. *Archives of Neurology and Psychiatry, 47*: 971–1008.

Bogen, J.E., & Gazzaniga, M.S. (1965) Cerebral commissurotomy in man: Minor hemisphere dominance for certain visuospatial functions. *Journal of Neurosurgery, 23*: 394–399.

Denny-Brown, D. & Banker, B.Q. (1954) Amorphosynthesis from left parietal lesions. *Archives of Neurology and Psychiatry, 71*: 302–313.

DeRenzi, E., Faglioni, P., & Scotti, G. (1970) Hemispheric contribution to exploration of space through the visual and tactile modality. *Cortex, 6*: 191–203.

Durso, F.T., & Johnson, M.K. (1979) Facilitation in naming and categorizing repeated pictures and words. *Journal of Experimental Psychology: Human Learning and Memory, 5*: 449–459.

Friedland, R.P., & Weinstein, E.A. (1977) Hemi-inattention and hemispheric specialization: Introduction and historical review. In E.A. Weinstein & R.P. Friedland (Eds.), *Hemi-inattention and Hemispheric Specialization*. New York: Raven Press.

Gazzaniga, M.S. (1970) *The Bisected Brain*. New York: Appleton-Century-Crofts.

Gazzaniga, M.S., Bogen, J.E., & Sperry, R.W. (1962) Some functional effects of sectioning the cerebral commissures in man. *Proceedings of the National Academy of Science, 48*: 1765–1769.

Gazzaniga, M.S., Bogen, J.E., & Sperry, R.W. (1965) Observations on visual perception after disconnection of the cerebral hemispheres in man. *Brain, 88*: 221–236.

Gazzaniga, M.S., Bogen, J.E., & Sperry, R.W. (1967) Dyspraxia following division of the cerebral commissures. *Archives of Neurology, 16*: 606–612.

Gazzaniga, M.S., & Freedman, H. (1973) Observations on visual process after posterior callosal section. *Neurology, 23*: 1126–1130.

Gazzaniga, M.S., & Hillyard, S.A. (1971) Language and speech capacity of the right hemisphere. *Neuropsychologia, 9*: 273–280.

Gazzaniga, M.S., Sidtis, J.J., Volpe, B.T. et al. (1982) Evidence of paracallosal verbal transfer after callosal section: A possible consequence of bilateral language organization. *Brain, 105*: 53–63.

Gazzaniga, M.S., & Smylie, C.S. Facial recognition and brain asymmetries: Clues to underlying mechanisms. *Annals of Neurology*, in press.

Gazzaniga. M.S., & Sperry, R.W. (1967) Language after section of the cerebral commissures. *Brain, 90*: 131–148.

Gazzaniga, M.S., Volpe, B.T., Smylie, C.S. et al. (1979) Plasticity in speech organization following commissurotomy. *Brain, 102*: 805–815.

Holtzman, J.D., Sidtis, J.J., Volpe, B.T. et al. (1981) Dissociation of spatial information for stimulus localization and the control of attention. *Brain, 104*: 861–872.

LeDoux, J.E., Wilson, D.H., & Gazzaniga, M.S. (1977) Manipulospatial aspects of cerebral lateralization: Clues to the origin of lateralization. *Neuropsychologia, 15*: 743–750.

Levy, J., & Trevarthen, C. (1977) Perceptual, semantic and phonetic aspects of elementary language processes in split-brain patients. *Brain, 100*: 105–118.

Levy-Agresti, J., & Sperry, R.W. (1968) Differential perceptual capacities in major and minor hemispheres. *Proceedings of the National Academy of Science, 61*: 1151.

Maspes, P.E. (1948) Le syndrome experimental chez l'homme de la section du splenium du corps calleux alexie visuelle pure hemianopsique. *Revue Neurologique, 80*: 100–113.

Meyer, D.E., & Schvaneveldt, R.W. (1976) Meaning, memory structure and mental processes. *Science, 192*, 27–33.

Milner, B., & Taylor L. (1972) Right hemisphere superiority in tactile pattern-recognition after cerebral commissurotomy: Evidence for non-verbal memory. *Neuropsychologia, 10*: 1–15.

Milner, B., Taylor, L., & Sperry, R.W. (1968) Lateralized suppression of dichotically presented digits after commissural section in man. *Science, 161*: 184–186.

Moscovitch, M., & Klein, D. (1980) Material-specific perceptual interference for visual words and faces: Implications for models of capacity limitations, attention, and laterality. *Journal of Experimental Psychology: Human Perception and Performance, 6*: 590–604.

Myers, R.E. (1956) Function of the corpus callosum in interocular transfer. *Brain, 79*: 358–363.

Myers, R.E. (1962) Transmission of visual information within and between the hemispheres. In V.B. Mountcastle (Ed.), *Interhemispheric Relations and Cerebral Dominance*. Baltimore: The Johns Hopkins University Press.

Myers, R.E., & Sperry, R.W. (1953) Interocular transfer of a visual form discrimination habit in cats after section of the optic chiasma and corpus callosum. *Anatomical Record, 115*: 351–352.

Nebes, R. (1972) Dominance of the minor hemisphere in commissurotomized man on a test of figural unification. *Brain, 95*: 633–638.

Patterson, A., & Zangwill, O.L. (1944) Disorders of visual space perception associated with lesions of the right cerebral hemisphere. *Brain, 67*: 351–358.

Perenin, M.T., & Jeannerod, M. (1975) Residual vision in cortically blind hemifields. *Neuropsychologia, 13*: 1–7.

Piercy, M., & Smyth, V.O.G. (1962) Right hemisphere dominance for certain non-verbal intellectual skills. *Brain, 85*: 775–790.

Posner, M.I., Snyder, C.R., & Davidson, B.J. (1980) Attention and the detection of signals. *Journal of Experimental Psychology, 109*: 160–174.

Schvaneveldt, R.W., & McDonald, J.E. (1981) Semantic context and the encoding of words: Evidence for two modes of stimulus analysis. *Journal of Experimental Psychology: Human Perception and Performance, 7*: 673–687.

Shulman, G.L., Remmington, R.W., & McClean, J.P. (1979) Moving attention through visual space. *Journal of Experimental Psychology: Human Perception and Performance, 5*: 522–526.

Sidtis, J.J. (1978) Dichotic listening following commissurotomy. Paper presented as part of a symposium entitled, *Human Split-Brain Research — The Second Decade*. Eastern Psychological. Association, Washington, D.C.

Sidtis, J.J., Holtzman, J.D., & Gazzaniga, M.S. (1981) Interhemispheric semantic interaction in split-brain man. Abstract presented to the annual meeting of the Body for the Advancement of Brain, Behavior and Linguistic Enterprises (BABBLE), Niagra Falls, N.Y.

Sidtis, J.J., Volpe, B.T., Holtzman, J.D. et al. (1981a) Cognitive interaction after staged callosal section: Evidence for transfer of semantic activation. *Science, 212*: 344–346.

Sidtis, J.J., Volpe, B.T., Rayport, M. et al. (1981b) Variability in right hemisphere language function after callosal section: Evidence for a continuum of generative capacity. *Journal of Neuroscience, 1*: 323–331.

Smith, K.U., & Akelaitis, A.J. (1942) Studies on the corpus callosum. I. Laterality in behavior and bilateral motor organization in man before and after section of the corpus callosum. *Archives of Neurology and Psychiatry, 47*: 519–543.

Sparks, R., & Geschwind, N. (1968) Dichotic listening in man after section of the neocortical commissures. *Cortex, 4*: 3–16.

Springer, S.P., & Gazzaniga, M.D. (1975) Dichotic testing of partial and complete split-brain subjects. *Neuropsychologia, 13*: 341–346.

Springer, S.P., Sidtis, J.J., Wilson, D.H., & Gazzaniga, M.S. (1978) Left ear performance in dichotic listening following commissurotomy. *Neuropsychologia, 16*: 305–312.

Sugishita, M., Iwata, M., Toyokura, Y. et al. (1978) Reading of ideograms and phonograms in Japanese following partial commissurotomy. *Neuropsychologia, 16*: 417–425.

Trescher, J.H., & Ford, F.R. (1937) Colloid cyst of the third ventricle. *Archives of Neurology and Psychiatry, 37*: 959–964.

Volpe, B.T., Sidtis, J.J., Holtzman, J.D. et al. (1982) Cortical mechanisms involved in praxis: Observations following partial and complete section of the corpus callosum. *Neurology, 32*: 645–650.

Weisenburg, T., & McBride, K.E. (1935) *Aphasia: A Clinical and Psychological Study*. New York: Commonwealth Fund.

Weiskrantz, L., Warrington, E.K., Sanders, M.D., & Marshall, J. (1974) Visual capacity in the hemianopic field following a restricted occipital oblation. *Brain, 97*: 709–728.

Zaidel, E. (1976a) Auditory vocabulary of the right hemishere following brain bisection or hemidecordication. *Cortex, 12*: 191–211.

Zaidel, E. (1977) Unilateral auditory language comprehension on the token test following cerebral commissurotomy and hemispherectomy. *Neuropsychologia, 15*: 1–18.

6

Dichotic Listening To CVs: Method, Interpretation, and Application

Robert J. Porter, Jr.
Larry F. Hughes

INTRODUCTION

Simultaneous presentation of different speech messages to the two ears does not result in a twofold gain in transmitted information. Instead, overall performance (relative to the 200% maximum) is only 125% to 150%. Broadbent (1954),[1] suggested that this limitation reflects a "bottleneck" in speech information processing; that is, below a certain level, both channels can be processed in parallel (or in a rapidly alternating, serial) fashion, but beyond a certain point, sensory/perceptual analysis is time and/or capacity limited and cannot process both signals together. As a result of the bottleneck, some of the information in one or both channels is lost.

The relative degree of information loss for each ear can be manipulated by varying the task. For example, asking the listeners to attend to sentences or digit sequences in one ear (while ignoring similar material in the other) can reduce recall of the unattended ear's material to virtually zero (Cherry, 1953; Norman, 1968). In addition, if the material in the two ears is semantically or syntactically related, and/or is spoken by the same voice, correctly attending to only one ear's message is especially difficult (Triesman, 1969). Such results suggest that the bottleneck occurs beyond basic sensory analysis, at a level of processing where perceptual, attentional, or cognitive mechanisms attempt to focus on and abstract the messages conveyed by the two ears' signals.

In one variant of the task, attentional factors are minimized (e.g., by requiring report of both messages) and messages of very similar type (e.g., strings of digits) are used. In this case, loss of information tends to be greatest for the left ear signal: That is, the left ear is up to 20% more poorly reported than the right. Kimura selected this ear bias as a topic of investigation in the early 1960s (Kimura, 1961, 1962). She speculated that it might reflect a poor linkage of the left ear transduction mechanisms to the ipsilateral left hemisphere mechanisms responsible for language decisions. This hypothesis rested upon the known prepondence of contralateral (as opposed to ipsilateral) cortical projections of afferent and efferent systems and upon the independently demonstrated (normal) specialization of the left hemisphere for language tasks. However, since both ears performed equally well for monaural presentations of language material, Kimura further proposed that the relative prepondence of contralateral projections could be observed only under conditions of simultaneous stimulation of the two ears by different signals (i.e., dichotic presentation). This notion was based on the electrophysiological work of Rosenzweig (1951) and others (Hall & Goldstein, 1968), who had shown that many cortical units that responded equally well to stimulation of either ear alone would not fire to ipsilateral ear stimuli in the presence of simultaneous contralateral ear stimulation. Generalizing these observations to dichotic speech listening, it is reasonable to propose that the right ear's signal might have direct, contralateral access to the left hemisphere, whereas the left ear's signal would be delivered to the right hemisphere before being interhemispherically transferred to the left. In some way, the more roundabout route of left ear signal could place it at a disadvantage at the processing bottleneck (Milner, 1962; Sparks & Geschwind, 1968).

If Kimura's speculation was correct, there were three important consequences:

> 1. Since ipsilateral suppression might be assumed to operate, regardless of which hemisphere possessed the limited capacity language processor, those rare individuals with right hemisphere speech dominance should show loss of information for the right ear signal,
> 2. Since ipsilateral suppression during dichotics might be assumed to occur for all sorts of simultaneous auditory events, signals requiring processing that was lateralized in the right hemisphere might be expected to yield right ear deficits,
> 3. Since the left ear signal was presumed to have access to the right hemisphere primarily via interhemispheric (corpus collosum) pathways, listeners without these pathways should show extremely poor left ear performance in dichotic speech tasks.

All of these predictions were confirmed in studies in which: right hemisphere lateralization of speech processing was independently determined via the Wada technique (Wada & Rasmussen, 1960); dichotic musical sequences were used (Kimura, 1964); or corpus collosum–sectioned patients were studied (Milner, Taylor, & Sperry, 1968). Thus, Kimura's interpretation received considerable early support (Bryden, 1967; Kimura, 1967). (See also Zaidel, this volume.)

Additional studies explored the generality of the dichotic effects across the language spectrum. Since most of the early experiments used word sequences, sentence material, or musical sequences, the question arose as to whether simpler language events might also show asymmetrical ear performance. More specifically, studies of the perception of nonsense syllables (e.g., stop consonant–vowel CVs) had suggested that some phonetic decisions might involve quite complex and language-specific cortical processing (Liberman, Cooper, Shankweiler, & Studdert-Kennedy, 1967). If such language-specific processing was involved, it might very well reside in the left hemisphere and such signals might yield ear asymmetries. With this in mind, Studdert-Kennedy and Shankweiler examined the perception of single dichotic pairs of nonsense syllables differing in consonants or vowels (Shankweiler & Studdert-Kennedy, 1967; Studdert-Kennedy & Shankweiler, 1970). Listeners were asked to report both members of the pairs immediately after presentation. Results revealed nearly the same degree of poor performance on left ear signals as had the results of tasks requiring the recall of sentences or digit sequences. In addition, the effect was greater for identification of the more linguistically complex consonants, with vowel identification showing a smaller, nonsignificant, left ear disadvantage. As a result of analysis of error patterns and of performance variations across stimulus types, Studdert-Kennedy and Shankweiler (1970) concluded, following Kimura (1961), that, "... the right ear advantages are to be attributed to the left cerebral dominance and functional prepotency of the contralateral pathways during dichotic stimulation.... We have tentatively concluded that while the general auditory system may be equipped to extract the auditory parameters of the speech signals, the dominant hemisphere is specialized for the extraction of linguistic features from those parameters. The laterality effect would then be due to the loss of auditory information arising from interhemispheric transfer of the ispilateral signal to the dominant hemisphere for linguistic processing" (pp. 592–593).

The Studdert-Kennedy and Shankweiler formulation generates two important questions. First, what is the exact nature of the loss for left ear information? Secondly, how does loss of information, together with the speech processing bottleneck, yield asymmetrical performance? Each of these questions is treated separately in the two following sections.

What is the Nature of the Loss of Left Ear Information?

In the context of the above formulation, one signal is presumed to have less direct access to a lateralized processor, but why does the less direct route of one ear's signal have the consequence of making it less accurately perceived?[2]

One possibility is that the longer route results in a relatively delayed arrival of one signal, compared with the other. In this case, the earlier (more directly transmitted) signal could tend to occupy the limited processor first and consequently be more often correctly perceived. Another possibility is that the longer route, perhaps because of the increased number of synaptic transfers, results in the delivery of a "noisier" signal to the lateralized processor. In this case, processing of the noisier signal would more often result in errors than would processing of the less noisy, more directly transmitted signal.

Studdert-Kennedy, Shankweiler, and Schulman (1970) investigated the temporal delay possibility by presenting the two speech signals asynchronously. They reasoned that the delivery of the left ear signal slightly before the right might counteract its possible temporal disadvantage. This manipulation turned out to have exactly the opposite effect; making the left ear lead the right by 15 to 60 msec resulted in it being more poorly perceived. (This phenomenon is discussed further in the section below on asynchronous presentation.)

The second possibility (that the less direct route results in a noisier signal) was first investigated in studies in which the relative intensity of the two signals was varied. Brady-Wood and Shankweiler (1973), for example, examined the effect of attenuating the right ear signal relative to the left. As would be consistent with the noise loss hypothesis, the difference between the performance on the two ears decreased as the left ear was made relatively more intense, that is, as it was made relatively more noise resistant. Similar results were reported by Thompson, Samson, Cullen, and Hughes (1974) (see also Cullen, Thompson, Hughes et al., 1974), who investigated the effects of making one ear's signal less intelligible by the addition of noise, by band-pass filtering, or by varying intensity. In all three cases, the relative difference between the ears increased or decreased (depending upon which ear's signal was manipulated) in a way consistent with the noise loss hypothesis.

There is an important aspect of the results of the noise loss studies that has not received as great an emphasis as it may deserve. This aspect can be illustrated by reference to the data of Thompson et al., shown in Figure 6-1. These data were obtained by asking listeners to identify both consonants in dichotic pairs of synthetic stop-vowel syllables. (The consonants were always different, and the vowels were always *a*). In a counterbalanced design, each ear's signal level was independently varied above and below the equal-level condition that is indicated by the 50-over-50 on the abscissa. Points on the abscissa to the right of the equal-level condition represent increases in one ear relative to the other; points to the left represent relative decreases. The ordinate is marked in terms of mean number correct. For this experiment, a mean of 30 represents the maximum possible (100%) correct for either ear. Each ear's score and whether that ear was varied or not is shown in the key.

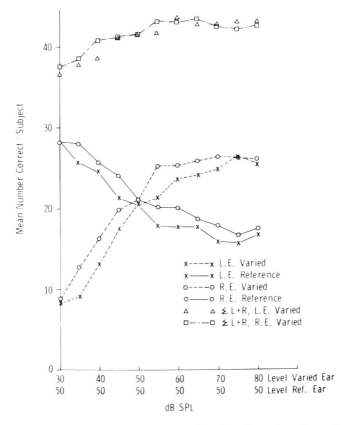

Figure 6-1. *Mean number of correct identifications of members of dichotic pairs of stop-vowel syllables presented at different interaural intensity levels; intensity conditions were blocked. See text for further discussion (L.E. = left ear; R. E. = right ear) (from Thompson et al., 1974; used with permission of the authors).*

Observe, in Figure 6-1, that the left ear's scores are lower than the right ear's scores in virtually all conditions; this is the typical asymmetry seen in dichotics. Of principal interest, however, are the effects of the manipulation of relative levels. It can be seen that, as one ear is made more or less intense, the performance on that ear increases (or decreases), but importantly, *performance on the other ear also decreases (or increases) by a corresponding amount.* This "trade-off" in performance between ears is seen in the symmetrical divergence of the ear's scores as levels change up or down. It can also be seen in the total performance curves represented at the top of the figure. These latter curves show a relatively constant level of performance across the intensity variations, particularly in conditions where both signals equal or exceed 50 dB. (When one ear is reduced below 50 dB, it approaches the single ear identification threshold of 30–40 dB. Because of this, performance on the more intense ear rises near 100% performance, whereas the less intense ear drops to chance; overall performance, therefore, drops.) This level of performance (an average of approximately 45 correct out of a maximum of 60 for both ears combined, i.e., 75% of total possible or 150% of a single ear's maximum) can be interpreted as reflecting the information processing capacity of the lateralized speech processor. That is, although the processor cannot handle both signals, it can handle about 1.5 times the information conveyed by a single channel alone. These results can be phrased in terms of the model proposed above, that is, the lateralized processor has a limited processing capacity that is less than the twofold maximum; when signals are presented dichotically, the signal having a less direct and consequently more noisy route is, on the average, less likely to be correctly processed, and a relative difference in ear scores results. However, the important point is that, except at extremely low levels (e.g., 30 dB), the difference in ear scores does not occur because one ear is at 100% and the other is at some lower level; instead, both ears scores are depressed, with one ear's score being slightly lower than the other's. Thus, dichotic listening, under the ordinary conditions of equal signal levels, and so forth can be seen to yield differences in ear performance because of preprocessor biases in signal quality produced by pathway differences, whereas the overall poorer perform-ance on both ears together represents the general loss of information that occurs for both signals, due to the limited information-processing bottleneck at the lateralized processor. This brings one to the second question posed above: how are the nature of processing at the bottleneck and ear differences related?

How are Processing Capacity and Differences in Performance of the Two Ears Related?

Capacity limitations are observed in a number of information-processing tasks (Shwartz, 1976). For example, simultaneous or rapidly sequential stimulus events can overload early "sensory storage" and preperceptual processing (e.g., Crowder & Morton, 1969). Limitations have also been seen for attentional processes. That is, selective attention to particular events or dimensions may be difficult in the presence of distractors, and dividing attention among events may not be possible if the number of events is large (Norman, 1968; Garner & Felfoldy, 1970). Short-term memory (STM) also appears limited in its capacity, with loss of information occurring when the number of events to be recalled exceeds seven plus-or-minus two (Miller, 1956).

It is not appropriate here to go into the details of these preperceptual, attentional, and STM processing limitations nor into the many varieties of processing models that attempt to characterized what is happening. What is important and particularly relevant for our purposes is that *such bottlenecks may influence the size of the ear differences seen in dichotics.* This is because these processes are sensitive to the relative "quality" of input events. For example, inputs with poor signal-to-noise ratios are (on the average) more susceptible to interference and may be less adequately analyzed during early processing (Miller & Nicely, 1955). Noisy signals would also presumably be more susceptible to loss in STM (Wickelgren, 1965). If a model of dichotics such as that proposed is generally correct, poor performance on one ear in, for example, a digit-sequence recall task might be, in part, the result of the relatively greater probability of loss of noisy (left ear) signal information in STM (Porter & Berlin, 1975). Even in this simple case, the size of the ear difference would depend both upon the sensitivity of the process to signal quality and upon the extent to which the signals resisted noise during transmission. An even more complex picture emerges if signals are presumed to require (because of task requirements) several different stages of processing (e.g., preperceptual processing, followed by attentional processing, followed by STM).[3] In this case the propagation of an originally noisy signal through each successive stage could place it at more or less of a disadvantage, depending upon how sensitive each processor was to "noise" and/or how well early processors handled the signal. Thus, ear differences in different tasks could be of different magnitudes, depending upon the depth of processing or the number of processes involved in each task. (Hellige, Cox, & Litvac, 1979, present an interesting discussion of similar issues in visual laterality studies; see also Hardyck, this volume).

An additional complexity is involved if one assumes that some of the processes required by a task are lateralized and others are not, or if some are lateralized in one hemisphere and others are lateralized in the other. That is, dichotic tasks requiring processing that is equally available in both hemispheres might not show ear differences. Similarly, tasks requiring a mixture of unilateral and bilateral processing could show different amounts of ear difference, depending upon the capacity limitations of the lateralized processes, the hemisphere of lateralization, and the degree to which the interhemispheric transfer from one processor to another added noise to the transferred information.

The problem is that relatively little of the nature of the processes involved in many dichotic tasks is known. Interpreting the magnitude and the direction of ear differences must, consequently, be done with extreme caution. Unfortunately, caution has not typically been exercised. Differences in the size and direction of ear advantages are often casually interpreted as reflecting differences in the degree or direction of *lateralization* of the mechanisms believed to be involved in the task. As discussed above, differences in the direction and the size of ear differences across tasks (or subjects) could be revealing less about the lateralization of mechanisms than they are revealing about the number of processing stages involved, the susceptibility of information processing to noise, or the differences in the pathways to and between the hemispheres.

What Might Dichotic Listening Results Tell Us?

One potential benefit of dichotics would be its ability to assess lateralization of information-processing mechanisms. Dichotics could then allow determination of abnormalities in the degree or direction of lateralization and help in understanding the distribution of function between the hemispheres. Given the present understanding of dichotics, however, the interpretation of asymmetry in performance is not so straightforward. This is because the size and direction of differences can depend upon the above-mentioned factors, and comparison of the degree of ear differences between tasks or individuals is meaningful only in those cases in which the levels of processing, processing capacities, and the kinds of processing involved are clearly understood.

This pessimistic picture may be partly responsible for the decrease in interest in dichotic listening over the last several years. (In addition, it is virtually impossible to do a complete literature search!) This is unfortunate, since dichotic listening may be helpful in telling something about language processing in the nervous system even if it does not always clearly reveal degree or direction of hemispheric laterality. For example, it may tell something about abnormal nervous systems. Given a simple task with careful control of tasks and stimulus parameters, and given a normative performance base, dichotic listening may be used to assess the viability of the auditory pathways and of the interhemispheric connections. Dichotics may also be able to provide some "basic science" information. That is, systematic manipulation of task and stimulus parameters can help in understanding which bottleneck is involved in a particular task and in telling something of the nature of the central processing that occurs there. Both of these advantages of dichotic listening can be combined, since determining something of the consequences of central nervous system injury will help in better understanding of the complex coordination of processes in the normal brain. Some of these optimistic possibilities will be discussed further following consideration of factors influencing the choice of tasks and stimuli.

CHOICE OF PROCEDURES AND METHODS

Stimuli

The type of stimuli chosen affect the magnitude and direction of the ear differences as well as overall performance. Stimuli with simple acoustic-phonetic structures (such as vowels or transitionless fricatives) tend to yield small ear differences (and, sometimes, relatively poorer right ear performance) as well as higher overall performance than do more complex signals such as stop-vowel syllables (e.g., Darwin, 1971; Shankweiler & Studdert-Kennedy, 1967; Studdert-Kennedy & Shankweiler, 1970). Stimuli that are meaningful (e.g., digits or words) or that are imbedded in context (e.g., in sentences) can also yield smaller differences and higher performance (Zurif, 1974; Zurif & Mendelsohn, 1972). Consequently, the use of more meaningful signals or of simpler acoustic-phonetic events can yield a narrow dynamic range of performance that is less sensitive to manipulations of independent variables than might be desired. A wider performance range can be achieved by making the task more "difficult." Examples of this are increasing the rate of stimulus presentation, presenting longer strings of stimuli, or asking subjects to order their responses in particular ways (Bartz, Satz, & Fennel, 1967; Bartz, Satz, Fennel, & Lally, 1967; Satz, 1968; Satz, Achenback, Pattishall, & Fennel, 1965). Unfortunately, the resulting increases in range and sensitivity may be bought at the expense of involving additional perceptual, cognitive, or mnemonic processes, which may preclude a direct interpretation of perform- ance variations in terms of either the lateralization of, or type of, processing involved. For these reasons, a convenient choice of stimuli has been single pairs of stop-vowel nonsense syllables (e.g., ba, da, ga, pa, ta, ka). This choice is presumed to minimize the involvement of memory and sematic processes while highlighting the central auditory mechanisms involved in extracting the phonetic message from the complex acoustic code. The choice of such signals also has the benefit of allowing for the comparison of several acoustic-phonetic dimensions (three places of articulation and two categories of voicing) and benefits from the literature concerned with the perception of such stimuli in tasks other than dichotic listening. In addition, computer-assisted synthesis and signal processing can be effectively used to manipulate the acoustic structure of such signals, thus allowing for precise control of signal similarities and differences and for alignment of pairs during dichotic presentation.

Tasks

The Use of Nonsense Syllable Pairs

The earliest studies used strings of dichotic pairs of words. As discussed previously, such tasks may involve mnemonic or other processes that can influence the overall level of performance and may influence the size and the direction of ear differences. An additional complication is the possiblity of variations in response strategies that lead to intersubject and interexperiment variability; for example, some subjects may elect to report all left ear stimuli first, whereas others may attempt to recall each pair. These different strategies can be manipulated somewhat by instructions but, particularly with special populations (e.g., children), the effectiveness of such control is difficult to assess. A third complication is statistical; unless the response set is restricted and the subjects are carefully instructed to identify all stimuli on each trial (even if they have to guess), it is not possible to model the effects of guessing nor is it possible to get a clear picture of between-subject differences in performance. The use of a small set of CV syllables, presented a pair at a time, minimizes these difficulties.

Even if single pairs of CVs are used, the question arises as to whether or not response bias or variations in attention may influence results. A number of studies have manipulated instructions in an attempt to evaluate these effects (see Note 2). Directed attention to one ear's signals tends to increase performance on that ear; however, performance on the other ear decreases in nearly direct proportion, with overall performance remaining nearly the same (e.g., Kirstein, 1971). If attentional instructions are counterbalanced and data from both directed attention conditions combined, the results are comparable to a condition in which both ears are attended to on each trial (Kirstein, 1971). Instructing listeners to attend to both ears' signals but to report the stimuli by ear seems to increase the variability somewhat but otherwise appears to have little effect (our own data, 1975).

In general, then, stable and statistically manipulatable data can be obtained by using single pairs of CVs drawn from a restricted set. It is important to note that the use of this procedure is coupled with careful instructions to the subjects that each trial consists of two different syllables selected from the restricted set and, although they may not always clearly hear both, they should always make two different responses.[4]

In some cases, variations in these procedures may be necessary to answer particular questions or to obtain different measures. One such variation is discussed in the next section.

The Target/ Challenge Paradigm

As discussed in the introduction, we believe that the less-than-perfect performance in dichotic listening stop-vowels results from two factors: the relatively greater noisiness of one signal, due to its indirect access to the lateralized, limited-capacity, central processor; and the loss of information during processing. Within the context of this interpretation, the procedures outlined above were concerned with measures presumed to reflect three aspects of processing: the *direction of ear difference* (in normal brains) is presumed to reflect the *lateralization* of the central processor; the *degree of difference* is presumed to reflect the *relative degree of noisiness* of the two signals; and *overall performance* is presumed to reflect *central processing capacity*.

Additional questions may be asked regarding the nature of the processing at the limited capacity processor (or processors) and concerning the nature of the loss of information during processing. For example, the probability that a particular left ear signal is correctly perceived is not independent of the right ear signal; a voiceless alveolar stop-vowel (ta) may be more often correctly identified at the left ear if paired with a da than when paired with a ba. Since the pathway-related loss for the ta may be assumed to be the same in both cases, the difference in performance is presumably due to differences in the "demand" placed on the processor and/or to differences in the way in which the neural representations of the two signals interact during processing. Viewed in this way, performance on a particular "target" syllable may be examined as a function of the nature of the dichotically paired "challenge" syllable. The dichotic procedures discussed above can be modified to examine such effects systematically. In this alternative procedure, listeners are asked to identify target CVs presented to a specified ear. These syllables are dichotically paired with other CVs or with various types of speech or nonspeech acoustic events. In this target/challenge procedure, only one response is required. Response measures obtained include overall performance on target items as well as the nature of response errors. Performance is analyzed as a function of the challenge structure (e.g., presence or absence of certain spectral cues) or type (e.g., stop-vowel vs. fricative-vowel).

Latency of response may also be measured using target/challenge procedures (Hughes, 1978). A large (126 msec +) difference in latency of response for left and right ear targets under this paradigm suggests that it is a sensitive measure of performance asymmetries. Furthermore, as performance levels increase, the efficiency of reaction-time measures increases; this is a problem in identification studies using percentage correct.

Asynchronous Presentation

Additional information concerning the nature of the processes involved in dichotic listening can be obtained by presenting the signals asynchronously. For example, as the onsets of a dichotic pair of stop-vowels are placed further and further apart in time, a point should be reached at which both are successfully perceived. The minimal separation yielding 100% for both ears may be interpreted as reflecting the temporal "window" for processing a stop-vowel.

Further information can be provided by observing how performance on the leading and lagging members of the dichotic pair changes as a function of increases in asychrony. Studdert-Kennedy et al. (1970) proposed that, if performance increased for a leading left ear signal, this would support the idea that poorer left ear performance at simultaneity was due to its relatively delayed transmission to the central processor. As previously discussed, the obtained results did not support this prediction; the data are shown in Figure 6-2. To the right are those conditions in which the left ear leads; to the left, the right ear leads. Correct performance on each ear's signal is presented parametrically.

At zero msec asynchrony (simultaneity), the right ear outperforms the left. If the poor left ear performance at simultaneity were due to a delay in its processing, then making the left lead should produce increased left ear performance. The result is just the opposite; left ear performance drops slightly with small asychronies, rising and approaches the right ear performance at the longest right ear "lags." A complimentary picture emerges for the right ear leading condition; right ear performance drops slightly and then rises toward left ear performance at long left ear lags. This advantage for the lagging stimulus has been referred to as the "lag effect" and may be described as revealing a greater "backward masking" of the leading signal by the lagging than "forward masking" of the lagging signal by the leading. Similar results are obtained in other sensory systems and have been interpreted as reflecting the effects that the rapidly propagated mask-related events have on the ongoing extraction of information in the leading target (May, Grannis, & Porter, 1980; Porter, 1974; von Bekesy, 1971).

The Studdert-Kennedy et al. (1970) results suggested that the temporal window for stop-vowel processing was 120 msec or slightly longer. Additional studies confirmed this suggestion, with performance on both ears reaching

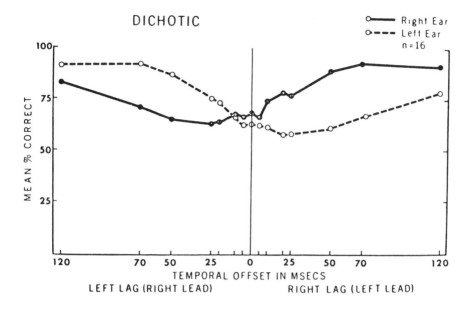

Figure 6-2. *Mean-number-correct identification of members of dichotic pairs of stop-vowel syllables presented at different stimulus-onset asynchronies. These data reveal the lag effect, that is, perceptual benefit that accrues to the temporally lagging member of a dichotic pair (from Studdert-Kennedy et al., 1970; used with permission).*

100% in the range of 120 to 150 msec (Porter, 1974). For the purposes of further discussion, this asymmetry value will be referred to as the "point of closure" in the lag-effect function.

Another type of perceptual information available when dichotic stimuli are presented asynchronously is the perceived order of occurrence. Hughes and Holtzapple (1979) have shown a large asymmetry in the accuracy of judgments of the temporal order of left and right ear CVs, which is not seen for pairs of nonspeech signals (right ear CVs are judged as occurring earlier than simultaneously presented left ear CVs).

Presentation Parameters and Control Procedures

Differences in intensity of as little as 3 to 6 dB SPL between ears can dramatically change (or even reverse) the differences in ear scores (see Figure 6-1). Similar effects occur if CV-syllable onsets are made asynchronously by as little as 10 or 15 msec (Figure 6-2). Overall presentation level and signal-to-noise ratio can also influence the dynamic range of effects as well as introduce variability. Variations among subjects in terms of their ability to identify isolated speech sounds or differences in their auditory sensitivity can also obviously influence results. Consideration of such factors leads to the following control procedures and presentation conditions.

> 1. All of the stimuli to be used in the experiment are presented monaurally to subjects in order to obtain identification performance as a function of presentation level and signal-to-noise ratio. These data are used to establish dichotic presentation levels by selecting values that place monaural performance at or near the knee of the identification function, thus assuring greatest sensitivity to transmission and processing loss (Berlin & Cullen, 1975).
>
> 2. Audiograms and monaural intelligibilities for the signals are obtained for all subjects before dichotic presentation in order to establish (equal) baseline performance for both ears.
>
> 3. Signal levels and presentation conditions are precisely controlled across trials and subjects. A convenient way to do this is to record calibration tones with amplitudes equivalent to the vocalic nucleus of the signals; tape recorder output levels and voltages at various points in the stimulus delivery system can be assessed to assure equal levels of presentation; an artificial ear can be used to assess transmission through the earphones.
>
> 4. Effects of residual differences in channel amplification, signal-to-noise ratios, and so forth can be minimized by running subjects twice under the same conditions, once with channel one presented to the right ear and once with channel one presented to the left ear.

Response Analysis and Scoring Issues

Laterality Indexes

Early dichotic studies required subjects to identify sets of items presented to both ears, and a laterality score was obtained by subtracting the correct responses for the left ear from those for the right ear (i.e., R–L). Since this score varies in size, depending upon the number of trials and overall performance levels, as well as underlying laterality differences, it was replaced by a relative measure of ear-performance difference: R–L/R + L. This "laterality index" has been referred to as "d" (not to be confused with signal detection theory's d') Repp (1977).

Figure 6-3 depicts the isolaterality contour for d. As can be seen, the index reaches its maximum value at an overall performance level of 50%; at all other performance levels, it is less. This correlation between performance level and the value of d was pointed out by Harshman and Krashen (1972), who argued that, because of this correlation, neither d nor the R–L procedure was an adequate measure of underlying perceptual laterality. They investigated two other indexes, the "proportion of corrects" (POC) and "proportion of errors" (POE). The POC was computed by taking the number of correct items for the right ear and dividing by the number of correct items for both ears combined, that is $R/R + L$. The POE was computed by taking the number of left-ear errors and dividing by the total number of errors for both ears combined, that is, $L(errors)/(L(errors) + R(errors))$. They evaluated the results of 45 published experiments in terms of the proportion of variance (r^2) held in common among each of the indexes, R–L, POC, and POE, and the overall performance level; for R–L, it was found to be 0.20; for POC, 0.56; and for POE, it was 0.04. They concluded that the POE was the preferable index since it appeared least influenced by overall performance.

Unfortunately the POE is, in fact, influenced by overall performance in a way that is complementary to that seen for the POC. The POC is relatively uninfluenced if overall performance level is less than 0.5 (small number of double corrects), whereas the POE is relatively uninfluenced by overall performance level as long as performance is greater than 0.5 (small number of double errors). Harshman & Krashen's observation of a low correlation was due to the overall high performance observed in many of the studies they examined.

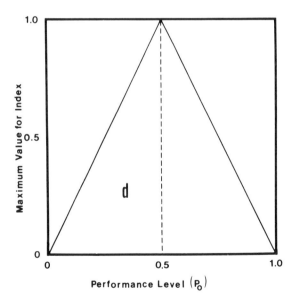

Figure 6-3. *The range of d as a function of overall performance level.*

Problems with POC and POE led to two proposals. One was to use POE and POC disjunctively, depending upon overall performance level (this was referred to as "e"). The second was to use POE and POC conjunctively by taking the square root of the product of linerally transformed POE and POC. This latter procedure yields the familiar ϕ coefficient.

All of the proposed measures have the objective of "decontaminating" ear-difference measures by adjusting for overall performance differences. We propose that these indexes are, however, only symptomatic treatments that do not address the etiology of the problem. The apparent "dependence" between overall performance level and ear differences can be traced to the failure to separate different outcomes of dichotic trials. Dichotic presentation of a stimulus pair gives rise to one of four possible outcomes: both items may be correctly identified, stimulus A is correctly identified while stimulus B is not; stimulus B is correctly identified while stimulus A is not; and neither stimulus is correctly identified. Three examples of different patterns of occurrence of these outcomes are presented in Figure 6-4.

The examples presume a double report procedure, using a 30-item test. The examples are hypothetical and, although extreme cases, the patterns chosen do represent situations that are seen to varying degrees in actual experiments. These examples will be used to demonstrate that the only unbiased information regarding laterality is obtained by utilizing trials in which one ear is correct and the other is in error. A similar argument was first made by Studdert-Kennedy and Shankweiler (1970), but has rarely been addressed since.

As indicated in Figure 6-4, different distributions of trial outcomes can yield the same total correct performance for the two ears. Thus, when the previously discussed laterality indexes are calculated (utilizing all correct responses), the indexes will be the same for all three examples. These indexes ignore important differences among the patterns of outcomes in the three instances.

Example I represents a case in which only six single-correct trials occur. The errors occur only on the left ear stimulus. This is a case in which 100% of the single-correct trials are right ear correct. The probability of obtaining a distribution of responses favoring the right ear this much or more by chance alone (given a sample of six single-correct trials) is 0.016. In other words, only 1.6% of the time will 100% of six, single-correct responses favor the right ear by chance alone. Clearly then, even though the sample of single corrects is small, the extremely asymmetric performance yields a reliable indication of asymmetry.

What happens as the single-correct sample size is increased while the absolute difference between ear scores is maintained? The relative advantage for the right ear decreases. This is seen in Example II, in which there are ten

I			II			III		
SC_l	0		SC_l	2		SC_l	12	
SC_r		6	SC_r		8	SC_r		18
DC	12	12	DC	10	10	DC	0	0
DE	12	12	DE	10	10	DE	0	0

$$SC_p \ 1.00 \qquad\qquad SC_p \ 0.80 \qquad\qquad SC_p \ 0.60$$

$$d = \frac{TC_r - TC_l}{TC_r + TC_l} = \frac{(DC + SC_r) - (DC + SC_l)}{2DC + SC_r + SC_l} = 0.2$$

$$POC = \frac{TC_r}{TC_r + TC_l} = \frac{DC + SC_r}{2DC + SC_r + SC_l} = 0.6$$

$$POE = \frac{TE_l}{TE_l + TE_r} = \frac{DE + SE_l}{2DE + SE_l + SE_r} = 0.6$$

Figure 6-4. *Three examples of different response patterns, using a double report procedure for a 30-trial test. The single correct trials for the left ear (SC_l), for the right ear (SC_r), double correct trials (DC), and double errors (DE) are depicted in the examples. The equations for d, POC, and POE are also expressed in terms of total correct (TC) or total errors (TE) for left and right ears. SC_p represents the proportion of the total single corrects accountable to the right ear.*

single-correct trials; eight of these favor the right ear and two favor the left. The probability of obtaining a distribution of responses favoring the right ear by 80% or more by chance alone is 0.055. Therefore, an 80%/20% split in performance, when based upon a sample size of 10, may be obtained, by chance, 5.5 percent of the time. This is a marginally significant difference.

In Example III, the right ear is favored 60% of the time. The single-correct sample size is now 30, and the probability of the responses favoring the right ear 60% or more of the time by chance alone is a nonsignificant 0.181.

The examples illustrate the way in which the relative number of right and left ear single-corrects and the single-correct sample size interact to determine significance of performance asymmetry. There are two important points. First, when the total corrects are composed entirely of single correct trials (Example III), all methods give the same value because there are no double-correct or double-error trials to influence the laterality measures. Second, the value of the single-correct index is independent of performance level, while the sample size for evaluating the index varies with performance level.

Figure 6-5 shows the incestuous relationship among the indexes POC, POE, the conjunctive use of the POC and POE, the phi-coefficient, and, lastly, the disjunctive use of the POC and POE in e. It is clear from these formulas that, since there are problems with the indexes d, POC, and POE, none of the other indexes will be satisfactory. A satisfactory index must be based upon single correct responses, the relative ear advantage being expressed by $(R/L+R) \times 100$ or $(L/L+R) \times 100$ with only single correct responses being utilized. (For additional discussion of laterality indexes, see chapters by Hellige, Sprott and Bryden, and Levy in this volume.)

$$POC' = 2POC - 1.0$$

$$POE' = 2POE - 1.0$$

$$\phi = \left[(POC)(POE) \right]^{1/2}$$

$$e = \begin{cases} POC' & \text{if } 0.0 \le P_0 \le 0.5 \\ POE' & \text{if } 0.5 \le P_0 \le 1.0 \end{cases}$$

Figure 6-5. *The relationship of POC and POE to the following indexes: POC', POE', ϕ, and e.*

Guessing

In the "standard" dichotic paradigm, the listeners are informed that they will always hear two different sounds from a restricted set and that they are required to produce two responses, even if one or both of the responses are guesses. First consider the set of responses expected if a listener received no information regarding the stimuli. Let n represent the number of stimuli in the response set. The probability of obtaining a correct answer on a subject's first response would be $2/n$. The conditional probability of obtaining a correct answer on his second response (conditional upon having made a correct answer on the first response) would be $1/(n-1)$, thus giving a joint probability of $2/n \times 1/(n-1) = 2/n(n-1)$ for a double-correct response. Likewise, $2/n \times [1-(1/(n-1))] = 2(n-2)/n(n-1)$ is the probability of obtaining a correct first response and an erroneous second response. Conversely, $[1-(2/n)] \times 2/(n-1) = 2(n-2)/n(n-1)$ is the probability of obtaining an erroneous first response and a correct second response. Finally, $[1-(2/n)] \times [(1-(2/(n-1)))] = (n-2)(n-3)/n(n-1)$ is the probability of neither the first n nor second response being correct. For a 30-trial dichotic randomization of 6 CVs, this would lead to the occurrence of 2 double corrects, 16 single corrects (8 from first responses and 8 from second responses) and 12 neither corrects.

It is apparent that complete loss of information leads to a set of responses for which the expected value of the probability of first and second responses being correct is not different. Thus, if ear of presentation is counterbalanced across stimulus channels, guessing will not introduce asymmetries in single-correct responses. Also, if the loss of information is not complete (e.g., the subject perceives some information concerning either the place or the manner of articulation of one or both stimuli), this would serve to further restrict the set of response alternatives but not to introduce ear differences. This is fortunate, since it would be extremely difficult to ascertain when subjects are making use of partial information and when they are not. Most importantly, even if there is a total perceptual asymmetry and the subject always correctly perceives, for example, the right ear stimuli, overall performance will increase since double corrects and single corrects will increase and neither correct will decrease. Correct guesses for the left ear stimulus (since the right is correct) will account for the increase in double corrects; this will occur with a frequency of $1/(n-1)$ of the trials. However, the single correct responses will still accurately reflect the underlying asymmetry. Changes in performance will alter single-correct sample size; hence, the reliability of the conclusions drawn, but this does *not* bias the asymmetry itself.

VARIATION IN MEASURES ACROSS CONDITIONS AND IN DIFFERENT POPULATIONS

Ear-Performance Differences

The direction of the ear difference varies with the type of stimuli used. Dichotic melodies, chords, and other musical stimuli often reveal poor right ear performance, that is, left ear advantage (Goodglass & Calderon, 1977; Kimura, 1964; Shankweiler, 1966; Spellacy, 1970). Some complex nonspeech sounds and the more "musical" aspects of speech (e.g., intonation) also yield left ear advantages (Curry, 1967; Halperin, Nachshon, & Carmon, 1973; Nachshon, 1973; Spellacy & Blumstein, 1970). These results are consistent with the independently observed lateralization of music abilities in the right hemisphere in most normal persons (Bogen & Gordon, 1971). It is presumed that the ear difference for music arises from differences in the ears' access to a lateralized, limited-capacity processor in a manner such as that presumed to occur with speech. In general, however, the differences between the ears for musical signals tend to be smaller and more labile than in the case of speech; this may be related to the fact that such stimuli are often acoustically redundant and, thus, may be more resistant to loss of information, either during transmission or during central processing. This hypothesis receives support from studies of the perception of dichotic vowels. Although speech sounds, these signals are also highly redundant acoustically and tend to yield small and labile ear advantages (Darwin, 1971; Shankweiler & Studdert-Kennedy, 1967). There is a need for musical or other stimuli that yield as large and stable a left ear advantage as stop-vowels do a right ear advantage.

Magnitude of ear differences may not be normally distributed across individuals. Early studies using CVs or CVCs (e.g., Studdert-Kennedy & Shankwiler, 1970) suggested a relatively platykurtic distribution of ear differences with a mode between 12 and 18 percentage points difference (right ear advantage, based on single corrects only). Our experience suggests the distribution to be both wide and, perhaps, at least bimodal; that is, there is some tendency for a clustering of right ear advantages near 0 and at approximately 12 to 20%. In addition, 1 out of every 10 to 15 right-handed listeners will show a left ear advantage of as large as 10 to 20%. The distribution may then be trimodal, with the largest peak at 12 to 20% right ear advantage, a smaller peak near 0, and an even smaller peak around 15% left ear advantage. Such a distribution would be consistent with the model discussed previously. That is, the direction of ear advantage for CVs would be primarily a consequence of the hemispheric lateralization of the limited capacity process, whereas the magnitude of the ear difference would be a consequence of variations in the "noiseness" of the transmission channels, together with variations in the efficiency of the lateralized processor.

A recent study by Lauter (1980) presents an interesting perspective on the possible distribution of ear advantages across individuals and across different types of sounds. She asked listeners to identify (via arbitrary, computer-monitered, response panels) left or right ear members of dichotic pairs of either speech (stop-vowel) or nonspeech sounds (tone or noise burst sequences). Figure 6-6 presents her data for seven listeners; the ordinate is relative accuracy, expressed as $R - L/R + L$ and calculated across counterbalanced conditions of targeting for each ear. The letter T, N, V, TR, and CV refer to the conditions, tone sequences, noise sequences, vowels, CV-transitions, or whole CV targets. The numbers (50 and 80) associated with T and N refer to the milliseconds duration of the component bursts. Overall, five listeners show a clear advantage for the right ear on CVs (three showing no advantage) and five show a clear left ear advantage for at least one of the nonspeech sequences. What is important to the current discussion is that each listener showed a continuum of ear advantages across the speech-nonspeech set. That is, listeners tended to show the "right-most" ear advantage for CVs or CV transitions and the "left-most" advantage for the nonspeech stimuli. Such a pattern is exactly what would be expected if the direction of ear advantage reflected (dichotomous) hemispheric specialization, whereas the degree of advantage reflected (continuous) variation in the degree of noise in interhemispheric transmission.

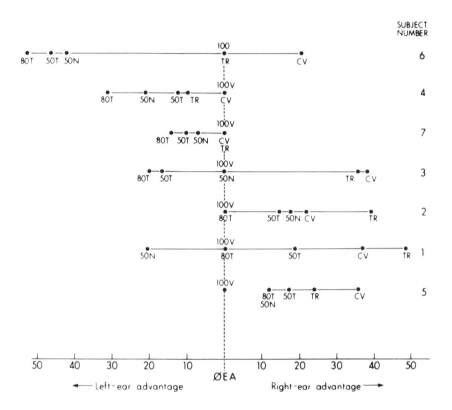

Figure 6-6. *Relative ear advantages for seven subjects and five different types of dichotic speech and nonspeech pairs. Note that the left-most ear advantages tend to occur for nonspeech events, with right-most advantages occurring for CVs and transitions; see text for additional explanation (from Lauter, 1980; used with permission).*

The largest variations in the size and the direction of ear differences occur for patient populations. Assuming normal peripheral-hearing function, lesions of the auditory pathways, primary cortical projection areas, or the corpus callosum can result in markedly poor performance on one ear's signal. A summary of these abnormal results is shown in Figure 6-7. In general, the ear contralateral to the sight of the lesion is the poorest. Note that these effects are independent of the lateralization of the processor and are consistent with the notion that the poorer performing ear has a (injury-related) less direct or noisier access to the limited capacity processor. It is also important to note that these abnormally large ear differences are not necessarily accompanied by grossly impaired monaural performance (Berlin, 1977). That is, dichotic presentation can dramatically reveal effects of lesions that otherwise have minimal effects on standard audiometric or speech intelligibility tests.

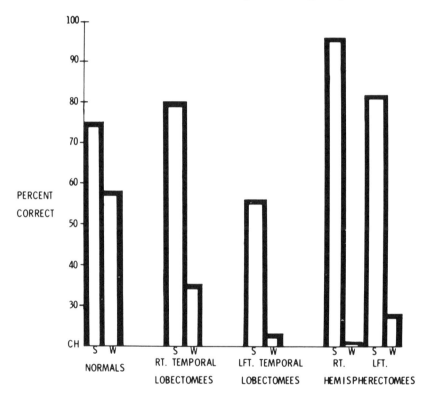

Figure 6-7. *Summary of correct performance, by ear, on CV syllables for normals and three groups of patients. S indicates left ear for normals and the ear ipsilateral to the lesions in patients (''strong ear''); W represents the contralateral (''weak'') ear (from Cullen, Tobey, Hughes, & Berlin, 1975; used with permission).*

In some relatively rare cases, cortical injury reveals poorer performance on the ear ipsilateral to a lesion in the language-dominant hemisphere (Sparks,

Goodglass, & Nickel, 1970). These interesting, "paradoxical" patients provide additional support for the proposed anatomical basis for signal routing in dichotic listening; the lesions in these patients appear to involve injury to regions that receive input from auditory areas in the nondominant (undamaged) hemisphere. These regions are separate from those (undamaged) dominant-hemisphere areas receiving contralateral ear signals. Since it is the interhemispheric linkage that is presumed to convey the ipsilateral signal to the lateralized processor, the observed lesion pattern can account for the paradoxical result (Damasio & Damasio, 1979).

Changes in the size of ear performance differences over age have been reported (Bryden & Allard, 1973; Satz, Bakker, Goebel, & Van der Vlugt, 1975), but other studies report nonsignificant variations (Berlin, Hughes, Lowe-Bell, & Berlin, 1973; Kimura, 1963). Resolving this issue is difficult, due to the large variation in the types of stimuli and tasks used (see Porter & Berlin, 1975). Representative results of two separate, large-sample studies, yielding nonsignificant variations in stop-vowel ear advantage with age are shown in Figure 6-8 (Berlin et al., 1973a; Mirabile, Porter, Hughes, & Berlin, 1978).

In Figure 6-8, correct performance is catagorized in terms of single corrects for the left ear, single corrects for the right ear, and occasions when both ears were correct. This presentation reveals an increasing number of double corrects, a relatively consistent performance level for right ear single corrects, and a tendency for the left-ear single corrects to diminish slightly with age. The change in double-correct performance over age can be interpreted as an age-related increase in information-processing capacity.

The change in single corrects suggests that the adult right ear advantage might stem from a progressively less efficient or noisier processing of left-ear stimuli with age. In any case, this method of analysis allows for the separation of questions regarding ear differences and processing capacity by focusing on either single- or double-correct responses.

These data also illustrate the importance of considering single-and double-correct performance in the evaluation of dichotic effects. As noted, there is a significant increase in overall performance with age. However, there is also an overall performance difference among the studies. The generally higher overall performance in the Mirabile et al. study was interpreted by the authors as due to higher overall intelligibility of the stimuli that they used. Thus, if experimental procedures or stimuli are such as to result in high overall performance in some conditions and not others, ear differences taken relative to total performance will be forced to vary in size, whereas differences based on single corrects vary in reliability. This can be seen in the Mirabile et al. data, where there is a nonsignificant trend toward decreases in the ear differences at the older, higher performing ages.

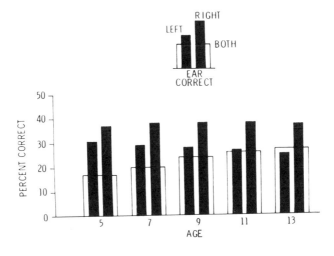

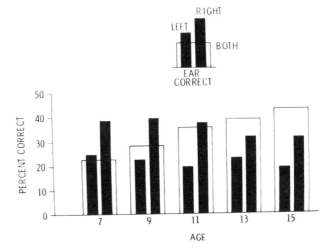

Figure 6-8. *Performance on dichotic step-vowel syllables in two different studies of change in performance over age; see text for discussion (from Mirabile et al., 1978; used with permission).*

Overall Performance and Point of Closure

As previously noted, overall performance on dichotic stop-vowels varies as a function of their signal-to-noise ratio and overall intensity level. As a consequence, consideration of these factors is important (as illustrated in the previous section) in comparing performance across conditions or experiments, particularly if judgments of differences in information-processing capacity are to be made. An additional factor contributing to variation in overall performance is practice (e.g., Porter, Troendle, & Berlin, 1976; Ryan & McNeil, 1974). The results of the Porter et al. study revealed that stability of overall performance can, apparently, be expected after 180 to 300 trials. It is interesting to note, however, that the overall increase in performance did not influence the difference between the ears' performance in the Porter et al. study. This suggests that the direction of laterality and the degree of ear difference stablizes in fewer trials and that, as long as overall performance remains at a relatively low level (150% or so), the absolute difference in performance between the two ears may be a suitable descriptive measure of asymmetry.

As noted in the previous section, overall performance (information-processing capacity) tends to increase with age. There are data that suggest that overall performance may also change with recovery from brain injury (Berlin & Cullen, 1975) or may be abnormally low for children with certain perceptual disorders (Tobey, Cullen, Rampp, & Fleischer-Gallagher, 1979).

Variation in overall performance has also been observed in conjunction with variations in the point of closure of the lag-effect function. The data in Figure 6-9 are from an investigation of the lag effects at various ages (Mirabile et al., 1978). The figure shows performance averaged over both ears as a function of whether the ears are leading or lagging. The "point of closure" for these curves is, therefore, that asynchrony at which performance asymptotes (or would be expected to asymptote, given the slope of the curve). The data reveal that the overall poorer performance of younger children is combined with a tendency for a slower rise to asymptote. This suggests that these children may have a less temporally efficient speech processor as well as one of lower overall capacity. An interesting comparison can be made between these data and those for auditory processing of disabled children of comparable ages (Figure 6-10). Not only do these children show poorer overall performance than their age-matched controls, the very slow rise in performance with asynchrony suggests a very long point of closure and, therefore, a very temporally inefficient processor (see also Tallal, 1976). Interestingly, both of these abnormal results are coupled with ear differences and general speech intelligibility scores that are normal. Such results suggest that these children's difficulties may be related more to decreased processing capacity or efficiency than to abnormalities in either their primary auditory pathways or their hemispheric laterality.

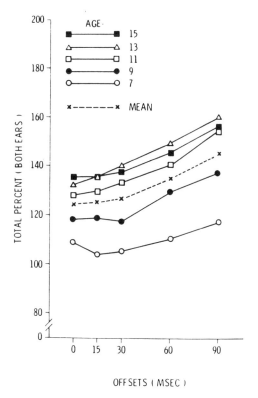

Figure 6-9. *Total correct perform-ance on dichotic stop-vowel syllable pairs presented at different stimulus-onset asynchronies. Data are combined over left and right ears. Overall performance increases with both age and offset; younger children show a slower rise with in-creased offset than do older children. (from Mirabile et al, 1978; used with permission).*

The point of closure is also abnormal in many patients. Figure 6-11 presents representative data from one patient with a right temporal resection (Berlin, 1977). As one would expect with such a patient, the lesion-contralateral left ear is abnormally depressed at simultaneity. The low performance persists, however, as the signals are made asynchronous. We attribute this general pattern of results to three factors: first, performance on the contralateral ear stimulus might be expected to be poor due to compromise of the auditory projection areas and/or of the pathways to and from it; second, such an already compromised signal might display an abnormally increased susceptibility to backward masking by a dichotically lagging signal and could, thirdly, itself produce less backward masking of a leading CV. Although these three factors might account for the overall depressed performance on the lesion-contralateral signal across the shorter asynchronies, it is unclear whether they can account for the reason that the performance stays at a low

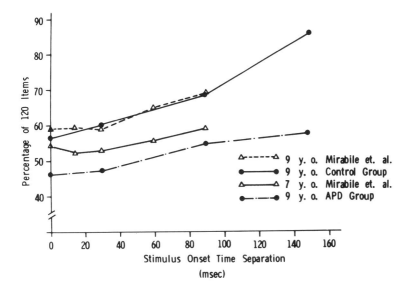

Figure 6-10. *Comparison of results for seven- and nine-year-olds in Figure 6-9 to those for nine-year-old auditory-processing disabled children and nine-year-old controls. The control data duplicate the earlier study; the nine-year-old APD children's data show lower overall performance and a slower rise with stimulus offset than both the controls and the seven-year-olds (from Tobey et al., 1979; used with permission).*

level over such a wide range of asynchronies or the reason that such long lags are required before performance on both ears reaches a common maximum. The pattern is somewhat similar to that for younger children and APD children; the listeners seem to require a long "temporal window" in order to process both signals. For the children, the long temporal window was interpreted as reflecting a less temporally efficient lateralized processor; this interpretation was consonant with the observation of diminished capacity (fewer trials with both ears correct) with simultaneous presentation. Given the similarity of children's and patients' data, a similar interpretation might be proposed. However, the situations are not comparable. In the case of the patients, the long point of closure can be associated with lesions in the nonlanguage hemisphere (as is the case for the patient in Figure 6-11). In such cases, the decreased temporal efficiency of the language processor would have to be an indirect consequence of the lesion. In this context, it is important to remember that these effects typically occur only dichotically; both normals and many patients can correctly perceive a monaural sequence of syllables presented at stimulus-onset asychronies of approximately 100 to 150 msec. The dichotic results with patients may be reminding us that dichotic presentation is an abnormal listening situation. As such, it may invoke a mode of operation that involves temporal coordination of neural processes not required by single ear presentation. The patients' abnormal lag-effect functions may, therefore, be revealing the inability of the damaged system to make required readjustments in the time domain.

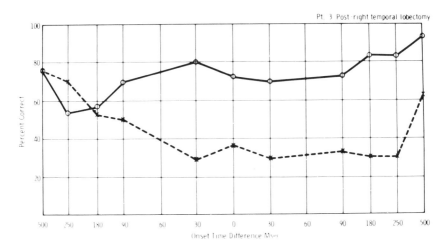

Figure 6-11. *Performance of a right temporal lobectomy on dichotic pairs of CVs projected at different stimulus-onset asynchronies. Note the severe depression of performance on the lesion-contralateral ear (dashed line) and the large size of the asynchrony required to bring both ears to a comparable performance level (from Berlin, 1977; used with permission).*

An additional perspective on possible changes in the temporal aspects of processing with brain injury is provided by the results of temporal order judgement (TOJ) tasks (Edwards & Auger, 1965; Efron, 1963; Hughes & Holtzapple, 1979; Swisher & Hirsh, 1972). Hughes and Holtzapple (1979) asked subjects to indicate which ear was stimulated first when presented with asynchronous dichotic pairs of stop-vowel syllables or (as a control) pairs of uncorrelated noise bursts. For noise pairs, normals typically reach 75% performance with asynchronies of about 10 msec. Pairs of syllables require a longer asynchrony (20 to 25 msec). In addition, syllables show an asymmetry of performance not seen for noise, the right ear (typically) being heard as leading the left even if the left actually leads the right by up to 13 msec. The results for patients are often dramatically different. Figure 6-12 compares the accuracy of TOJs of temporal lobe lesion patients with summary data collected from normals. The patients show chance accuracy across all asynchronies. We have found, in fact, that many of these patients may require the syllable stimuli to be presented with asychronies of approximately 300 msec before they can accurately judge the order of ear stimulation: These results provide additional evidence in support of the suggestion that such patients are having difficulty marshaling processes in the time domain. Since the dichotic situation appears to be sensitive to interhemispheric transfer, it may be the temporal coordination of the two hemispheres that is impaired. In this regard, it is interesting to note that not all brain-damaged patients show the abnormal TOJ or dichotic-lag functions. Several studies suggest that the most severe disruption takes place for temporal lobe lesions; patients with damage elsewhere, even if extensive, produce normal or near normal performance (Hughes & Holtzapple, 1979).

The previous two sections have illustrated how different dichotic measures can allow one to investigate the lateralization of processing, the viability of auditory pathways, and the integrity of central auditory areas. It was also suggested that these measures might allow for the assessment of central processing capacity and temporal efficiency. However, these measures provide only indirect information concerning the nature of the central processing or its limitations. Information of this latter sort can be provided via the target/ challenge procedure.

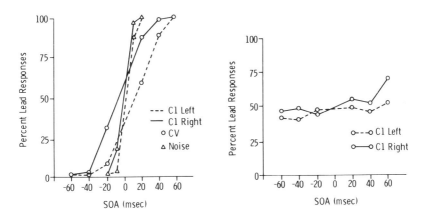

Figure 6-12. *The percentage of responses for which the subject indicated that channel 1 (C1) preceded channel 2 for speech (CV) and noise stimuli, as a function of the onset asynchrony of channel 1 relative to channel 2. The left panel depicts data from normals; the right from temporal lobe lesion patients. The patients were not tested with the noise stimuli.*

Results of Target/Challenge Studies

The target/challenge procedure has been used to assess the nature of the competition occurring at the limited capacity processor as well as something of the way that speech is represented at the central point. For example, if the target is a stop-vowel syllable, the challenge need not be another stop-vowel for a decrement in target performance to occur. The disrupted processing thus appears to have some "general" auditory nature. However, challenges that cause decrements must apparently have some acoustic characteristics in common with stop-vowels. Figure 6-13 presents a summary of performance on stop-vowel targets when they are paired with a variety of challenges that have the acoustic structures schematically represented at the bottom of the figure. These data suggest that a challenge with a well-defined transition followed by a steady state is sufficient to produce interference nearly as great as a CV-syllable challenge itself. These non-CV signals, which are produced by synthesizing only the second and/or third formant resonances of stop-vowels, have been called "bleats." In spite of the fact that they are part of a speech signal, they have a decidedly nonspeech perceptual quality. The fact that such signals can disrupt the perception of a stop-vowel suggests that the processing being disrupted may be that involved in interpreting the resonance patterns contained in speech.

The results shown in Figure 6-13 are for simultaneous presentation of target and challenge. The same variation in effects occurs, however, for asynchronous presentation (Porter & Mirabile, 1977), suggesting that simultaneous, forward, and backward effects may all involve the same processes (Porter, 1974).

The spectral content of a challenge does not seem to be a critical factor influencing its disruptive effect. This is demonstrated by the observation that variations in transition-onset frequency of a single, second-formant, "bleat" challenge minimally influence its disruptive effect on a target (Porter & Whittaker, 1980). Similarly, varying the steady-state center frequency of the bleat, while keeping the transition in the same relative position, has little effect (Miller, Ralston, & Porter, 1980). These results are interesting in that: they suggest that the central "masking" that is occurring for these signals is like other forms of central masking that are also relatively insensitive to spectral structure (Elliot, 1962; Wright, 1964; Zwislocki, Buining, & Glatz, 1968); and this form of central masking is very different from monotic masking, which is very sensitive to the spectral structure of target and challenge, presumably because of peripheral interference with frequency resolution (Porter & Whittaker, 1980).

Although varying spectral properties of bleat challenges has minimal effect, varying the time-by-frequency patterns has dramatic effects; transitions

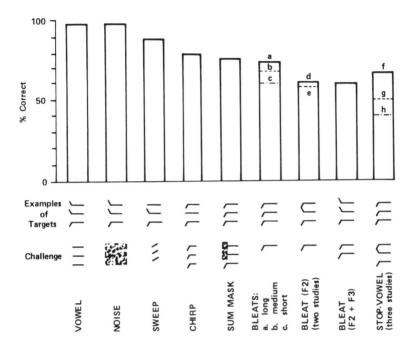

Figure 6-13. *Performance on stop-vowel targets as a function of the acoustic structure of a dichotic challenge. The acoustic structures (formant center frequencies) are shown schematically. Challenges that produce the biggest decrement in performance are often stop-vowels or "bleats"; see text for further discussion.*

with very short or absent steady states or steady states without transitions both yield smaller effects than challenges with both transitions and steady states (see Figure 6-13). Two studies recently examined these effects more closely by independently varying the lengths of either the steady states or the transitions of challenges. The largest interference occurs when the steady state of a bleat approached the length of the steady state of the target and when the challenge transition was longer than that of the challenge (Cullen et al., 1975; Porter, Cullen, Whittaker, & Castellanos, 1981). In a fashion contrasting to that for spectrum variation, these dichotically important temporal variations had minimal effects when varied in monotic listening.

The target/challenge results lead to the tentative conclusion that the central interference between target and challenge occurs at a point in processing where the time-by-frequency pattern of the signals is being extracted, perhaps in preparation for a linguistic decision.

An additional perspective on target/challenge effects can be obtained by varying the relative intensity of the signals. Figure 6-14 shows the results of varying the overall level of three types of right ear challenges on the perception of stop-vowel targets presented to the left ear (Berlin, Porter, Lowe-Bell et al., 1973). Again, stop-vowel challenges and second formant bleats extracted from stop-vowels provide the greatest interference, with vowels and noise bursts providing minimal effects. Note that the bleats actually provide more interference than stop-vowels at high relative presentation levels. This is presumably because, at these levels, the second formant bleats have higher per-bandwidth energy than do the information-bearing second formants embedded in the stop-vowel targets. This would give the second-formant bleat a better signal-to-noise ratio at the central processor than the second formant of the target. This conclusion is supported by an analysis of errors that reveals that the bleat cues "intrude" in responses, producing erroneous identifications that are consistent with the second formant pattern represented by the bleat challenge. On first examination, this sort of result seems to suggest that the interaction between target and challenge is occurring during those linguistic processes responsible for the phonetic interpretation of the acoustic patterns. Upon closer examination, however, such a conclusion is not supported. Although the listeners' responses can reflect phonetic cue characteristics of the challenge, both the presence of interference and its degree appear to be more dependent upon the pattern of acoustic cues than upon any actual or possible phonetic message conveyed by them. This was seen in a study where bleats from phonetically ambiguous syllables were found to provide nearly as high a degree of interference as those from unambiguous syllables (Porter & Whittaker, 1980). It was also seen in the previously noted studies of variations in challenges' transition and steady-state durations, where the degree of interference was predicated on variations in the durations of the segments, even though the variations did not produce changes in the phonetic identity of the challenges. Such findings suggest that "phonetic intrusion" effects observed in dichotic listening result from a phonetic interpretation being forced upon the consequence of what seems to be a complex form of central "masking."

The presence of brain damage can increase the susceptibility of targets to central masking by bleats and vowels. Figure 6-15 shows the results for patients, paralleling those for normals shown in Figure 6-14. The patients received the targets in the ear contralateral to their lesions ("weak ear") with the challenges in the other ("strong ear"). Although the overall pattern of results is similar in both normals and patients, the magnitude of interference is

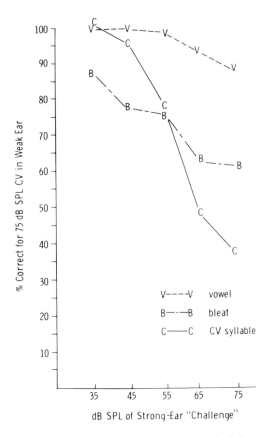

Figure 6-14. *Performance on stop-vowel, left ear targets as a function of the level of three types of dichotic challenges in the right ("strong") ear. The challenge level is equal to that of the target at 55 dB SPL (from Berlin et al., 1973b; used with permission).*

generally greater, and perhaps importantly, the vowels and bleats seem to produce relatively greater effects in the patients. Whether these increased effects simply reflect a general lability of processing in this population, or whether they instead reflect a change in the character of processing remains to be determined. However, it is interesting to recall that these patients also showed both an overall decrease in processing capacity and changes in the temporal character of processing (as shown by lower overall performance and by a longer point of closure in the lag-effect function). All of the patient results together suggest that complex changes in the coordination of central processing, in addition to loss of function, may occur in some types of brain injury. Dichotic listening procedures may provide an important first insight into the nature of the reorganization and, thus, may provide clues to the question of how the brain's component parts normally coordinate their shared responsibilities.

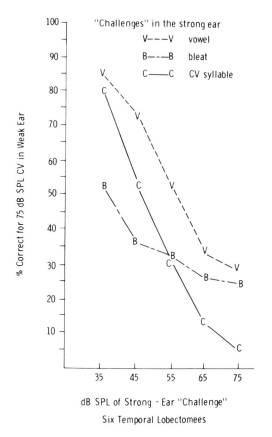

Figure 6-15. *Performance of six temporal lobectomies in the same task as described in Figure 6-14. Note the overall greater depression of performance, relative to the normals in Figure 6-14 (from Berlin et al., 1973b; used with permission).*

ACKNOWLEDGMENTS

We wish to acknowledge many thought-provoking and thought-clarifying discussions with our colleagues, C. I. Berlin, J. Cullen, E. Tobey, and C. J. Miller. Many of the formulations included have stemmed directly from their work and insights. Errors of omission or commission we must, unfortunately, acknowledge as our own. We wish to particularly thank Judy Knight for her patient help in manuscript preparation and Rich Launey for help with the figures.

Support for preparation of the manuscript was provided by federal grant, USPHS PO1 NS-11647. Support for facilities was provided by the Kresge Foundation and the Greater New Orleans Lions' Eye and Ear Foundation.

Please address correspondence to Kresge Hearing Research Laboratory of the South, LSU Medical Center, 1100 Florida Ave., Bldg. 147, New Orleans, La. 70119.

NOTES

1. Due to the vastness of the dichotic literature, we have elected to include only seminal references and representative studies rather than to attempt a comprehensive review. Reviews of dichotic listening are available in Berlin and McNeil (1976) and Bradshaw and Nettleton (1981).

2. There are other points of view. It might be that it is not the indirectness of the route to the processor that leads to poorer performance but, rather, biases of the processor itself. Kinsborne, for example, has suggested that perceptual asymmetry, in general, may reflect a natural biasing of each hemisphere's mechanisms toward stimuli entering from the contralateral sensory field (e.g., Kinsborne, 1970, 1973). Thus, if language processors are located in the left hemisphere, language stimuli presented to the right ear (or, more generally, presented to the right side) might be preferentially treated. A similar attentional-bias mechanism has been proposed by Morais (Hublet, Morais, & Bertelson, 1976; Morais, 1975; Morais & Bertelson, 1973, 1975). Several studies suggest that such biases may play a role in ear differences but that they do not explain all the effects. For example, identification of fused speech stimuli, which yield a single perceptual event subjectively located in the midsagittal plane, can show a bias in favor of the right ear information (Repp, 1977). In an experiment addressing attentional effects more directly, Kallman (1978) used dichotic pairs of musical and speech sounds randomly intermixed. The subjects were required to press a button whenever a prespecified target sound was detected at either ear. A right ear advantage was found for the speech and a trend for a left ear advantage was found for the music targets, suggesting that an attentional explanation based upon expectancy may not fully explain ear asymmetries.

3. The serial nature of processing is not a necessary component of the following discussion. Either parallel or serial processing stages could have the proposed effect on ear differences. In any case, we are not intending to invoke the serial/parallel controversy.

4. Other procedures have been suggested to minimize the effects of memory factors, and so forth. For example, Repp (1977) proposed the use of dichotically "fusable" signals. Here, either a part of the spectral information of a single stimulus is put in one ear and the remainder in the other, or two different utterances with identical fundamental frequencies are dichotically presented, such that a single fused event is perceived. Ear differences are then assessed by determining which ear's information is more instrumental in determining the subjects' responses. The technique is much more complex than is apparent in this description but may be a useful tool in addressing some questions. Repp also argues for the use of single responses, in that requiring one response is more consistent with listeners' subjective impressions of a "single event" and thus may yield less variable results. Using fusable signals and/or a single report procedure does not reveal, however, those occurrences where both signals are perceived, nor does it always allow for guessing-corrections.

REFERENCES

Bartz, W. H., Satz, P., & Fennel, E. Grouping strategies in dichotic listening: The effects of instruction, rate and ear asymmetry. *Journal of Experimental Psychology*, 1967, *74*, 132–136.

Bartz, W. H., Satz, P., Fennel, E., & Lally, J. R. Meaningfulness and laterality in dichotic listening. *Journal of Experimental Psychology*, 1967, *73*, 203–210.

Berlin, C. I. Hemispheric asymmetry in auditory tasks. In S. Harnad (Ed.), *Lateralization in the nervous system*, New York: Academic Press, 1977.

Berlin, C. I., & Cullen, J. K., Jr. Dichotic signs of speech mode listening. Paper presented at the Symposium on Dynamic Aspects of Speech Perception, Einhoven, Netherlands, August, 1975.

Berlin, C. I., & McNeil, M. R. Dichotic listening. In Norman J. Lass (Ed.), *Contemporary issues in experimental phonetics*. New York: Academic Press, 1976.

Berlin, C. I., Hughes, L. F., Lowe-Bell, S. S., & Berlin, H. L. Dichotic right ear advantage in children 5 to 13. *Cortex*, 1973a, *9*(4), 394–402.

Berlin, C. I., Porter, R. J., Lowe-Bell, S. S. et al. Dichotic signs of the recognition of speech elements in normals, temporal lobectomees, and hemispherectomees. Institute of Electrical and Electronics Engineers, Inc., *Transactions on Audio and Electroacoustics*, 1973, *AU-21*(3), 189–195.

Bogen, J. E., & Gordon, H. W. Musical tests for functional lateralization with intracarotid amobarbital. *Nature*, 1971, *230*, 524–525.

Bradshaw, J. L., & Nettleton, N. C. The nature of hemispheric specialization in man. *The Behavioral and Brain Sciences*, 1981, *4*, 51–91.

Brady-Wood, S., & Shankweiler, D. Effects of one of the two channels on perception of opposing pairs of nonsense syllables when monotically and dichotically presented. Paper presented at the eighty-fifth meeting of the Acoustical Society of America, April 10–13, 1973, Boston, Mass.

Broadbent, D. E. The role of auditory localization in attention and memory span. *Journal of Experimental Psychology*, 1954, *47*, 191–196.

Bryden, M. P. An evaluation of some models of laterality effects in dichotic listening. *Acta Otolaryngology*, 1967, *63*, 595–604.

Bryden, M. P., & Allard, F. Dichotic listening and the development of linguistic processes. Paper presented at the International Neuropsychology Society, 1973, New Orleans, La.

Cherry, E. E. Some experiments on the recognition of speech, with one and with two ears. *Journal of the Acoustical Society of America*, 1953, *25*, 975–979.

Crowder, R. G., & Morton, J. Precategorical acoustic storage (PAS). *Perception and Psychophysics*, 1969, *5*, 365–373.

Cullen, J. K., Thompson, C. L., Hughes, L. F. et al. The effects of varied acoustic parameters on performance in dichotic speech perception tasks. *Brain and Language*, 1974, *1*, 307–322.

Cullen, J. K., Jr., Tobey, E. A., Hughes, L. F., & Berlin, C. I. Dichotic performance for temporally altered consonant-vowel tokens. *Journal of the Acoustical Society of America*, 1975, *57*(1):S52.

Curry, F. K. W. A comparison of left-handed and right-handed subjects on verbal and non-verbal dichotic listening tasks. *Cortex*, 1967, *3*, 343–352.

Damasio, H., & Damasio, A. "Paradoxic" ear extinction in dichotic listening: Possible anatomic significance. *Neurology*, 1979, *29*, 644–653.

Darwin, C. J. Ear differences in the recall of fricatives and vowels. *Quarterly Journal of Experimental Psychology*, 1971, *23*, 46–62.

Edwards, A. E., & Auger, R. The effect of aphasia on the perception of precedence. Proceedings of the seventy-third Anniversary Convention of the American Psychological Association, Washington, D. C., 1965, pp. 207–208.

Efron, R. Temporal perception, aphasia, and deja vu. *Brain*, 1963, *86*, 403–424.

Elliot, L. L. Backward and forward masking of probe tones of different frequencies. *Journal of the Acoustical Society of America*, 1962, *34*, 1116–1118.

Garner, W. R., & Felfoldy, G. Integrality and separability of stimulus dimensions in information processing. *Cognitive Psychology*, 1970, *1*, 225–241.

Goodglass, H., & Calderon, M. Parallel processing of verbal and musical stimuli in right and left hemispheres. *Neuropsychology*, 1977, *15*, 397–407.

Hall, J. L., & Goldstein, M. H. Representation of binaural stimuli by single units in primary auditory cortex of unanesthetized cats. *Journal of the Acoustical Society of America*, 1968, *3*, 456–461.

Halperin, Y., Nachshon, I., & Carmon, A. Shift of ear superiority in dichotic listening to emporally patterned nonverbal stimuli. *Journal of the Acoustical Society of America*, 1973, *53*, 46–50.

Harshman, R., & Krashen, S. An "unbiased" procedure for comparing degree of lateralization of dichotically presented stimuli. *UCLA Working Papers in Phonetics*, 1972, *23*, 3–12.

Hellige, J. B., Cox, P. J., & Litvac, L. Information processing in the cerebral hemispheres: Selective hemispheric activation and capacity limitations. *Journal of Experimental Psychology: General*, 1979, *108*(2), 251–279.

Hublet, C., Morais, J., & Bertelson, P. Spatial constraints on focused attention: Beyond the right-side advantage. *Perception*, 1976, *5*, 3–8.

Hughes, L. F. Effects of varied response modes upon dichotic consonant-vowel identification latency. *Brain and Language*, 1978, *5*, 301–309.

Hughes, L. F., & Holtzapple, P. Temporal-order judgments of speech and noise stimuli by normal and brain-injured subjects. In J. J. Wolf & D. H. Klatt (Eds.), *Speech Communication Papers*. Acoustical Society of America: New York, 1979, pp. 583–586.

Kallman, H. J. Note: Can expectancy explain reaction time ear asymmetries? *Neuropsychologia*, 1978, *16*, 225–228.

Kimura, D. Cerebral dominance and the perception of verbal stimuli. *Canadian Journal of Psychology*, 1961, *15*, 166–171.

Kimura, D. Perceptual and memory functions of the temporal lobe: A reply to Dr. Inglis. *Canadian Journal of Psychology*, 1962, *16*, 18–22.

Kimura, D. Speech lateralization in young children as determined by an auditory test. *Journal of Comparative Physiology and Psychology*, 1963, *56*, 899–902.

Kimura, D. Left-right differences in the perception of melodies. *Quarterly Journal of Experimental Psychology*, 1964, *16*, 355–358.

Kimura, D. Functional asymmetry of the brain in dichotic listening. *Cortex*, 1967, *3*, 163–178.

Kinsbourne, M. The cerebral basis of lateral asymmetries in attention. In Sanders, A. F. (Ed.), *Attention and performance, III*. Amsterdam: North-Holland, 1970, pp. 192–201.

Kinsbourne, M. The control of attention by interaction between the cerebral hemispheres. In Kornblum, S. (Ed.), *Attention and performance IV*. New York: Academic Press, 1973, pp. 239–256.

Kirstein, E. F. Temporal factors in perception of dichotically presented stop consonants and vowels (Doctoral dissertation, University of Connecticut, 1971). *Dissertation Abstracts, International*, 1971, *32*, 3035-B.

Lauter, J. Dichotic identification of complex sounds: Absolute and relative ear advantages. Unpublished doctoral dissertation, Washington University, St. Louis, 1980.

Liberman, A. M., Cooper, F. S., Shankweiler, D., & Studdert-Kennedy, M. Perception of the speech code. *Psychological Review*, 1967, *74*, 431–461.

May, J. G., Grannis, S., & Porter, R. J., Jr. The "lag effect" in dichoptic viewing. *Brain and Language*, 1980, *11*: 19–29.

Miller, C. J., Ralston, J. R., & Porter, R. J., Jr. Dichotic competition and target-challenge center frequency disparities. Paper delivered to the fifty-sixth annual convention of the American Speech-Language-Hearing Association, Detroit, Michigan, November, 1980.

Miller, G., & Nicely, P. An analysis of perceptual confusions among some English consonants. *Journal of the Acoustical Society of America*, 1955, *27*, 338–352.

Miller, G. A. The magical number seven, plus or minus two. *Psychological Review*, 1956, *63*, 81–97.

Milner, B. Laterality effects in audition. In Mountcastle, V. B. (Ed.), *Interhemispheric relations and cerebral dominance*. Baltimore: The Johns Hopkins University Press, 1962, pp. 177–195.

Milner, B., Taylor, S., & Sperry, R. W. Lateralized suppression on dichotically presented digits after commissural section in man. *Science*, 1968, *161*, 184–185.

Mirabile, P. J., Porter, R. J., Jr., Hughes, L. F., & Berlin, C. I. Dichotic lag effect in children 7 to 15. *Developmental Psychology*, 1978, *14*(3), 277–285.

Morais, J. The effects of ventriloquism on the right side advantage for verbal material. *Cognition*, 1975, *3*, 127–139.

Morais, J., & Bertelson, P. Laterality effects in diotic listening, *Perception*, 1973, *2*, 107–111.

Morais, J., & Bertelson, P. Spatial position versus ear of entry as determinant of the determinant of the auditory laterality effects: A stereophonic test. *Journal of Experimental Psychology: Human Perception and Performance*, 1975, *1*, 253–262.

Nachshon, I. Effects of cerebral dominance and attention on dichotic listening. *T.I.T. Journal of Life Sciences*, 1973, *3*, 107–114.

Norman, D. A. *Memory and Attention*. New York: Wiley, 1968.

Porter, R. J., Jr. The dichotic lag effect: Implications for the central processing of speech. *Proceedings of the Speech Communication Seminar*, Stockholm (Speech Transmission Laboratory, Department of Speech Communication, KTH, Stockholm, Sweden), 1974, *3*, 21–30.

Porter, R. J., & Berlin, C. I. On interpreting developmental changes in the dichotic right-ear advantage. *Brain & Language*, 1975, *2*, 186–200.

Porter, R. J., Jr., Cullen, J. K., Jr., Whittaker, R. G., & Castellanos, F. X. Dichotic and monotic masking of CV syllables by CV-second-formants with different steady-state durations. *Phonetica*, 1981, *38*, 252–259.

Porter, R. J., Jr., & Mirabile, P. J. Dichotic and monotic interactions between speech and nonspeech sounds at different stimulus onset asychronies. *Perception Psychophysics*, 1977, *21* (5), 408–412.

Porter, R. J., Jr., Troendle, R., & Berlin, E. I. Effects of practice on the perception of dichotically presented stop-consonant-vowel syllables. *Journal of the Acoustical Society of America*, 1976, *59*(3), 679–682.

Porter, R. J., & Whittaker, R. G. Dichotic and monotic masking of CV's by CV second formants with different transition starting values. *Journal of the Acoustical Society of America*, 1980, *67*(5), 1772–1780.

Repp, B. H. Measuring laterality effects in dichotic listening. *Journal of the Acoustical Society of America*, 1977, *62*(3), 720–737.

Rosenzweig, M. R. Representation of the two ears at the auditory cortex. *American Journal of Psysiology*, 1951, *167*, 147–158.

Ryan, W. I., & McNeil, M. Listener reliability for a dichotic task. *Journal of the Acoustical Society of America*, 1974, *56*, 1922–1923.

Satz, P. Laterality effects in dichotic listening. *Nature*, 1968, *218*, 277–278.

Satz, P., Achenback, K., Pattishall, E., & Fennel, E. Order of report, ear asymmetry and handedness in dichotic listening. *Cortex*, 1965, *1*, 377–396.

Satz, P., Bakker, D. J., Goebel, R., & Van der Vlugt, H. Developmental parameters of the ear asymmetry: A multivariate approach. *Brain and Language*, 1975, *2*, 171–185.

Shankweiler, D. Effects of temporal-lobe damage on perception of dichotically presented melodies. *Journal of Comparative and Physiological Psychology*, 1966, *62*, 115–119.

Shankweiler, D., & Studdert-Kennedy, M. Identification of consonants and vowels presented to left and right ears. *Quarterly Journal of Experimental Psychology*, 1967, *75*, 49–55.

Shwartz, S. P. Capacity limitations in human information processing. *Memory and Cognition*, 1976, *4*(6), 763–768.

Sparks, R., & Geschwind, N. Dichotic listening in man after section of neocortical commissures. *Cortex*, 1968, *4*, 3–16.

Sparks, R., Goodglass, H., & Nickel, B. Ipsilateral versus contralateral extinction in dichotic listening resulting from hemisphere lesions. *Cortex*, 1970, *6*, 249–260

Spellacy, F. J. Lateral preferences in the identification of patterned stimuli. *Journal of the Acoustical Society of America*, 1970, *47*, 574–578.

Spellacy, F., & Blumstein, S. The influence of language set on ear preference in phoneme recognition. *Cortex*, 1970, *6*, 430–439.

Studdert-Kennedy, M., & Shankweiler, D. Hemispheric specialization for speech perception. *Journal of the Acoustical Society of America*, 1970, *48*, 579–594.

Studdert-Kennedy, M., Shankweiler, D., & Schulman, S. Opposed effects of a delayed channel on perception of dichotically and monotically presented CV syllables. *Journal of the Acoustical Society of America*, 1970, *48*, 599–602.

Swisher, L., & Hirsh, I. J. Brain damage and the ordering of two temporally successive stimuli. *Neuropsychologia*, 1972, *10*, 137–152.

Tallal, P. Rapid auditory processing in normal and disordered language development. *Journal of Speech and Hearing Research*, 1976, *19*, 561–571.

Thompson, C. L., Samson, D. S., Cullen, J. K., & Hughes, L. F. The effect of varied bandwidth, signal-to-noise ratio, and intensity on the perception of consonant-vowels in a dichotic context: Additivity of central processing. Paper presented at the eighty-sixth meeting of the Acoustical Society of America, October 29–November 2, 1973, Los Angeles, Calif. *Journal of the Acoustical Society of America*, 1974, *55*(2), 435(A).

Tobey, E. A., Cullen, J. K., Jr., Rampp, D. L., & Fleischer-Gallagher, A. M. Effects of stimulus-onset asychrony on the dichotic performance of children with auditory-processing disorders. *Journal of Speech and Hearing Research*, 1979, *22*, 2.

Treisman, A. M. Strategies and models of selective attention. *Psychological Review*, 1969, *76*, 282–299.

von Bekesy, G. Auditory backward inhibition in concert halls. *Science*, 1971, *171*, 529–536.

Wada, J., & Rasmussen, T. Intracarotid injection of Sodium Amytal for the lateralization of cerebral speech dominance. *Journal of Neurosurgery*, 1960, *17*, 266–282.

Wickelgren, W. A. Acoustic similarity and retroactive inhibition in short-term memory. *Journal of Verbal Learning and Verbal Behavior*, 1965, *4*, 53–61.

Wright, H. N. Backward masking for tones in narrow-band noise. *Journal of the Acoustical Society of America*, 1964, *36*, 2217–2221.

Zurif, E. B. Auditory lateralization: Prosodic and syntatic factors. *Brain and Language*, 1974, *1*, 391–404.

Zurif, E. B., & Mendelsohn, M. Hemispheric specialization for the perception of speech sounds: The influence of intonation and structure. *Perception and Psychophysics*, 1972, *11*, 329–332.

Zwislocki, J., Buining, E., & Glantz, J. Frequency distribution of central masking. *Journal of the Acoustical Society of America*, 1968, *43*, 1267–1271.

Seeing Each Other's Point of View: Visual Perceptual Lateralization

Curtis Hardyck

In a review of language and cognition, George Miller began his commentary by stating that the only person he knew who would feel comfortable discussing as broad a topic as "Language and Cognition" was a physicist friend of his who enjoyed giving talks with titles such as "The Universe and Other Things." Somewhat similar feelings occurred to me after the initial enthusiasm with which I approached this task—an analysis of visual perceptual lateralization research—I began to grind against reality and found myself wishing that I could pass this burden on to Miller's physicist friend.

A comprehensive review and integrative summary of work in this area would require a volume by itself, if the task could be accomplished at all. Some of this has been done, for example, Harcum's (1978) encyclopedic compilation of perceptual lateralization studies from the pioneer work of Heron through the state of research as of 1969. The recent review by Bradshaw and Nettleton on "The Nature of Hemispheric Specialization in Man" (1981) is an impressive attempt to summarize and integrate the now enormous body of work on human cerebral asymmetry into a meaningful framework.

I will attempt no such heroic task. The material covered herein is limited to visual perceptual studies, almost without exception on normally functioning individuals. Studies on dichotic listening, haptic perception, and patient studies have not been included and will hopefully have been dealt with by those more competent to evaluate them (see other chapters in this volume).

There is also no determined attempt made to include all work. Meehl (1978) has satirized the typical process of writing a review article as that of counting up experiments, listing those who support and fail to support a particular position, and completing it with a table of asterisks indicating the size of the significance. Assuming that theory X has nine experiments in support and seven against, the reviewer can conclude that theory X has some support, but that more research is needed to reach a decision. Meehl regards this as a "simply preposterous way to reason," and I find myself in considerable sympathy with his views.

The approach used here is admittedly arbitrary. Studies that seemed seriously methodologically flawed to me were ignored. (The absence of a particular study does not automatically connote such a judgment, since I make no claim to have found every appropriate or relevant study published between 1978 and 1981, the years covered in this review.) I sought to develop coherence in given areas and to try to obtain some overall picture of where research in a given area was going and the current status that it had reached. Above all, I sought theoretical positions and evidence that could be evaluated from a theoretical position. [1]

APPROACHES TO THE STUDY OF HEMISPHERE DIFFERENCES

Approaches to the understanding of hemisphere differences can perhaps best be described as the search for a unifying principle. Several such principles have been suggested, and numerous attempts exist to apply these principles to existing sets of research findings. As an overall classification, most of these approaches can be described as difference models, classification systems that seek to develop unifying principles through an analysis of the differential qualities of the cerebral hemispheres. Within a difference approach, systems can be characterized as oriented toward hemisphere differences or task/ conceptual differences. Although the distinction between these two approaches is somewhat arbitrary, the difference may have some heuristic value.

Hemisphere Differences: Anatomical Locus Models

Classification systems based upon hemisphere differences take as their starting point the observed differences found in data coming from a patient population. The basic technique of inference is the process of establishing brain-behavior relationships through the examination of deficits or loss of skills or abilities in individuals suffering from injury or stroke, incapacitating given areas of the cortex, or individuals who have undergone surgical interventions, such as the commissurotomy patients studied by Sperry (1974) or the infantile hemispherectomy patients studied by Smith and Sugar (1975) and by Kohn and Dennis (1974).

The basis of inference is that these events constitute experiments in nature and that through the repeated examination of these experiments as they occur, there will be a systematic accumulation of information about both the functional and anatomical relationships of areas of the brain to given aspects of behavior.

Such an approach has much to recommend it and can lead to a powerful accumulation of information (witness the monumental contributions of Luria, 1962, 1976, to human neuropsychology). Data for such approaches has been accumulating literally for centuries, and the development of new techniques such as computed axial tomography and positron-emission scanning have done much to improve the precision of observation. The problem remains that such an approach is, with some exceptions, necessarily post hoc; the experimenter is nature, and the interpreter is the passive observer of the events that have taken place. Such an approach may run the risk of an accumulation of observations serving as blinders, narrowing the field of inquiry and perhaps "choking off" lines of investigation that would otherwise have proved useful and informative. An illustration of such difficulties is easily provided by comparing some of the early conclusions about the severe limitations of right hemisphere language capability in commissurotomy patients with the later findings of Zaidel (1978) on the language capabilities of the right hemisphere. (See also chapters by Zaidel and by Sidtis & Gazzaniga, this volume.)

Perhaps the most serious criticism that can be leveled against the hemisphere approach is that frequently insufficient care is taken in generalizing from a patient population to a normally functioning group. Whitaker and Ojemann (1980) have pointed out the limitations of the commissurotomy patients as a model for normal hemisphere functioning, reviewing with considerable precision the limitations on inferences from this patient population to a normal group. In a similar manner, Chiarello (1980), in her review of cases of agenesis of the corpus callosum, points out the striking differences in performance abilities between individuals with agenesis and individuals who have had surgical intervention to sever the callosum.

Such approaches generally lead to a set of conclusions that can best be described as "strict localization." A patient with left perisylvan damage will, depending upon the nature and extent of the lesion, show deterioriation of verbal abilities. The statistics are quite stable for this phenomenon: approximately 95% of all individuals so afflicted will display a deterioration of language abilities.

While findings such as these constitute an excellent descriptive model of brain-behavior relationships for the population of the brain injured, the model does not seem applicable to normally functioning individuals. Subjects tested with a variety of language tasks performed under conditions for which language information is initially input to one cerebral hemisphere through display within the corresponding visual field show an astonishing versatility for both accuracy and speed of response. Within a given experiment, subjects selected at random may show a strong right visual field–left hemisphere (RVF-LH) advantage; no particular advantage; or, more rarely, a left visual field–right hemisphere (LVF-RH) advantage for language functions. Despite these considerable variations, the accumulation of centuries of evidence leads to the conclusion that 95% of these individuals would show language impairment if left perisylvan damage were to occur.

It has been the usual practice to suggest that such discrepancies between findings on normal and patient populations reflect errors of measurement in the study of normals or perhaps insufficiently developed research techniques. Such explanations do not take into account the fact that this variability seems astonishingly persistent and stable across a great many experiments, using a wide variety of techniques, stimuli, and subjects. Stable and reliable errors of measurement are not a believable phenomenon. The determination of such variability and the demonstration that such variability is reliable over repeated measures on the same subjects have led to several suggestions (Chiarello, Dronkers & Hardyck, 1982; Kirsner & Brown, 1981) that generalizations from patient populations to normally functioning individuals seem inappropriate and frequently misleading, given the current state of knowledge about the flexibility of normal functioning in the performing of cognitive tasks.

Task Differences: Polarity Models

It is only slightly unfair to describe the task-difference approach to the understanding of cerebral differences as the search for the perfect pair of polar descriptive adjectives. Examples abound: digital-analog (Bateson & Jackson, 1964), propositional-appositional (Bogen, 1969), serial-parallel (G. Cohen, 1973), and focal-diffuse (Semmes, 1968). One of the most favored, analytic-holistic, was originally proposed by Levy-Agresti and Sperry (1968) and has most recently been used by Bradshaw and Nettleton (1981) in their extensive review and analysis of hemispheric specialization. Although Bradshaw and Nettleton make an impressive and well-documented argument, the limitations of such a classification principle are still evident, as outlined in Bertelson's (1982) thoughtful critique:

The analytic/holistic distinction is however a vague one. Like most terms borrowed from everyday language, it carries a number of different meanings. This is not a reason to prohibit such importations, but the danger exists that terms of that kind be taken more seriously than they deserve, leading to unwarranted generalizations from some of their meanings to the others. It has been suggested above that this has happened in the case of the verbal-visual distinction. If one tries to translate the analytic/holistic dichotomy into more operational terms, which would allow testable predictions, one finds that it is compatible with several not necessarily equivalent translations such as focal attention vs. pre-attentive segmentation of the sensory field, attention to local detail rather than overall configuration, serial classification vs. parallel testing of several features (or template matching), attention to high frequency vs. low frequency Fourier components. Hence, as several commentators of the Bradshaw & Nettleton paper pointed out, many apparent explanatory successes of the analytic/holistic dichotomy are actually post-hoc. Marshall (1981) took the example of the task consisting of choosing among several circles the one of which a particular arc is a part, and which work with split-brain patients has shown to be better accomplished by the isolated RH (Nebes, 1974). Bradshaw & Nettleton describe the task as involving "the ability to form a complete Gestalt (e.g. a circle) from incomplete information (e.g. arcs of a circle)." And Marshall comments: "Had the data gone the other way, we can be sure that the task would have been described as implicating the ability to decompose circles into their constituent arcs (an analytic operation) . . ." (Bertelson, 1982, 197–198)

Bertelson's (and Marshall's) point seems well taken. As long as the descriptive terminology is its own referent, this ambiguous state of understanding will remain. Until an external referent can be supplied, the kind of semicircular reasoning pointed out above will continue. The physicist can indulge in discussions of "charm" or "quarks" and any other type of fanciful and idiosyncratic language he wishes since he is able to specify the physical parameters about which he is talking. (In this context, it is interesting to speculate what kinds of definitions lateralization workers would develop should they decide to investigate which hemisphere has more charm!)

On a more serious level, such classification systems all have to postulate the existence of some specialized structures within the cortex—a variant of what is commonly referred to as the structural-pathways model—the conceptualization that specialized structures exist in the brain and that given types of tasks are done better or faster because they are input to nerve pathways leading directly to those specialized structures. (Such a model is implicit in the hemisphere differences classificatory approach, but its limitations did not need to be dealt with there, in view of the other limitations of such a classification system.) In such a model, specialized stimuli, such as language, are processed more accurately and in less time if sent initially along those nerve pathways that lead more directly to language processing areas. Thus, verbal material shown in the RVF-LH will be processed more quickly and accurately because the LH is postulated as having specialized "hardware" for such processing. As G. Cohen (1982) has pointed out, there are several subspecies of this model; an absolute model, in which stimuli sent to the wrong hemisphere cannot be analyzed and no response is possible; a relative model in which information is rerouted from an incorrect location such as the LVF-RH to the correct area for analysis, suffering a little "wear and tear" during the long journey; and the efficiency model, which says that both hemispheres can do things but that one is much more efficient.

Some variants of this model can be dismissed rather quickly. An absolute model is completely without any support. There is not a single report on normal individuals of any task that can be performed only when input is to one visual field, leading to only one hemisphere.

The problem of interhemispheric transfer is more complex. We know that interhemispheric comparisons of information are more efficient than intrahemispheric comparisons (Davis & Schmit, 1971, 1973; Hardyck, Tzeng, & Wang, 1978). A favored explanation of visual field differences is to argue that information received in an area of the brain other than that specialized for its analysis is promptly rerouted to the appropriate area. Such problems as lower accuracy rates or longer reaction times than are consistent with the transmission time expected in the nervous system are dealt with by suggesting that information transferred within the brain suffers degradation during the transfer process. The most appropriate answer to such explanations seems to be that of G. Cohen (1982), who argues that it is difficult to conceive of a system that permits accurate transmission of signal information from a sense organ to a given area of the brain but does not permit accurate transfer of this information from one area of the cortex to another without serious loss of fidelity.

There is another aspect of this position regarding interhemispheric transmission that has not, to my knowledge, been examined. The corpus callosum supposedly has the function of transmitting information from one hemisphere to another. If the signal-degradation hypothesis is to be supported, it seems appropriate to ask why the corpus callosum does its job so poorly, as compared with the rest of the forebrain. Is it necessary to return to the era of Lashley (1950) and McCulloch (1944), who considered the corpus callosum the largest single unimportant structure in the brain?

Another variant or subspecies of the structural-pathways models is the selective activation system, such as that originally proposed by Kinsbourne (1970, 1973, 1975). In such a system, specialized hardware exists, just as in the structure pathways models, but the processing system is rendered more versatile by a condition known as selective activation. In such a condition, an area having specialized processing abilities, such as language, may also at a given time process material for which it is not specialized simply because it is actively functioning as a processor at the moment, while the other areas normally specialized for such processing are not active. Such a model does provide a good deal more flexibility than a limited structural-pathways model in that each hemisphere seems to have more capability to process a variety of input stimuli on its own without having to resort to the process of interhemispheric transfer to explain findings.

However, the problems of the activation model are numerous. Perhaps the major problem is an apparent lack of replicability, as illustrated rather strikingly by Boles's (1979) ten attempted replications without a single success. The experiments of Hellige and Cox (1976), Hellige, Cox, and Litvac (1979), and Moscovitch and Klein (1980) all illustrate the limitations of such a formulation. As the Hellige et al. experiments point out, an activation system that works only within very narrow load limits can scarcely serve as a general operating principle for cognitive-cortical relationships.

Similarity Models

Recent attempts at conceptual solutions to hemisphere functioning have taken a radically different orientation from previous approaches that tended to concentrate on explaining differences and hunting for unifying principles that would provide an acceptable taxonomy of differences in function. These other approaches, which can be described as similarity models, have their roots in such fields as vision and information theory rather than the cortical damage data, which served as the information base for hemisphere and task differences approaches.

To grossly oversimplify, similarity models are variations of the position that the two cerebral hemispheres are duplicate processors of limited and similar capacity, with relatively few differences. The implications of such models are numerous and should be developed at some length, but their principal immediate advantage is that they allow some specific predictions and testing of observed findings that, until now, rested only on post hoc justifications and similar sorts of conceptual-tinkering explanations.

Two such models have been developed in sufficient detail to allow their evaluation in relation to current sets of data: the model proposed by Sergent (1982b), which argues that the hemispheres differ in speed of analysis of visuospatial frequencies; and the model of Friedman and Polson (1981), proposing that the hemispheres act as separate limited-capacity processors with similar capacities and with extremely limited sharing of resources and capacities. Both models represent a provocatively new approach and will be outlined in some detail before being examined for their ability to account for the current sets of perceptual laterality data.

The Visuospatial Frequency (VSP) Model

The explanatory system offered by Sergent (1982b) developed rather directly from her attempts to systematize the research on face recognition (Sergent, 1982a, b; Sergent & Bindra, 1981). An analysis of the experimental parameters found in current face recognition experiments suggested to Sergent that a great majority of this work, yielding both right and left hemisphere superiorities, could be explained on the basis of responses dependent upon specifiable characteristics of stimulus presentation:

> . . . in general a left visual field (right hemisphere) advantage is obtained when (a) stimulus information is degraded; (b) faces to be compared are highly discriminable; (c) a set of unfamiliar faces is used; and (d) task requirements allow a lax criterion of recognition. These conditions seem to make holistic processing adequate for the task; if the conditions require analytic judgments, then a right visual field (left hemisphere) advantage may be obtained. Thus no hemifield has an inherent or absolute advantage. . . .(Sergent & Bindra, 1981, p. 541).

This point of view, as presented in Sergent (1982b), can be summarized as follows. In general, verbal and visuospatial stimulus patterns have little in common. Verbal patterns are overlearned, have sharply defined features communicating a considerable amount of information and with these features and their relationships well known. By contrast, visuospatial patterns are usually new, with features having little or no known relationship to each other, an extensive variation in perceptual saliency, and with an almost infinitely large set of features.

Given these possibilities for variation, it does not seem an extreme step to postulate differential abilities to code sensory representations in the brain. It is also not an extreme step to argue that differential mechanisms may exist to process sensory representations differing as widely as the examples given earlier. A convenient way to separate such differing demands for stimulus processing and task demands may be by differential hemispheric sensitivity to sensory components. Thus, Sergent, on the basis of these assumptions, suggests the following: hemisphere differences will not exist when both verbal and visuospatial patterns have similar task demands and similar visual representation states. The argument is made that the hemispheres differ in sensitivity to sensory components, specifically the ability to analyze visuospatial frequencies. The right hemisphere is specialized for the fast analysis of low-spatial frequencies and the left hemisphere for the analysis of higher-spatial frequencies.

An immediate implication of this position that Sergent emphasized is that the basic conditions under which one studies lateralization differences—very brief exposures and lateral presentation—become central to any conceptualization. In general, as Sergent points out, these factors have been overlooked in the evaluation of results, as if they were somehow irrelevant, inconsequential, or of little importance in the visual system. They are of importance, as is known, and being intrinsic to the study of lateralization in normals, have achieved a kind of experimental invisibility in the analysis and interpretation of experiments, as if they had no effect at all. These viewing conditions are central to analysis and interpretations and undoubtedly deserve more attention than is usually accorded to them.

The relationship of such a model to the analysis of hemisphere differences is relatively straightforward. As support for her framework, Sergent reports two experiments with verbal material, similar to the global-local processing experiments carried out by Navon (1977) and Robertson (1980).

Although the manipulation of visuospatial frequencies is a complex undertaking (see De Valois & De Valois, 1980; Graham, 1981), an effective manipulation for behavioral research can be done by varying the size of the stimuli. As the visual angle subtended by a stimulus is doubled, the spatial frequency is halved. Sergent used this approach to determine the size of stimuli used in the experiments reported in support of her model.

In her experiments, Sergent (1982b) first demonstrated that response time to a global-local processing task (specifically, large letters made up of smaller letters that may or may not be the same as the large letters) will change systematically as a function of the processing task (global or local) and the visual field (RVF-LH or LVF-RH). For a global task, the RH is clearly superior in speed of response. In fact, the response times are not increased for global processing by having the local elements made up of nontarget letters. Sergent interprets this finding to mean that global processing may be complete, allowing a response before local processing is finished. Her second experiment provided a few refinements to the argument by showing that, as exposure time was decreased, only global processing could be carried out and with a RH superiority. Sergent's second experiment provided evidence for the differential rate at which the components of a visual form are extracted, indicating that brief exposure durations allow only the extraction of the lower visuospatial frequencies. The immediate implication of such a finding is that, in any brief exposure experiment, the only frequencies that can be extracted to provide information are the low frequencies, a process strikingly similar to what Broadbent (1977) has called "The Hidden Preattentive Process." Sergent interprets these results (and the results of her earlier analysis of face recognition) as evidence for the position that hemisphere differences, as observed, are a function of both achieved sensory resolutions—the extent to which the sensory information received has been processed—and the sensory resolution required for efficient processing, that is, the amount of information needed to make an effective analysis.

Given this rather condensed account of Sergent's framework, what kinds of conclusions can be drawn? Sergent points out a major implication of her model: physical parameter differences considered unimportant in relation to more global distinctions such as verbal-visuospatial may be much more important in producing hemispheric differences that had been thought in the past:

> Any factor susceptible of influencing the quality of the stimulus representation has to be controlled and, due to the properties of the visual system, one cannot select the duration of exposure, the size of the stimulus, its visual angle from fixation, the delay between target and test presentation. . . without examining how they affect the characteristics of the representation achieved in the brain. Similarly, the requirements of the tasks to be performed have to be analyzed, and one must realize that detection, discrimination, recognition, identification. . .do not make the same demands in terms of processing and of stimulus features to be considered. Then, our understanding of the intact brain may progress with less confusion. (Sergent, 1982b, p. 270)

This is a concern that has probably lurked in the background of consciousness of many researchers when attempting to summarize and evaluate research on a given problem or area of study. Technology in visual-perceptual research on hemifield differences has considerable variation, to say the least, and the possibilities range from sophisticated computer-generated displays to primitive tachistoscopes. While there is no evidence that technical differences per se can account for a substantial proportion of experimental variance, the possibility, especially in view of Sergent's formulations, cannot be overlooked. (It should be pointed out, as Sergent did, that state-of-the-art technology may not necessarily be superior. Computer-controlled displays are frequently dot-matrix displays, while old-fashioned hand-loaded tachistoscopes may provide superb visual contrast displays. Anyone doubting this should spend a few hours reading dot-matrix copy and compare for reading ease with a typeset version.)

At the very least, the implications of this model suggest that a more precise set of specifications needs to be developed for the reporting of research data.

The Dual Processor (DP) Model

At the beginning of this chapter, comments were made to the effect that trying to summarize findings in an area such as visual-perceptual lateralization was more than a mildly frustrating task. Friedman and Polson (1981) seem to have experienced similar frustrations in the development of their model, judging from some of their introductory remarks:

> . . . it could be argued that the most frequent findings to emerge in well over 100 years of research are (a) the apparent capriciousness of the phenomena, that is, the ease with which relatively superficial changes of stimuli, instructions or other task parameters can switch a performance advantage from one hemisphere to the other; (b) the large amount of data that defy replication across laboratories and paradigms; (c) the wide range of individual performance differences observed on tasks that are supposed to be lateralized one way or another, even among populations suspected to be relatively homogeneous in their degree of lateralization of function such as right-handed males; (d) the lack of consistency within individuals in the degree of lateralization they show across time and tasks; and finally (e) the absence of a global theory that can adequately explain the factors underlying even the existing regularities that have been observed.

Although there are some remarkable similarities between the model proposed by Sergent and the model of Friedman and Polson, comparisons will be delayed until the dual processor model is outlined. The DP model has its origins in the multiple capacity model of resource allocation originally formulated by Kahneman (1973) and Norman and Bobrow (1975) and generalized to a multiple resource model by Navon and Gopher (1979). The limiting case of such a model is one that is isomorphic (in a very general sense) to the anatomical structure of the human brain. Friedman and Polson propose that the two human cerebral hemispheres can be regarded as two independent pools of resources, each with finite processing capacity. In their model, the resource supply of each hemisphere is inaccessible to the other hemisphere; there is no shared pool of resources.

Each hemisphere is capable of performing any task required of it by using its own mechanisms and resources, but performance differences may be present between the hemispheres. For Friedman and Polson, the hemispheres differ not in amount of resources but in the possible composition of those resources and the efficiency of their utilization. These differences may be characterized as differences in performance-resource functions. Performance-resource functions may be affected either by resource limitations (there are either insufficient resources allocated to the task or the resources available are insufficient to improve performance on the task) or data limitations (regardless

of the amount of resource available, the data received are such that performance cannot be improved).

Friedman and Polson provide specifications for the conditions under
which particular sets of resource compositions are requested and allocated.
Basic to their formulation are the following conditions:

1. Each hemisphere has the same total resource capacity, and the amount of
resources available to each hemisphere is always equal. The idea that hemispheres
differ in amounts of resources or in differential activation or arousal is, in their
words, "specifically disallowed."

2. The resource allocation within a given hemisphere is constant; if attention
is increased for whatever reason, the amount of increased resource allocation is
constant for both hemispheres, even if the task demands are primarily on one
hemisphere.

Therefore, in a single-task situation, hemispheric differences in performance
are a function of the demand for resources at a particular intended level of
performance and differences in the efficiency of those resources, rather than
being a function of differences in the available supply, which is assumed to be
equal in both hemispheres. (Friedman & Polson, 1981, p. 1043).

The DP model is evaluated on a variety of data. Perhaps the best
illustration of the effectiveness of their model is the use of the Hellige and Cox
(1976) and Hellige et al. (1979) dual-task experiments. Hellige and Cox
(1976) found that noun naming combined with a noun-memory load caused a
decrement in correct noun naming for both hemispheres as the memory load
increased. In the Hellige et al. (1979) experiment, where the memory task was
a dot-pattern recall, noun naming was unaffected by increasing the memory
load for dot patterns. Friedman and Polson interpreted these results as
evidence for their formulation, arguing that a task such as vocal naming places
a relatively heavy demand for mechanisms that are specific to the left
hemisphere, such as motor speech. Consequently, when the memory load, also
postulated as a left hemisphere task, becomes too great, there is a deterioration in performance for both hemispheres, not because the right hemisphere is
overloaded by its demands, but because the left hemisphere is unable to handle
the input from the right hemisphere and still carry out the vocal naming tasks.

They concluded their presentation with a detailed discussion of problems
involved in the replication of results in the study of hemisphere differences,
stating the positon that tasks that can be performed with a variety of resource
compositions drawn from the two hemispheres may account for the difficulties
in replication. They urge that investigators use populations that show the
largest and most consistent hemispheric differences; try to use, whenever
possible, within-subjects design; and pay very close attention to the types of

task situations used, detecting patterns of interference whenever possible and testing for their effects:

> We urge that investigators of cerebral specialization adopt the strategy of (a) using populations that have shown the largest and most consistent performance differences between the hemispheres (e.g., right-handed males with no familial history of left-handedness who use a normal rather than an inverted writing posture, . . . (b) using within-subject designs, (c) carefully controlling resource allocation in both single and dual-task conditions through various payoff schemes, (d) carefully controlling resource demands by adding tasks or increasing their difficulty in the dual-task situations, and (e) looking at patterns of interference or noninterference across carefully chosen sets of task pairs.
>
> With respect to the last point, we feel that investigators should try to use tasks that either logically or empirically have resource compositions that draw primarily from one or the other hemisphere and for which the processing options are few. Otherwise, when two tasks whose resource compositions draw from both hemispheres are paired, the results may be difficult or even impossible to interpret. (Friedman & Polson, 1981, p.1055)

COMMENTARY

Before beginning any commentary, it should be pointed out that the summarizations given here of Sergent's and of Friedman's and Polson's positions are rather condensed, and for a full appreciation of their accomplishments the original papers deserve careful study.

There are a good many similarities in the positions, as stated. Both viewpoints argue a "separate but equal" status for the two hemispheres as processors of equal ability, given certain requirements: similarity of stimulus parameters or resource composition and effiency of utilization. Both models are in agreement that processing is carried out in the hemisphere where information is received and that hemispheric interchange is an exchange of processed information and not a rerouting of raw sensory information. Given an equivalence of conditions, either hemisphere can do any task—a position quite in accord with many current experimental results, but one at considerable variance with the position that would be developed from a study of patient populations.

Both models call for better control of experiments, but interestingly, there is almost no overlap in what is considered important. Sergent proposes that very precise control of physical parameters is essential if the replicability of results is to be improved; Friedman and Polson argue for restricted subject selection and for careful choices of tasks.

Similarly, both positions have some omissions of note. Emphasis on physical parameters is perhaps overly strong in Sergent's position, leading her to the position that a right hemisphere superiority may be obtained for almost any type of task by reducing exposure duration. Regardless of how qualified, such a position is difficult to defend. It is extremely difficult to produce a right hemisphere advantage for a complex language task. In addition, Sergent's formulation has no obvious way to account for individual differences, other than the suggestion of better control of physical stimulus parameters. If the implication is that the individual differences that complicate interpretation of current work are removable or controllable through better control of physical parameters, such a position needs to be more precisely specified than is the case at present.

Exactly the same problem is present for the model of Friedman and Polson. Their formulation contains either an implicit equality or an unspecified hope. It is not clear how the careful subject selection that they advocate will control for the problems of subjects using different resource compositions in order to achieve solutions to the tasks, unless they mean to imply that right-handed males with normal writing posture are homogeneous with regard to utilization of resource composition. I suspect than an examination of individual differences within right-handed properly writing males on almost any perceptual lateralization experiment would quickly refute that hope.

A similar difficulty exists for the problems of specifying resource composition. What criteria does one use to ensure that the tasks chosen draw primarily on one hemisphere? This is not an easy job, as the results of the attempted hemisphere-specific task analysis of Tomlinson-Keasey and Kelly (1979) show. All too frequently, one finds out after the fact where the hemispheric advantages lie and has to develop a post hoc explanation of why a particular task turned out to be a right/left hemisphere task. Thus, one returns to the criticisms of Bertelson (1982) given earlier in this chapter, with reference to the polar-adjective approach.

Friedman's and Polson's specifications of resources plus effiency of utilization are flexible enough to allow exactly the type of ad hoc solution that has plagued such dichotomies as analytic-holistic or propositional-appositional. Unless the task in question can be anchored to some externally definable criterion, the results for any given set of data can be interpreted as making particular demands on a hemisphere-specific set of resources. Sergent, tying her model to certain stimulus parameter–visuospatial frequencies, has no such escape route and thus may have a more powerful formulation, simply because it is capable of being disproved. [2]

RECENT EMPIRICAL STUDIES

In the remaining sections of this chapter, an examination will be carried out of much of the visual lateralization research appearing between 1978 and the present. Following as coherent a summarization as can be managed, given the diversity of current research, some attempts will be made to evaluate current work in the light of the possible theoretical perspectives. Any division of research into categories becomes arbitrary and the division used here, language and visuospatial research, is no exception, the only justification being that any taxonomic sorting possible has some advantages over treating visual-perceptual lateralization research as an undifferentiated mass.

Visuospatial Studies

At least four studies have appeared, offering as a group, convincing evidence that hemispheric differences are not present at simple sensory coding levels. Di Lollo (1981) tested subjects on a 4 × 4 dot matrix that appeared dot by dot within visual fields with plotting times of 50, 100, and 150 msec. Satisfactory resolution of the problems required perceptual integration of the stimulus display. He found no differences in visual fields and concluded that previously reported accounts of LVF superiority were due to the requirement that stimuli had to be retained in memory; with a continuously visible display, no differences were present. Similar results were reported by Marzi, Di Stefano, Tassinari, and Crea (1979), who found no differences in iconic storage between visual fields. Birkett (1978), in a similar study, showed random shapes within visual fields for a 10-msec interval, reporting no differences in visual fields.

Bevilaqua, Capitani, Luzzati, and Spinnler (1979) presented abstract visual patterns within visual fields for 100 msec, with subsequent delays of 0, 5, 15, 30, and 60 seconds. Subjects had to recognize the item presented out of six alternatives. They found an LVF superiority at a 15-second delay and an RVF superiority at a 60-second delay, a result that offers support for the conclusions of Di Lollo.

Another type of argument, displacement of stimuli from the visual midline, was examined by Harvey (1978), who found no evidence for bilateral pathways near the visual midline. It appears that stimuli can be placed as close as 0.25 degrees of visual angle, with no evidence of dual representation.

Pitblado (1979) presented random-dot stereograms within visual fields and found no visual field differences in ability to resolve the stereograms but a substantial interaction between visual fields and dot size. Pitblado's findings are of considerable interest, since his interaction was precisely the reverse of what would have been predicted by the Sergent model. In Pitblado's work, smaller dots (higher spatial frequencies) were more effective in the LVF and large dots (lower spatial frequencies) in the RVF, a circumstance that urges a replication of the Pitblado study, in view of considerable supporting evidence for possible spatial frequency differences.

Within visuospatial studies, numerous experiments concerned with various aspects of face recognition were carried out. Sergent and Bindra (1981) and Sergent (1982a, 1982b) have already been mentioned, in relation to the hemispheric functioning model proposed by Sergent. Emphasis in this group of studies seems to be more on various aspects of face recognition by hemispheric specialization, rather than on the earlier obsession over the cerebral locus of the ability.

Reuter-Lorenz and Davidson (1981) showed six faces with happy and sad expressions, using relatively long times for the maintenance of fixation (328 msec) and found that left hemispheres prefer (are faster at recognizing) happy faces and right hemispheres, sad faces. Overriding this unexplained difference in emotional preferences, an overall RVF superiority was present.

Galper and Costa (1980) carried out an interesting manipulation of verbal orientations or outlooks in relation to a face recognition task, presenting either physical or personality descriptions of faces. They hypothesized that personality descriptions lead to holistic processing and physical descriptions to an analytic mode of recognition. They found this hypothesis to be correct for some subjects and reversed for others. When a second experiment was done, with no verbal descriptions, their subjects displayed a more consistent hemispheric advantage, with wide individual differences still present. When these subjects were shown the same faces in a repetition of the recognition task with verbal descriptions, the diversity of response found in the first experiment was again present.

Strauss and Moscovitch (1981) examined the ability to discriminate expressions, using 18 photographs of three males and three females, each with three different expressions, and exposure times of 800 msec. They found small (but statistically significant) differences in favor of the LVF for same expressions but not for different expressions. A second experiment also reported an LVF advantage, and a third experiment allowed the subjects to examine the pictures prior to the tachistoscopic procedure, resulting in an RVF advantage. Unlike Reuter-Lorenz and Davidson, these subjects had no emotional preferences related to visual fields.

Safer (1981) carried out an emotion recognition study, using empathic and labeling instructions for faces first presented in central vision and then shown laterally. He found no differences between exposure times of 50 and 150 msec and an LVF advantage for both times, for same-different judgments of same face and same expression. A second experiment had subjects make identity judgments, using exposure times of 30 and 50 msec, again with an LVF advantage.

Ley and Bryden (1979) used cartoon line drawings of five adult male faces, portraying different emotional expressions. The paradigm was the reverse of the Safer study, with a face presented in a visual field for 85 msec and then with a central presentation. Same-different judgments were made for emotions and for faces, a large LVF advantage being found for both judgments.

Leehey and Cahn (1979), in a combined verbal-face recognition study, showed familiar words, familiar faces, and unfamiliar faces, using verbal response for the words and recognition from a panel of 12 faces for the faces. As might be expected, they found an RVF advantage for words and an LVF advantage for faces. In a second experiment, using only familiar faces and a naming response, an LVF advantage was again found. Leehey, Carey, Diamond, and Cahn (1978), using a similar paradigm, showed words, upright faces, and inverted faces, finding an LVF advantage for the upright faces and no VF difference for the inverted faces.

Hay (1981) presented subjects with line drawings of faces, with rearrangements of features such that the nose could appear in the appropriate location for the mouth and so forth. Four drawings were used with four rearrangements, exposed for 175 msec and with yes-no judgments, producing an LVF advantage.

St. John (1981) reported two experiments on facial recognition. The first experiment was a same-different judgment task. He found an RVF advantage in both accuracy and reaction time. In a second experiment, two male and two female faces, normal and mirror images, were compared with photographs of four different shoes, photographed with four different orientations. This type of comparison produced an LVF advantage for faces and no visual field differences for the shoe photographs. (The lateralized location of the organ of shoe recognition has yet to be discovered.)

Two experiments exist in the nonlanguage category that will not fit conveniently into any of the subtypes discussed thus far. Beaton (1979) compared digit detection within visual fields while performing a manual sorting task. His first experiment indicated no differences in VF accuracy. In a second experiment, using a more difficult sorting task, he found that, with right-hand difficult sorting, there were identical decrements in digit detection in both visual fields. When difficult sorting was done with the left hand, there was no RVF drop in accuracy but a drop in LVF accuracy.

Goldberg, Vaughan, and Gerstman (1978) put forth the argument that the left hemisphere processes stimuli in terms of existing descriptive systems and that the right hemisphere processes stimuli for which no descriptive systems exist, a resurrection of an earlier hemisphere typology of language-nonlanguage. To test their formulation, they showed nonsense figures of different shapes and textures and found an RVF advantage in recognition of shapes, as compared with textures, with LVF performance equal for both categories. They interpreted this result as supportive of their hypothesis, although it is difficult to see how the obtained result is supportive. It would have been of interest to know if their subjects had attempted any verbal coding of their stimuli. In this context, the authors report that two of their subjects had art and design backgrounds and that these two subjects showed strong RVF advantages on this task. Although not stated by the authors, such a result implies the presence of a well-developed verbal descriptive system for shape and texture for these two subjects.

Language Studies

Given the diversity of studies found between 1978 and 1981, even such a broad conceptual label as "language" is scarcely adequate as a covering category, given the complexity of some current work.

Kirsner (1980) reported a series of experiments on retrieval processes in language. Using a bilateral probe in a name-identity, physical-identity, letter-matching task with differing set sizes, he found a slower response time of 20 msec per item in the RVF. A second experiment was able to eliminate this difference by using a unilateral probe, and a third experiment eliminated intertrial intervals as a possible explanation. Kirsner argues that retrieval processes occur at an advanced stage of cognitive processing and that the hemispheres are qualitatively different in their retrieval processes.

Kirsner and Brown (1981) continued the study of retrieval processes in a series of four experiments examining hemispheric differences in recognition memory for letters. Their first experiment systematically varied combinations of letters, digits, random dot arrays, and blank fields. They found that response to a probe of one of two sequentially presented items produced a visual-field-by-position interaction only for the condition of two letters presented serially; reaction time was longer for the first serial item only in the RVF, a replication of the earlier findings of Kirsner (1980).

A second experiment contrasted stimulus category (digits vs. letters) and memorization, finding that memorization is the critical factor, again producing the interaction between visual field and serial position found in their first experiment. A third experiment contrasted verbal stimuli (letters) with random forms, finding that the interaction of visual field and serial position occurs only when both target stimuli are letters.

A fourth experiment required subjects to generate verbal codes from visual stimuli, using dot patterns where the number of dots represented the digit to be remembered. The same interaction with visual field was found, indicating that mental process rather than stimulus class was the critical element.

Their work is an impressive demonstration of the complexity of visual-field-by-task interactions. Their subjects carried out the same task on every trial, the only difference being the recency of the target information. They concluded that many visual field differences may be a function of the recency of presentation—a conclusion that raises doubts about the use of main effects in the study of lateralization in normals and the use of patient data to interpret functioning in normals. They also pointed out that such a conclusion implies that hemispheric differences may be, in part, a function of those processes active at the moment information is received.

An ingeniuous demonstration of how language effects can be manipulated was reported in a series of experiments by Jonides (1979). Using a response–no response paradigm for the letters, C, E, F, and G, he was able to show that, when a response was to be made to C or E as compared with E or F, the visual field advantage changed, an LVF advantage being present for CE as targets and an RVF advantage for EF as targets. In a second experiment, using F as the target with E and T as frequent distractors and C as an infrequent distractor, an overall LVF advantage was present. Reversing the similarity process in a third experiment, using F as a target and G, Q, and C as distractors, an RVF advantage appeared.

Jonides argued that his results indicate that a language task will be done as a language task, regardless of instructions or other considerations, unless the task cannot be done efficiently by language-processing methods. When stimuli are discriminable as language, as in the easy discrimination of F as compared with GQC, language processing will be used. If finer discriminations are needed, as in F from ET, other processing methods will be used, the characteristics of the task determining the hemisphere most effective.

Hellige and his colleagues have reported a series of experiments on verbal processes. Hellige et al. (1979) carried out a series of five experiments. The first experiment, showing no interaction between memory for a dot matrix and a naming task, regardless of hemisphere, has already been reviewed in the discussion of the Friedman and Polson (1981) model of hemispheric functioning. Their second and third experiments demonstrated a strong visuospatial memory by visual field interaction, as compared with a minimal interaction for early visuospatial processes. Experiments four and five were variations on the dual-task paradigm used by Hellige and Cox (1976), demonstrating that with no memory load, responses to a letter-naming task are faster in the RVF, and for memory set sizes of two, four, and six letters, an LVF advantage is present.

They interpreted their results as evidence for the hemispheres acting as separate limited capacity processors.

Hellige and Webster (1979) reported an experiment on letter recognition with forward and backward masking, using masks with features similar and dissimilar to the target letters. They found an overall LVF superiority that was enhanced when the features were similar to the target and concluded that the right hemisphere is superior at extracting information from degraded displays, a conclusion quite in accord with the model proposed by Sergent.

In a related experiment, Hellige (1980) used a Sternberg paradigm for single letters shown in visual fields with set sizes of two, three, four, or five letters. For positive trials, degradation of the stimulus probe increased the slope of the memory set size function for LVF trials but not for RVF trials. Hellige offered this as further evidence for a LVF-RH visuospatial memory process, as compared with a more abstract process in the RVF-LH.

Hellige and Webster (1981) presented pairs of letters varying in name and case and obtained reaction times to appropriate key-press choices of same-different. For stimuli appearing in the LVF, reaction time was faster to same-name items than to different-name items of the same case. Similarly, RT was faster for same items when case differed than for different items of different case but with no name-by-case interaction. In the RVF, a strong name-by-case interaction was found, with large RT differences between same name–same case and same name–different case. However, the conditions of different name–same case and different name–different case had almost identical reaction times. Hellige and Webster interpret their findings as evidence for a two-stage analysis process in which gross physical characteristics are analyzed first, followed by a finer analysis if the gross analysis reveals any discrepancies. Their data indicate that right hemisphere analysis of the condition with two discrepancies, different name and different case, takes considerably longer than the same analysis in the left hemisphere, another result quite compatible with the VSF model of Sergent (1982b).

Hannay, Dee, Burns, and Masek (1981) reported a series of six experiments in which subject selection was used to provide an experimental manipulation. They selected subjects who displayed a strong LVF advantage in a random-form recognition task. In the first experiment, a form–verbal label, paired-associates training was able to reverse the visual field advantage. In the second experiment, the P-A training was done, but a verbal response was not required in the experiment, attenuating the LVF effect. In the third experiment, the subjects were allowed to become familiar with the forms prior to the experiment but with no labeling explicitly provided, again resulting in an attenuation of the LVF advantage. The fourth experiment varied time intervals between stimulus and test, showing that a longer time interval again attenuated the LVF advantage. A final experiment selected subjects who initially showed an RVF advantage on the forms recognition task and gave them the paired associates training used in the first experiment, the effect being to increase the size of the RVF advantage. Relatively few lateralization experiments utilize individual differences and the Hannay et al. experiments are an excellent illustration of the power that appropriate use of such subject variables can bring to an investigation.

Moscovitch and Klein (1980) examined the possibility that interference effects could be demonstrated among items processed by one hemisphere. Using a central display with lateralized probe presentation and words and faces, they found a central-peripheral interference pattern with a face followed by laterally presented faces, requiring more processing time than a word presented centrally followed by faces. When a shape was used centrally rather than a face, similar interference effects were found. Naming the faces did not remove the interference effect, leading the authors to argue that stimulus attributes are more important than the output response mode. A comparision of interference effects with a central shape that subjects were told to ignore, as compared with a blank central display, produced some interference in the ignored shape condition. Moscovitch and Klein interpreted their results as evidence for the hemispheres operating as relatively independent, limited capacity processors, where performance drops as competition for resources increases—a summary formulation remarkably similar to that proposed by Friedman and Polson.

Niederbuhl and Springer (1979) displayed single letters for 100 msec, using four target letters and four distractors. Subjects operated under naming and shape instructions, with no response to curved lines. They found that name instructions produced an RVF advantage over shape instructions. In the LVF, response time was faster overall than for the RVF, with a relative advantage present for shape instructions.

Segalowitz and Stewart (1979) had subjects perform a matching task on upper and lowercase letters, reporting that name matches produced a large RVF advantage, with a much smaller LVF advantage for physical matches.

Martin (1979) carried out a global-local processing experiment, finding a local-processing advantage in the RVF and a global-processing advantage in the LVF, a result identical to that reported by Sergent (1982b) as evidence for her model of hemispheric functioning.

Madden and Nebes (1980) used a Sternberg paradigm in a search for digits within visual fields, finding an RVF advantage as the set size increases for positive trials and no visual field differences in slope or intercept for negative trials.

Day (1979) compared nouns, adjectives, and verbs of high and low imagery, in a lexical decision task, finding an RVF advantage for low-imagery nouns and adjectives and high- and low-imagery verbs, but no advantage for high- and low-imagery nouns and adjectives. Koff and Reiderer (1981) carried out an experimental test of the Gazzaniga (1970) hypothesis of hemispheric differentiation relative to syntactic class. They used pure nouns, verb-derived nouns, category-ambiguous words, and adjectives, with categories matched for word frequency. After seeing 40 words for 80 msec each, subjects were given a list of 80 words and asked to identify those 40 just seen. They found a strong RVF advantage in recall, with nouns more easily recalled and with no category differences for the LVF, leading them to conclude that syntactic categories are irrelevant to hemisphere differences.

Two experiments used clock faces in an assessment of verbal coding. Hatta (1978) first showed clock faces, asking for verbal reports of time and found an LVF advantage. In a second condition, the subjects were required to either subtract or add one hour to the time displayed, according to a fixation cue; with this additional activity, an RVF superiority was reported. Berlucchi, Brizzolara, Marzi et al. (1979) displayed clock faces for a 100-msec interval, with vocal reaction time responses, and found a significant LVF advantage, concluding that verbal coding is not sufficient to automatically provide a left hemisphere advantage. Since they discarded one quarter of their subjects for overly long reaction times or irrelevant or incorrect responses, it is difficult to interpret their findings. A similar comment can be made of the Hatta study, which did not report exposure times.

CONCLUSIONS

At this point, what can be made of the current status of theory and research in visual lateralization work? As a start, some comments can be made about the impressive level of sophistication that characterizes the great majority of current experimental work. It is not an overenthusiastic comment to state that sophistication in experimentation has kept pace with increasing sophistication in theory.

As a beginning, it seems appropriate to ask what kinds of support for theoretical positions can be marshaled from the work reviewed here. It seems clear that structural-pathways models have little relevance or use for current thinking about hemisphere function. As an explanatory concept within a wider framework, the notion of specialized mechanisms seems alive and well, although only in the perspective of a broader framework, such as the similarity models provide.

There also seems little left of activation models; the current set of experimental results are simply not supportive. In particular, the work reported by Hellige and his colleagues (Hellige, 1980; Hellige et al., 1979;

Hellige & Webster, 1981), by Jonides (1979), by Kirsner (Kirsner, 1980; Kirsner & Brown, 1981), by Moscovitch and Klein (1980) and by Hannay et al. (1981) all generate results that are at variance with predictions drawn from an activation model. In fact, the last formulation of activation theory (Kinsbourne & Hicks, 1978) has the net effect of limiting the explanatory ability of the theory to those specialized areas for which motor-cognitive interference problems can be examined.

Similarity models, specifically those of Sergent (1982b) and Friedman and Polson (1981), by contrast, fare very well and are much more in accord with the results of current experimentation. The possibility of systematic testing is present for both formulations, and the models should provide an excellent basis for thinking about current sets of data and for the design of new experiments. Perhaps the most important aspect of what are undoubtedly signal contributions to neuropsychology lies in the fact that both Sergent's and Friedman's and Polson's models place the study of cerebral lateralization within the larger framework of human cognition and information-processing work. If there is one aspect of current work that is common to an astonishing diversity, it is the realization that cortical processes are more flexible and versatile than earlier, specialized-mechanisms formulations would admit.

At this point it seems appropriate to review the visuospatial frequency and dual processor models in light of the current set of experimental data. How well do these models compare with current results?

One comment was already made about the VSF model when the Pitblado (1979) experiment was reviewed. Clearly, this experiment should be replicated since the results that Pitblado found are the exact opposite of those predicted by Sergent. Given a Popperian outlook (1968), one would have to discard the VSF model immediately, but with the complexities of research, particularly on such tasks as random-dot stereograms, a second opinion would be helpful.

How well does the VSF model fare otherwise? Given the specificity that Sergent has provided for her model, it seems to do rather well when examined in relation to the experiments reviewed here. Figure 7-1 is a plot of visual field advantages versus exposure time for all the appropriate face recognition experiments reviewed in this chapter. If the VSF model is to be supported, we would expect left hemisphere advantages to increase as exposure time increases. We would also expect those experiments with very short exposure times to have right hemisphere advantages.

Given the data shown in Figure 7-1, at least two comments can be made. The first is that there is nothing overpoweringly in support but there is also nothing overpoweringly against the formulation. The results tend to offer mild support for Sergent's formulation. In evaluating these data, it should be pointed out that many of these studies were focused on secondary aspects of facial recognition, such as emotional changes and states, rather than on a strict recognition paradigm.

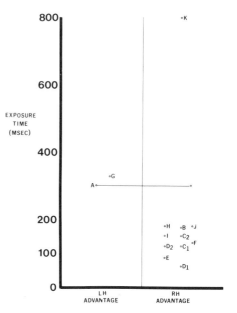

Figure 7-1. *Hemisphere Superiority by Exposure Time: Face Recognition. A. Galper & Costa, 1980; B. Hay, 1981; C1. Leehey, Carey, Diamond, & Cahn, 1978; C2. Leehey, Carey, Diamond, & Cahn, 1978; D1. Leehey & Cahn, 1979; D2. Leehey & Cahn, 1979; E. Ley & Bryden, 1979; F. Moscovitch & Klein, 1980 (FF and FW conditions only); G. Reuter-Lorenz & Davidson, 1981; H. Reynolds & Jeeves, 1978 (adult data only); J. St. John, 1981; K. Strauss & Moscovitch, 1981.*

A second comment deals specifically with the Galper and Costa study (1980), shown in Figure 7-1 A. The distinctions present in the Galper and Costa study illustrate the effects of verbal instruction on task differences in a powerful fashion. The VSF model at present has no explanatory framework that can account for these differences, since Galper and Costa, using only a physical versus personality description of the faces, were able to manipulate hemispheric differences by means of these instructions, holding physical parameters constant. Clearly, some allowance for the volitional control of the subject has to be added to the VSF formulation to account for results such as these.

Another kind of summary comparison relevant to the parameters of the VSF model can be done by examining the language experiments reviewed here. If spatial frequency differences have the effect indicated by the experiments of Sergent, one might be able to determine this by examining the sizes of the displays of letters and words used in the experiments reviewed earlier. Table 7-1 lists those experiments and when provided or calculable, the size of the letters (or the letters in the word stimuli) used in these experiments.

TABLE 7-1.
Stimulus Parameters: Verbal Visual Field Experiments

	VD	VA	DISP	TYPE	SIZE
Hellige, 1980	75	0.9	4.3	letters	1.2
Moscovitch & Klein, 1980	75	2.5	1.6	words	3.3
Koff & Reiderer, 1981	75	1.2	1.1	words	1.5
Hellige, 1976	75	1.0	1.5	words	0.3
Kirsner, 1980	40	0.8	3.0	letters	1.8
Kirsner & Brown, 1981	40	0.8	3.0	letters	1.8
Niederbuhl & Springer, 1979	75	NA	2.2	letters	NA
Jonides, 1979	75	NA	2.0	letters	0.8
Hatta & Dimond, 1980	50	NA	6.8	6 digits	1.2
	50	9.8	13.9	forms	NA
Day, 1979	85	3.2	1.5	words	1.2
Segalowitz & Stewart, 1979	75	NA	2.7	letters	1.3
Hellige & Webster, 1979	75	1.2	5.2	letters	1.5
Hellige & Webster, 1981	75	1.9	6.6	letters	2.4

Note: VD = viewing distance; VA = visual angle; DISP = displacement from fixation point; TYPE = stimulus type; SIZE = stimulus size; NA = not available.

There are two findings from Table 7-1, the first being that everyone seems to do the same experiment when selecting the size stimuli to use. This is not particularly surprising when one considers that tachistoscopes, slide projection systems, and computer-generated display systems all have much in common with regard to display size and that the size of a display, given the restrictions of visual angle, viewing distance, and so forth is going to be within fairly narrow limits. The second finding is that, if there were important differences related to spatial frequencies, one would not discover them from examining any of the current group of experiments nor probably from a historical review. Just as lateral displacement and brief exposures are part of the research environment, and as such, partially invisible, so is the size of the displays used. A study offering directly contradictory evidence to the VSF formulation has been carried out by Jonides (1979). To illustrate the direct opposition of the theory and the results, the following quotation from Sergent (1982b) is offered:

> The emergence of an LVF superiority with large letters should not be considered independently of the particular task demands involved in these experiments. A small set of fairly dissimilar letters was used, and the recognition of the letters may not have required a high level of discrimination. This may indicate that the low frequency components of the large letter were

sufficient for an efficient processing, whereas more similar letters (e.g., O and Q, E and F), a larger stimulus set, and more demanding requirements (e.g., identification or discriminating vowels from consonants) would have involved a finer discrimination of the stimuli, making the processing of higher frequency components necessary for an efficient performance.

The results found by Jonides are exactly the reverse of that predicted by Sergent. Using a response/no-response paradigm to the letters CEFG, he was able to show that the visual field advantage changed as a function of the response to the target; when CE was to receive a response, an LVF advantage was present; when E or F was to receive a response, an RVF advantage was found. In a second experiment, using F as a target and E and T as frequent distractors, an overall LVF advantage was present. When F was a target and G, Q, and C were the distractors, an RVF advantage was found.

Given the formulation offered by Sergent, exactly the reverse should have been found. However, in Jonides's experiment, the low-frequency advantages seem to be present for the left hemisphere. Unless some explanation can be offered that can account for this reversal, the VSF formulation is difficult to support. (It is, of course, possible that the frequency differences present in this experiment are so minimal that one would not expect hemispheric processing differences among letters that are all the same size. It would be of interest to repeat the Jonides experiments with substantial changes in size to see if a hemisphere-by-size interaction is found.) Jonides offers as an explanation the idea that language stimuli will be processed as language stimuli, regardless of other considerations, unless language-processing methods are not appropriate or efficient. Such a formulation seems testable, and it would be of considerable interest to see the outcome of such a test.

Can similar evaluations be made on the DP model of Friedman and Polson? Not to the same extent that the model of Sergent, using the specifiable parameters given, could be tested. Within the experiments reviewed, there were no specific studies such as those of Pitblado (1979) and Jonides (1979) that, even though done independently of the models, were applicable to testing them. The formulations of Friedman and Polson are simply too general to allow this type of comparison. The only work directly relevant to their model has not been reviewed here since it has not as yet been published. Prior to the publication of the DP model, I had begun work on the ability to orient attention within visual fields. This work, based upon some research by Bryden (1980), sought to manipulate attention within visual fields. The paradigm used was a lexical decision task—deciding whether a letter string was or was not an English word. Subjects viewed the stimuli while having eye position monitored by an eye movement monitor linked to a computer that controlled the stimulus display. If fixation was not at the defined point and stable, the stimulus did not appear until fixation was registered. This system allowed the use of various priming and informational conditions while insuring that fixation was controlled.

The stimuli used were common, imageable, concrete nouns, and pronounceable nonwords constructed in accordance with the rules of English orthography. To begin, subjects made decisions about a set of 200 stimuli presented randomly to the left or right of fixation. Following this, the subjects were instructed to try to improve their accuracy score on those items appearing to the left/right of the fixation point. The subjects were not told to ignore items in the other visual field but only to try and improve their scores in the designated field.

From the formulations of the DP model, the following predictions can be made: given the fact that different mechanisms may exist within the hemispheres, differences in visual fields under conditions of random presentation may be expected; given that the DP model specifically states that attention cannot be increased within one hemisphere without a corresponding increase in the other hemisphere, any increase in attention resulting in improved performance in one hemisphere should result in a proportional increase in performance in the other hemisphere; and since allocation of resources across hemispheres is specifically disallowed within the DP model, the circumstances in which performance improves within one hemisphere following instructions to increase attention cannot result in a decrement in performance in the other hemisphere.

In our results, we found that a great majority of subjects had a strong RVF advantage in the random presentation condition. When instructed to improve performance in the RVF, the net improvement was zero, as compared with the performance level achieved in the random presentation condition. When instructed to improve performance in the LVF, the net improvement was 10%, accompanied by a decrement in performance in the RVF of 7%. The orienting instructions for the RVF produced a performance that was in accord with the predictions made from the DP model, but the orienting instructions for the LVF produced a result of the type that would be specifically disallowed, since there was no additional demand placed on the left hemisphere by the instructions to improve performance in the LVF.

These results are from work still in progress and do not represent as much of a damaging criticism to the Friedman and Polson model as do the Pitblado and the Jonides results to the Sergent formulation, although the same sorts of questions can be raised. Clearly, some precisely defined studies need to be carried out with respect to these models.

Whether these formulations survive or not, the benefits that they have provided to the study of lateralization cannot be minimized. Both theories have provided new outlooks and have highlighted some changes that are needed if knowledge is to advance. Another useful property of a theory—and one present in both the Friedman and Polson and Sergent formulations—is the highlighting of limitations and the changes that need to be made for knowledge to advance. Both Friedman and Polson and Sergent have offered specific suggestions for changes in experimental procedures that deserve not only serious consideration but immediate examination and where necessary, implementation.

It is only a slight exaggeration to state that the research reported here, despite experimental sophistication and clear communication, is inadequately reported. Two aspects of this have been raised within the contexts of the Sergent and the Friedman and Polson formulations and should be emphasized. Sergent points out in her presentation that stimulus parameters may be much more important than generally realized and that some systematic examination of this area is badly needed.

Anyone questioning the importance of this point should examine carefully the face recognition studies reviewed in this chapter. Trying to evaluate face recognition work and to compare results is equivalent to having to award first prize in a mixed media art festival. There is simply no way to evaluate informational displays of this sort, given the current requirements on reporting. Humans are such flexible organisms at information processing that they are able to cope with almost any whimsicality of display that an experimenter can conceive and to provide responses within reasonable limits. Technological advances in display techniques have not been followed thus far with advances in reporting standards. How are computer-generated dot-matrix displays presented as a white or pale green display comparable to black lettering on a white background shown in a tachistoscope? How do these physical parameters differ and what effects do they have on the kinds of judgments that subjects make? These are aspects of research that have tended to be minimized in the eagerness to understand hemisphere functioning. It might be quite informative to show some experiments to a colleague working in the appropriate area of sensory psychology and to ask that individual what kinds of descriptive parameters need to be specified in describing the research so that an exact replication of the physical stimulus parameters can be done.

It would seem entirely appropriate to devote a conference or a series of meetings to discussion of the stimulus parameters to be reported and the form of such reportage. Such topics are rather dull and not nearly as much fun as reporting new results, but the alternative is the continued inability to compare results from different laboratories, to replicate findings, and to provide efforts with greater precision.

A similar point with a different emphasis has been made by Friedman and Polson, in their suggestions that experiments concentrate on eliminating extraneous variation by selecting only (for example) right-handed male subjects with no family history of left-handedness and with normal writing postures. They also recommend, among other things, a careful analysis of task demands—a difficult problem, as the attempts of Tomlinson-Keasey and Kelly (1979) illustrate.

From a personal and what may be an idiosyncratic point of view, an information-processing neuropsychology based entirely upon right-handed males with defined family history, specified writing posture, and perhaps numerous other things seems equivalent to a carefully prepared gastronomic delight with all the seasoning missing. Clearly it is necessary to know about subject variance and the extent to which handedness, sex, and other such considerations produce related effects on data. However, rather than eliminating such a large portion of the human race from studies, it would seem more appropriate to examine them specifically. For example, can systematic differences be found between a set of data collected on right-handed males with etc., etc. and a sample of whatever is around, including left-handed women with inverted writing postures? Experimental emphasis has centered either around investigation of a particular phenomenon, in which circumstances subject variance is carefully controlled, or investigations of subject differences in which individual differences are the focus, and the process or phenomenon has a secondary role. To complicate the matter, the accepted procedures for reporting such data are, by their very nature, inappropriate for comparisons.

As a final point, it should be emphasized that the process of reporting data in terms of statistically significant differences does more to obfuscate and obscure knowledge than any other process. Statistically significant differences, especially in relation to within-subject experiments are probably the ideal way to obscure the meanings of results, a condition that is only exacerbated by journal practices of publishing only p values. Had it been possible with the experiments reviewed in this chapter, an evaluation of effect sizes would have been provided. For those studies providing sufficient data to calculate statistics such as omega-square (Hays, 1963) or d (Cohen, 1977), the magnitude of the effects were, in most cases, rather small, as seems appropriate for measures collected within the same person. Progress in neuropsychological research would be greatly facilitated if, coordinate with the development of standards for the reporting of stimulus parameters, the reporting of data were expanded to allow the reporting or at least the possible computation of such statistics as effect sizes. Meehl (1978) has discussed at some length the limitations of significance testing, and his conclusions seem applicable to the problems of lateralization research. The area of cerebral lateralization research is a fascinating one, loaded with interesting findings and with well-designed and executed experiments; it would be helpful to know more about them than is currently possible in our reporting of results.

It does not seem appropriate to end on what may seem a pessimistic note. Certainly, work in visual lateralization would benefit from greater precision in reporting of parameters and from fewer space and style limitations in the reporting of results. Such suggestions do not alter the fact that research in this area has made remarkable advances, both in theory and experimentation, and is well on the way to becoming an integral part of research on human cognition.

ACKNOWLEDGMENTS

I would like to thank Christine Chiarello, Nina Dronkers, and Hilary Naylor for their comments on drafts of this work. Special thanks are due Joseph Hellige, not only for his comments, but also for his almost saintly patience in waiting for me to finish this.

1. When I began this task, I initially tried a new approach to evaluating work in this area, a technique borrowed from social psychology known as "policy capturing." I wrote to about 50 individuals working in the area of cerebral asymmetry and asked them to nominate those papers that they felt represented the most significant contributions to the area and to indicate why they held that opinion. No other restrictions were placed on the nominations, and people were free to nominate their own work. As is usual with surveys of this sort, I did not get 100% return. I am grateful to those individuals who answered my requests, but will have to state that not much has come of it. As an attempt to discover communality of opinion about research in cerebral asymmetry, it was an unambiguous disaster. There is almost no agreement in this field as to what is important, significant, or "good." If a "champion" in this field were to be selected on the basis of my results, the winner would be selected on the basis of having perhaps *one* more nomination than several other people. Clearly, this field (or perhaps this researcher) is not ready for social techniques.

2. The argument has been made that Sergent's formulation is nothing more than a recasting of the analytic-holistic formulation. This criticism overlooks the fact that she has specified physical parameters for the proposed differences. Thus, she is entitled to use whatever language she wishes, since the distinctions are definable in physical terms, just as the physicists' "charm" is definable.

REFERENCES

Bateson, G., & Jackson, D.D. Some varieties of pathogenic organization. *Research Publications of the Association for Research on Nervous and Mental Diseases*, 1964, *42*, 270–283.

Beaton, A.A. Hemisphere function and dual task performance. *Neuropsychologia*, 1979, *17*, 629–635.

Berlucchi, G., Brizzolara, D., Marzi, C.A. et al. The role of stimulus discriminability and verbal codability in hemispheric specialization for visuospatial tasks. *Neuropsychologia*, 1979, *17*, 195–202.

Bertelson, P. Lateral differences in normal man and lateralization of brain function. *International Journal of Psychology*, 1982, *17*, 173–210.

Bevilaqua, L., Capitani, E., Luzzati, C., & Spinnler, H.R. Does the hemisphere stimulated play a specific role in delayed recognition of complex abstract patterns? A tachistoscopic study. *Neuropsychologia*, 1979, *17*, 93–97.

Birkett, P. Hemisphere differences in the recognition of nonsense shapes: Cerebral dominance or strategy effects? *Cortex*, 1978, *14*, 245–249.

Bogen, J.E. The other side of the brain: An appositional mind. *Bulletin of the Los Angeles Neurological Societies*, 1969, *34*, 135–162.

Boles, D. Laterally biased attention with concurrent verbal load: Multiple failures to replicate. *Neuropsychologia*, 1979, *17*, 353–361.

Bradshaw, J.L., & Nettleton, N.C. The nature of hemispheric specialization in man. *The Behavioral and Brain Sciences*, 1981, *4*, 51–91.

Broadbent, D.E. The hidden preattentive process. *The American Psychologist*, 1977, *32*, 109–118.

Bryden, M.P. Attentional factors in the detection of hemispheric asymmetries. In G. Underwood (Ed.), *Strategies of information processing*. New York: Academic Press, 1980.

Chiarello, C. A house divided? Cognitive functioning with callosal agenisis. *Brain and Language*, 1980, *11*, 128–158.

Chiarello, C., Dronkers, N.F., & Hardyck, C. Choosing sides: Some questions concerning the apparent instability of language lateralization in normal as compared to clinical populations. 1982, in press.

Cohen, G. Hemispheric differences in serial vs. parallell processing. *Journal of Experimental Psychology*, 1973, *97*, 349–356.

Cohen, G. Theoretical interpretations of lateral asymmetries. In J.G. Beaumont (Ed.), *Divided visual field studies of cerebral organization*. London: Academic Press, 1982.

Cohen, J. *Statistical power analysis for the behavioral sciences*. New York: Academic Press, 1977.

Davis, R., & Schmit, V. Timing the transfer of information between hemispheres in man. *Acta Psychologica*, 1971, *35*, 335–346.

Davis, R., & Schmit, V. Visual and verbal coding in the interhemispheric transfer of information. *Acta Psychologica*, 1973, *37*, 229–240.

Day, J. Visual half-field word recognition as a function of syntactic class and imageability. *Neuropsychologia*, 1979, *17*, 515–519.

De Valois, R.L., & De Valois, K.K. Spatial vision. In M.R. Rosenzweig & L.K. Porter (Eds.), *Annual Review of Psychology*. Palo Alto, Calif.: Annual Reviews, 1980.

Di Lollo, V. Hemispheric symmetry in duration of visible persistence. *Perception and Psychophysics*, 1981, *29*, 21–25.

Friedman, A., & Polson, M.C. Hemispheres as independent resource systems: Limited-capacity processing and cerebral specialization. *Journal of Experimental Psychology: Human Perception and Performance*, 1981, *7*, 1031–1058.

Galper, R.E., & Costa, L. Hemispheric superiority for recognizing faces depends upon how they are learned. *Cortex*, 1980, *16*, 21–38.

Gazzaniga, M.S. *The bisected brain*. New York: Appleton-Century-Crofts, 1970.

Goldberg, E., Vaughn, H.G., & Gerstman, L.J. Nonverbal descriptive systems and hemispheric asymmetry: Shape versus texture discrimination. *Brain and Language*, 1978, *5*, 249–257.

Graham, N. Psychophysics of spatial-frequency channels. In M. Kubovy & J.R. Pomerantz (Eds.), *Perceptual organization*. Hillsdale, N.J.: Erlbaum, 1981.

Hannay, H.J., Dee, H.L., Burns, J.W., & Masek, B.W. Experimental reversal of a left visual field superiority for forms. *Brain and Language*. 1981, *13*, 54–66.

Harcum, E.R. Lateral dominance as determinant of temporal order of responding. In M. Kinsbourne (Ed.), *Asymmetrical function of the brain*. London: Cambridge University Press, 1978.

Hardyck, C., Tzeng, O.J.L., & Wang, W. S-Y. Cerebral lateralization of function and bilingual decision processes: Is thinking lateralized? *Brain and Language*, 1978, *5*, 56–71.

Harvey, L.O., Jr. Single representation of the visual midline in humans. *Neuropsychologia*, 1978, *16*, 601–610.

Hatta, T. Visual field differences in a mental transformation task. *Neuropsychologia*, 1978, *16*, 637–641.

Hatta, T. & Dimond, S.J. Comparison of lateral differences for digit and random form recognition in Japanese and Westerners. *Journal of Experimental Psychology: Human Perception and Performance*, 1980, *6*, 368–374.

Hay, D.C. Asymmetries in face processing: Evidence for a right hemisphere perceptual advantage. *Quarterly Journal of Experimental Psychology*, 1981, *33*, 267–274.

Hays, W.L. *Statistics for psychologists*. New York: Holt, Rinehart & Winston, 1963.

Hellige, J.B. Effects of perceptual quality and visual field of probe stimulus presentation on memory search for letters. *Journal of Experimental Psychology: Human Perception and Performance*, 1980, *6*, 639–651.

Hellige, J.B., & Cox, P.J. Effects of concurrent verbal memory on recognition from the left and right visual fields. *Journal of Experimental Psychology: Human Perception and Performance*, 1976, *2*, 210–221.

Hellige, J.B., Cox, P.J., & Litvac, L. Information processing in the cerebral hemispheres: Selective hemispheric activation and capacity limitations. *Journal of Experimental Psychology: General*, 1979, *108*, 251–279.

Hellige, J.B., & Webster, R. Right hemisphere superiority for initial stages of letter processing. *Neuropsychologia*, 1979, *17*, 653–660.

Hellige, J.B., & Webster, R. Case effects in letter and name matching: A qualitative visual field difference. *Bulletin of the Psychonomic Society*, 1981, *17*, 179–182.

Jonides, J. Left and right visual field superiority for letter classification. *Quarterly Journal of Experimental Psychology*, 1979, *31*, 423–439.

Kahneman, D. *Attention and effort*. Englewood Cliffs, N.J.: Prentice-Hall, 1973.

Kinsbourne, M. The cerebral basis of lateral asymmetries in attention. *Acta Psychologica*, 1970, *33*, 193–201.

Kinsbourne, M. The control of attention by interaction between the cerebral hemispheres. In S. Kornblum (Ed.), *Attention and performance IV*. New York: Academic Press, 1973.

Kinsbourne, M. The mechanism of hemispheric control of the lateral gradient of attention. In P.M.A. Rabbitt & S. Dornic (Eds.), *Attention and performance V*. New York: Academic Press, 1975.

Kinsbourne, M., & Hicks, R.E. Functional cerebral space: A model for overflow, transfer, and interference effects in human performance. In J. Requin (Ed.), *Attention and performance VII*. Hillsdale, N.J.: Erlbaum, 1978.

Kirsner, K. Hemisphere-specific processes in letter matching. *Journal of Experimental Psychology: Human Perception and Performance*, 1980, *6*, 167–179.

Kirsner, K., & Brown, H. Laterality and recency effects in working memory. *Neuropsychologia*, 1981, *19*, 249–261.

Koff, E., & Riederer A. Hemispheric specialization for syntactic form. *Brain and Language*, 1981, *14*, 138–143.

Kohn, B. & Dennis, M. Patterns of hemispheric specialization after hemidecortication for infantile hemiplegia. In M. Kinsbourne & W.L. Smith (Eds.), *Hemispheric disconnection and cerebral function*. Springfield, Ill.: Charles C. Thomas, 1974.

Lashley, K.F. In search of the engram. In *Proceedings of the Society for Experimental Biology*. Cambridge, Mass., 1950.

Leehey, S.C., & Cahn, A. Lateral aymmetries in the recognition of words, familiar faces and unfamiliar faces. *Neuropsychologia*, 1979, *17*, 619–628.

Leehey, S., Carey, S., Diamond, R., & Cahn, A. Upright and inverted faces: The right hemisphere knows the difference. *Cortex*, 1978, *14*, 411–419.

Levy-Agresti, J., & Sperry, R.W. Differential perceptual capacities in major and minor hemispheres. *Proceedings of the U.S. National Academy of Sciences*, 1968, *61*, 1151.

Ley, R.G., & Bryden, M.P. Hemispheric differences in processing emotions and faces. *Brain and Language*, 1979, *7*, 127–138.

Luria, A.R. *Higher cortical functions in man*. New York: Basic Books, 1962.

Luria, A.R. *The neuropsychology of memory*. New York: John Wiley & Sons, 1976.

Madden, D.J., & Nebes, R.D. Hemispheric differences in memory search. *Neuropsychologia*, 1980, *18*, 665–673.

Martin, M. Hemispheric specialization for local and global processing. *Neuropsychologia*, 1979, *17*, 33–40.

Marzi, C., Di Stefano, M., Tassinari, G., & Crea, F. Iconic storage in the two hemispheres. *Journal of Experimental Psychology: Human Perception and Performance*, 1979, *5*, 31–41.

McCulloch, W.S. Cortico-cortical connections. In P. Bucy (Ed.) *The pre-central cortex*. Chicago: University of Illinois Press, 1944.

Meehl, P.E. Theoretical risks and tabular asterisks: Sir Karl, Sir Ronald and the slow progress of soft psychology. *Journal of Consulting and Clinical Psychology*, 1978, *46*, 806–834.

Moscovitch, M., & Klein, D. Material-specific perceptual inference for visual words and faces: Implications for models of capacity limitations, attention and laterality. *Journal of Experimental Psychology: Human Perception and Performance*, 1980, *6*, 590–604.

Navon, D. Forest before trees: The precedence of global features in visual processing. *Cognitive Psychology*, 1977, *9*, 353–383.

Navon, D., & Gopher, D. On the economy of the human processing system. *Psychological Review*, 1979, *86*, 214–255.

Niederbuhl, J., & Springer, S.P. Task requirements and hemispheric asymmetry for the processing of single letters. *Neuropsychologia*, 1979, *17*, 689–692.

Norman, D.A., & Bobrow, D.G. On the analysis of performance operating characteristics. *Cognitive Psychology*, 1975, *7*, 44–64.

Pitblado, C.B. Cerebral asymmetries in random-dot stereopsis: Reversal of direction with changes in dot size. *Perception*, 1979, *8*, 683–690.

Popper, K.R. *The logic of scientific discovery*. New York: Harper, 1968.

Reuter-Lorenz, P., & Davidson, R.J. Differential contributions of the two cerebral hemispheres to the perception of happy and sad faces. *Neuropsychologia*, 1981, *19*, 609–613.

Reynolds, D., & Jeeves, M.A. A developmental study of hemispheric specialization for recognition of faces in normal subjects. *Cortex*, 1978, *14*, 511–520.

Robertson, L. *Global processes and the perception of disoriented figures*. Unpublished doctoral dissertation, University of California, Berkeley, 1980.

St. John, R.C. Lateral asymmetry in face perception. *Canadian Journal of Psychology*, 1981, *35*, 213–223.

Safer, M.A. Sex and hemisphere differences in access to codes for processing emotional expressions and faces. *Journal of Experimental Psychology: General*, 1981, *110*, 86–100.

Segalowitz, S.J., & Stewart, C. Left and right lateralization for letter matching strategy and sex differences. *Neuropsychologia*, 1979, *17*, 521–525.

Semmes, J. Hemispheric specialization: A possible clue to mechanism. *Neuropsychologia*, 1968, *6*, 11–26.

Sergent, J. About face: Left-hemisphere involvment in processing physiognomies. *Journal of Experimental Psychology: Human Perception and Performance*, 1982a, *8*, 1–14.

Sergent, J. The cerebral balance of power: Confrontation or cooperation? *Journal of Experimental Psychology: Human Perception and Performance*, 1982b, *8*, 253–272.

Sergent, J., & Bindra, D. Differential hemispheric processing of faces: Methodological considerations and reinterpretations. *Psychological Bulletin*, 1981, *89*, 541–554.

Smith, A., & Sugar, O. Development of above normal language and intelligence 21 years after left hemispherectomy. *Neurology*, 1975, *25*, 813–818.

Sperry, R.W. Lateral specialization in the surgically separated hemispheres. In F.O. Schmitt & F.C. Worden (Eds.), *The neurosciences: Third study program*. Cambridge, Mass.: MIT Press, 1974.

Strauss, E. & Moscovitch, M. Perception of facial expressions. *Brain and Language*, 1981, *13*, 308–332.

Tomlinson-Keasey, C., & Kelly, R.R. A task analysis of hemispheric functioning. *Neuropsychologia*, 1979, *17*, 345–351.

Whitaker, H.A., & Ojeman, G.A. Lateralization of higher cortical functions: A critique. In S.J. Dimond & D.A. Blizard (Eds.), *Evolution and lateralization of the brain*. New York: New York Academy of Sciences, 1980.

Zaidel, E. Lexical organization in the right hemisphere. In P.A. Buser & A. Rogeul-Buser (Eds.), *Cerebral correlates of conscious experience*. Amsterdam: North-Holland, 1978.

8

Asymmetries of
Dual-Task Performance

Marcel Kinsbourne
Merrill Hiscock

This chapter deals with consequences of attempting to perform two activities simultaneously. In particular, it deals with situations in which the interaction between concurrent activities is lateralized, that is, situations in which a person's ability to perform the two tasks depends upon whether one of the tasks involves a left limb or the corresponding right limb. If the interaction is lateralized, for example, if speaking interferes to a greater degree with right-hand performance than with left-hand performance, certain inferences may be drawn about the way in which the respective activities are represented in the brain (Kinsbourne & Hicks, 1978).

BACKGROUND

Divided Attention

The dual-task method to be discussed belongs to a larger family of simultaneous-task methods used to study attention (Posner, 1982). Different concepts of attention lead to contradictory expectations about performance on tasks to be carried out simultaneously. If the human being is like a single channel device (such as a computer that processes information from only one terminal at a time), attention to one task should always impair performance on a concurrent attention-demanding task (Welford, 1952, 1959). Since attention is indivisible, multiple-task performance could be achieved only through repeated switching of attention from one channel to another. Alternatively, if the human being possesses several discrete pools of processing capacity (multiple channels), one would expect that, under at least some circumstances, a task could be as well performed together with another one as in isolation (Allport, 1980). A viewpoint intermediate between single channel theory and multiple capacity models, portrays people as limited capacity processors with the ability to allocate processing capacity in a flexible manner (Kahneman, 1973; Moray, 1967, Norman & Bobrow, 1975, Posner & Boies, 1971). According to the allocatable capacity viewpoint, attention may be divided among channels but the performance of multiple tasks requires more capacity than the performance of any one of them. Performance of one attention-demanding task will interfere with performance of a second such task only if the total capacity demand (workload) exceeds the available capacity.

A comprehensive evaluation of the different models is beyond the scope of the present chapter (see Kinsbourne, 1981), but some of the conditions favoring each model can be specified. In general, dual-task performance improves as a person becomes more practiced; as the temporal pattern of task demands becomes more predictable; as stimuli and responses become more compatible; and as components of the respective tasks become less similar (Allport, 1980; Fitts & Posner, 1967; Posner, 1982). Judicious selection of task parameters or intensive training of subjects (see Spelke, Hirst, & Neisser, 1976) reveal a remarkable capacity for performing two activities concurrently with little or no mutual interference. There are many everyday instances of this ability to time-share dissimilar and highly practiced tasks—for example, people singing while playing a piano or driving an automobile while engaging in conversation. Such evidence favors a multichannel interpretation. Under other conditions single-channel or allocatable capacity models, both of which imply limited capacity for multiple-task performance, are more satisfactory than multiple-channel models (e.g., Kerr, 1973; Klapp, 1979; Noble, Trumbo, & Fowler, 1967; Trumbo & Noble, 1970; Trumbo, Noble and Swink, 1967). To resolve the contradiction between outcomes, it is usually postulated that different organizational principles obtain at different levels of processing (e.g., Posner, 1978). Automatized activities are exempt from capacity limitations because they do not require attention (e.g., Bahrick, Noble, & Fitts, 1954; Bahrick & Shelly, 1958). Multiple channels could process information in parallel while a limited central attentional resource is switched serially or divided among channels.

Functional Cerebral Distance

The application of multiple-task methods to questions of cerebral lateralization is guided by an attribute of brain organization that has been termed the functional cerebral distance principle (Kinsbourne & Hicks, 1978). This principle stems from an understanding of the brain as a differentiated neural network (Kinsbourne, 1982; Sherrington, 1906). The brain contains localized networks, which are specialized for different functions, and these networks are connected with all other local networks. A pattern of activation in any one region may spread throughout much or all the cerebral cortex via the dendritic network, or neuropil, that unifies the entire cortex (Purpura, 1967). It is through particular spatiotemporal patterns of activation, generated in one local network and spread to others, that behavior is controlled. As an activation pattern spreads through the cortex, it becomes altered and perhaps attenuated. Each synapse slows the neurally transmitted message a little and, in some instances, mixes the message with others that originate in other local networks. Also, since some synapses are inhibitory, they serve to limit the spread of activation and to protect other local networks from being influenced by what may for them be an irrelevant message.

On the basis of the functional distance principle, it is possible to explain some of the major findings from multiple-task studies. First, differences in the ability to time-share between more and less similar tasks can be understood if it is assumed that categorically similar operations are represented in highly connected regions. Localization of function in network terms refers to the fact that particular parts of the cortex are better able than others to generate specific patterns of neuronal firing. Presumably, regions that generate similar neuronal activity patterns are highly interconnected. This interconnection allows for economical and efficient representation of the countless variations within a category, but it is also this interconnection among similar local networks that makes it difficult to perform two similar activities concurrently. Either one activity will preempt the other because its neural pattern of activity overrides that of the other, or else neither activity will be accomplished efficiently because of mutal interference, or cross talk. To the extent that two regions are only sparsely interconnected, as is generally the case of regions that are specialized for dissimilar tasks, the reciprocal influence of one region upon the other decreases. Consequently, the two regions are better able to control their respective behaviors concurrently.

Divided attention research suggests that, if the degree of similarity between two concurrent tasks is held constant, the ability to perform both tasks decreases as the difficulty of one or both tasks increases (Hiscock, Kinsbourne, Samuels, & Krause, 1982b; Johnston, Greenberg, Fisher, & Martin, 1970; Keele, 1967; Michon, 1964, 1966). According to the functional distance model, difficult tasks involve more cortical mass than easier tasks, and the spread of activation is accordingly more extensive. A particular region therefore might interfere with the functioning of regions that would lie outside its sphere of influence under conditions of less extensive activation. These are the tasks that, in subjective terms, are relatively demanding of attention. Conversely, actions that are very simple, highly automatized, or biologically preprogrammed are represented in much less cortical territory and consequently generate much less spread of activation to other regions.

The functional distance principle provides a parsimonious account of the findings from divided attention experiments; a single organizing principle can be applied to different levels of processing. It obviates the necessity to assume that there are discontinuities in the brain, whether between one "channel" and another or between automatic and attention-demanding processes. The notion of discrete channels can be translated into the concept of functionally distant regions and the distinction between automatic and attention-demanding processes reduces to a difference in the extensiveness of the activated cortical region. Task-similarity effects can be attributed to differences in the degree of connectedness between the respective regions. It follows from the model that attempts to overcome the effects of network interactions, that is, to perform two tasks concurrently, will lead to three possible outcomes (Kinsbourne, 1982). First, when the timing of the tasks is predictable, staggered processing may alleviate the interference. Spreading activation will not interfere as only one activity is being performed at that instant. In fact, it may even facilitate insofar as it "primes" the region responsible for performance of the second task (Boners & Heilman, 1976; Kinsbourne, 1970). Second, the person learns to segregate the tasks—in neural terms to establish an inhibitory barrier between the cortical regions involved in generation of the concurrent activities. This inhibitory barrier is a neuropsychological construct that corresponds to Navon and Gopher's (1979) term "concurrence cost" and Duncan's (1979) "emergent" third task. The addition of a second task imposes a necessity for keeping the two neural programs from intermingling. If the respective cortical regions are functionally close, then forming an inhibitory barrier will be difficult and it may not be completely effective. Third, when the inhibitory barrier is absent or ineffective there is cross talk between the respective regions, and interference is observed.

Lateralized Interference: Implications of the Functional Distance Principle

As a rule, one would expect neuronal connectivity to be greater within a hemisphere than between hemispheres. There is, nevertheless, one important exception: mirror-image loci in opposite hemispheres are so closely connected via the corpus callosum that the greatest interaction seems to occur between homologous sites rather than between physically closer sites within a hemisphere (see Kinsbourne & Hicks, 1978). For example, a movement or movement sequence performed by one limb tends to generate similar movements in the other limbs, and the amplitude of these "overflow" movements is greatest in the contralateral homologous limb (Cernacek, 1961; Clare & Bishop, 1949; Lundervold, 1951). Electromyographic (EMG) overflow to other limbs also is most marked in the case of the contralateral homologous limb (Davis, 1942a, b). Unilateral stimulation of sensory nerves elicits cortical responses not only from the contralateral hemisphere but also from the homologous region of the ipsilateral hemisphere (Dawson, 1947, 1954). Conditioned stimuli generalize readily from one somatic site to the mirror-image site on the opposite side of the body (Anrep, 1923; Gibson, 1939). Movement of one limb can serve to decrease the latency of movement with another limb, and the facilitation is greater when mirror-image pairs of limbs are involved than when diagonally paired limbs are involved (Blyth, 1962). Finally, training with one limb generalizes more completely to the contralateral homologous limb than to either the ipsilateral limb or to the diagonally opposite limb (Ammons and Ammons, 1970; Cook, 1933a, b, 1934).

Reviewing the studies cited above in the light of predictions of the functional cerebral distance principle, one finds that when one limb is being used, the limb movement has the greatest influence on the mirror-image limb; a lesser degree of influence on the ipsilateral limb; and the least influence on the diagonal limb. The nature of the influence—whether facilitative, disruptive, or irrelevant—depends on the nature of the tasks. Kinsbourne and Hicks (1978) describe an experiment in which interference between limbs was measured in an attempt to confirm the previously reported differences in the degree to which pairs of limbs interact. Adult subjects performed a two-limb, step-tracking task that required independent goal-directed movements by the various possible pairings of limbs working concurrently. Since it was likely that each of the two participating limbs would have to move by different amounts and in different directions on any particular trial, the situation was one in which any interaction among limbs was maladaptive. The outcome conformed to expectation: performance was worst when contralateral homologous limbs were performing; better when ispilateral limbs were performing; and best when diagonally crossed limbs were performing.

Between- versus within-hemisphere comparisons represent a special case of the more general principle of functional distance. The mirror-image locus apart, a given cortical region should be more highly interconnected with other regions within the same hemisphere than with loci in the opposite hemisphere. This difference is reflected in the greater interaction between ipsilateral limbs than between diagonally opposite limbs in several of the studies cited above. The logic underlying predictions of lateralized effects in dual-task experiments can be illustrated as follows. Consider the typical experiment, in which a cognitive process, C takes place concurrently with either left- or right-hand performance. Assume that C is controlled by activity in the corresponding region C of the left hemisphere only. Of the cortical regions for hand control, the left-hemispheric region will receive the greater amount of activation from region C. Consequently, if the activation in region C disrupts manual activity, right-hand activity should be disrupted more than left-hand activity.

Alternatively, it is possible that activation associated with cognitive processing presumably also spreads across the corpus callosum to homologous regions as does activation associated with manual activity. In that case, region C′ of the right hemisphere would be highly activated by activation of region C. However, as C′ has no motor function activation of C′ will have no direct influence on hand performance (although some of the activation in region C′ may spread to the right hemisphere hand area). Even if the right hemisphere hand area receives activation from C via both the left hemisphere hand area and region C′, the evidence reviewed subsequently in this chapter suggests that the right hemisphere hand area is less affected than the left hemisphere hand area.

Input Interference

The focus of this chapter is on experimental paradigms of two kinds: those entailing competition between two output processes (e.g., speaking and finger tapping) and those entailing competition between an output process and a cognitive process (e.g., finger tapping and memory encoding). Other dual-task paradigms involve competition between two inputs or interaction between an input process and a cognitive process. In fact, the most common measures of perceptual laterality may be regarded as divided attention tasks. Broadbent (1954) developed dichotic listening as a means of studying divided attention, and it was not until Kimura's (1961) application of the technique to patients with known speech representation that dichotic listening gained popularity as a measure of laterality. Similarly, many studies of visual half-field asymmetry are divided-attention studies insofar as they involve simultaneous presentation of competing stimuli into the left and right half-fields. Though most investigators currently prefer to present stimuli unilaterally, if a fixation stimulus at midline has also to be repeated, this makes the unilateral procedure a divided-attention task with competition between the midline and lateral stimuli. In the realm of tactile laterality, Witelson's (1974) dichaptic test is a divided-attention task that entails competition between left- and right-hand perception.

Besides perceptual tasks that involve competition between two different inputs, there have been attempts to bias perception (or attention) toward the left or right side by introducing a concurrent cognitive task that is either nonverbal or verbal in nature. For example, Kinsbourne (1970) reported that a concurrent memory load of six words caused subjects to show a right-sided advantage in the detection of gaps in a briefly exposed square. Without the verbal memory load the likelihood of failing to detect gaps on the right side of the square did not differ significantly from the likelihood of failing to detect gaps on the left side. Thus, the presumed activation of the left hemisphere seemed to facilitate perception of stimuli from the right side of space. Similar results were obtained in a subsequent series of gap-detection experiments (Kinsbourne, 1973, 1975), and other studies suggested that concurrent musical activity can bias perception (or attention) to the left (Gardner, Eagan, & Branski, 1973; Goodglass, Shai, Rosen, & Berman, 1971; Bruce & Kinsbourne, cited in Kinsbourne, 1975). Nevertheless, there have been several failures to find biases of this kind (Allard & Bryden, 1979; Boles, 1979; Gardner & Branski, 1976). It is clear from the work of Hellige and his colleagues (Hellige, 1978; Hellige & Cox, 1976; Hellige, Cox, & Litvac, 1979). that the influence of a concurrent task upon a visual perceptual task may be quite complex. For instance, it appears that the biasing effect of a verbal memory load upon form recognition changes in a nonmonotonic fashion as the memory load increased from zero to six nouns. The effect emerges as the set size increases from zero to two nouns and it remains substantial at four nouns, but it dissipates completely at a set of size of six nouns (Hellige & Cox, 1976). These findings imply that a memory load may fail to generate a laterality shift either because the load is insufficient or excessive. Moreover, biasing effects seem to differ between visual half-fields and as a function of whether or not the stimuli to be recognized are verbal (Hellige & Cox, 1976; Hellige, Cox, & Litvac, 1979)

Standard perceptual measures of laterality are less than ideal for testing predications of the functional distance model, although the results often can be explained in terms of the model. In dichotic listening, for example, increasing the similarity between competing stimuli tends to enhance the difficulty of the task (Berlin, Porter, Lowe-Bell et al., 1973; Cullen, Thompson, Hughes et al., 1974; Deatherage and Evans, 1969), and this similarity effect may be attributed to activation of identical or functionally close cortical regions by the similar signals. In most cases, investigators have focused their attention on right versus left differences without exploring the factors that control performance on one side or the other, or overall performance. Performance on all perceptual laterality tasks may entail shifting of attention from one stimulus to another. With the possible exception of the dichaptic task, in which such shifts may be observed in the pattern of palpation, these attentional shifts usually are covert. Consequently, a potentially important source of variation is uncontrolled and unmeasureable. In the auditory modality, it is possible to designate one input as the target and to vary the competing input along dimensions such as acoustic, phonetic, and semantic similarity to the target. This research strategy has been used in the past (e.g., Berlin et al., 1973), but experiments of this nature have not been designed specifically to test implications of the functional distance principle.

With the addition of a concurrent task to a perceptual task, certain predictions of the functional distance model can be evaluated. Studies of this nature require careful design and parametric variation of the independent variables. The main difficulty lies in the capacity of secondary tasks to have both facilitative and disruptive effects on perception. When the primary (perceptual) task is easy, the secondary task is likely to facilitate perception because arousal is heightened. The facilitation may be general or it may apply only to the side of space contralateral to the hemisphere being activated (Kinsbourne, 1970, 1973). As the secondary task becomes more difficult, its arousing properties may be offset by the maladaptive cross talk that it generates and at an even higher level of difficulty the interference may override the enhancement. Thus, as the secondary task is varied in difficulty, recognition of stimuli from the side of space contralateral to the activated hemisphere (and perhaps overall recognition performance as well) may assume the form of a Yerkes-Dodson function, with increasing facilitation giving way to interference at the highest level of difficulty (Hellige & Cox, 1976). The function, however, will not necessarily persist as the perceptual task or the secondary task is changed (Hellige & Cox, 1976; Hellige, Cox, & Litvac, 1979). Only after extensive examination of interactions among perceptual tasks and secondary tasks at various difficulty levels will it be possible to specify the precise way in which a concurrent task may alter visual perception and perceptual asymmetry.

COMPETITION BETWEEN TWO MOTOR
PROCESSES

There are several advantages in using ouput tasks to measure laterality. First, output processes appear to be more distinctly lateralized in the human brain than are input processes (LeDoux, Wilson, & Gazzaniga, 1977; Searleman, 1977). Secondly, the components of task performance tend to be more observable in output tasks than in perceptual tasks. For instance, if measuring finger tapping, one can measure speed, regularity, speed of downstroke, speed of upstroke, speed of up-down reversal, fatigue, and force modulation (Peters, 1980). Attentional trade-offs are less likely to bias laterality in output tasks than in input tasks. In dichotic listening, for example, an attentional shift toward the right ear implies a shift away from the left. Thus, the effect of the shift on measured laterality is likely to be relatively great. In a situation requiring concurrent performance of cognitive task and a manual task, the left and right hands usually will be tested separately. The subject may shift attention from the cognitive task to the hand or vice versa, but that shifting of attention will not affect performance with the other hand. It is likely that, when the other hand is tested, there will be similar shifts of attention from the cognitive task to that hand. Finally, with output tasks, the investigator is unlikely to encounter instances of facilitation. As a rule, the concurrent performance of output tasks yield a decrement in the performance of one or both tasks, even if the tasks are relatively undemanding (Kahneman, 1973; Kinsbourne, 1981; Welford, 1968).

The literature dealing with dual-task laterality will be divided into studies of interference between two output processes and studies of interference between an output process and a cognitive process. Studies within each category will be further divided according to whether the subjects were adults or children.

Motor-Motor Interference in Adults

Numerous findings, as summarized in Table 8-1, confirm Kinsbourne's and Cook's (1971) claim that speaking interferes more with right-hand than with left-hand performance in normal, right-handed adults. The kinds of manual performance that show lateralized interference include dowel-rod balancing (Hicks, 1975; Johnson & Kozma, 1977; Kinsbourne & Cook, 1971), typing letter sequences (Dalby, 1980; Hicks, Bradshaw, Kinsbourne, & Feigin, 1978; Hicks, Provenzano, & Rybstein, 1975), repetitive finger tapping (Bowers, Heilman, Satz, & Altman, 1978; Hellige & Longstreth, 1981), sequential finger tapping (Lomas, 1980; Lomas & Kimura, 1976), tapping keys sequentially by moving the arm (Lomas, 1980; Lomas & Kimura, 1976), and visuomotor tracking (Briggs, 1975). Despite a few failures to find lateralized interferences (e.g., Lomas & Kimura, 1976, Experiment 3; Wolff & Cohen, 1980), the preponderance of evidence shows clearly that speaking disrupts right-hand performance more than left-hand performance on a wide assortment of manual tasks.

This collection of experiments raises two questions of fundamental importance. First, at what level does the interference between speech and manual performance occur? Does the disruption of manual performance reflect interferences at the level of motor programming, or is lateralized cognitive activity (verbal thinking) sufficient to account for the effect? Second, is it possible to demonstrate the opposite effect, that is, selective disruption of left-hand performance from concurrent execution of a nonverbal motor task?

Two studies from Table 8-1 (Hellige & Longstreth, 1981; Hicks et al., 1975) address the first of these questions directly and do so by examining verbal-manual interference with and without overt vocalization. In the Hicks et al. study, verbal rehearsal was performed concurrently with either bimanual (Experiment 1) or unimanual (Experiment 2) typing. Prior to each dual-task trial, a string of eight letters each was presented on a memory drum. Each string was a zero-, first-, second-, or fourth-order approximation to English. The presented string was to be rehearsed during the dual-task trial, after which the subject was asked to write the eight letters in the correct (left-to-right) order. On half of the trials at each level of letter-string difficulty, the letters were rehearsed aloud; on the other trials, rehearsal was silent. In both experiments, silent rehearsal disrupted typing to a lesser degree than did vocal rehearsal, but the difference was additive across hands, that is, the asymmetry of interference did not vary with the mode of rehearsal. Neither the hand used for typing (the hand leading the sequence in the case of bimanual typing) nor mode of rehearsal had a significant effect on recall of letter strings. These findings by Hicks et al. imply that, although some of the interference between speech and manual activity takes place at the output (motor) level, asymmetries of interference do not depend on output-output competition. A similar but slightly different conclusion may be derived from the Hellige and Longstreth study. In the first of their two experiments, Hellige and Longstreth required subjects to read a paragraph for 15 seconds while tapping a telegraph key with the index finger on either the left or right hand. A different paragraph was used for each of four dual-task conditions, that is to say, reading aloud with left-hand tapping, reading aloud with right-hand tapping, reading silently with left-hand tapping, and reading silently with right-hand tapping. When tapping rate in the concurrent-task conditions was compared with baseline tapping rate with the same hand, it was found that reading aloud was more disruptive than silent reading. That is, the reduction in tapping rate, averaged across hands, was greater in the reading aloud conditions than in the reading silently conditions. This is analogous with what Hicks et al. found; generalized interference was greater with vocal rehearsal than with silent rehearsal. Nevertheless, in the Hellige and Longstreth experiment, the effect for reading mode and the effect for hand was not additive. A silent versus aloud × hand interaction indicated that the asymmetry of interference was greater in the reading aloud conditions than in the reading silently conditions. From this finding, one can conclude that both the congnitive and the motor components of reading aloud contribute not only to generalized interference with concurrent manual activity but also to the lateralization of interference. Alternatively, since the overall interference in the silent reading conditions was only 4.9% (as opposed to 8.7% in the reading aloud conditions), the degree of asymmetry may have been constrained by a floor effect.

The second experiment of Hellige's and Longstreth's study approaches the level-of-interference question in a different manner. In their first experiment, as in the two Hicks et al. experiments, the effects of motor activity were isolated by contrasting the effects of motor-plus-cognitive activity with the effects of cognitive activity alone. In the second Hellige and Longstreth experiment, the effects of cognitive activity were isolated by contrasting the effects of motor-plus-cognitive activity with the effects of motor activity alone. Subjects in the second experiment used their free hand to solve Block Design problems from the Wechsler Intelligence Scale for Children-Revised while concurrently tapping a telegraph key for 15 seconds with the index finger of either the left or right hand. Insofar as the Block Design task entailed both cognitive and motor components, the investigators included control conditions in which subjects handled the blocks in a way that presumably required little cognitive processing. Half of the subjects continuously rotated a single block in a clockwise direction during the 15-second dual-task trial, and the other half of the subjects placed blocks, one by one, into a box and removed them again if time permitted. As these two motor activities had equivalent effects on tapping, data for both tasks were pooled in the authors' main analyses. It was found that block manipulation per se slowed tapping rate, irrespective of hand, by 14% relative to the baseline tapping rate, but this reduction was significantly less than that associated with solution of Block Design problems. Manipulation of blocks per se, as well as solution of Block Design problems, disrupted left-hand tapping more than right-hand tapping. However, there was a significant motor only versus block design × hand interaction, which shows that the asymmetry of interference was greater in the combined motor-plus-cognitive conditions than in the motor-only conditions. The inference, then, is that output-output interference may be lateralized, but introduction of a cognitive component to one of the motor tasks adds lateralized as well as generalized interference.

Any of several differences between the Hicks et al. study and that of Hellige and Longstreth might account for the different outcomes with respect to the lateralized or nonlateralized nature of interference at the motor level. For instance, Hicks et al. compared the number of letters typed in the silent rehearsal conditions with the number typed in the vocal rehearsal conditions, whereas Hellige et al. based their comparison on ratios reflecting the percentage reduction in tapping rate, relative to the control conditions. This difference in statistical treatment potentially could affect the silent versus aloud X hand interaction, as the existence of interaction effects sometimes depends upon the scale of measurement (Tukey, 1949). The results of the two studies, however, are more notable for their similarities than for their differences. In particular, both studies show that asymmetries of interference between verbal and manual tasks may occur in the absence of vocalization. Several other studies, which will be discussed below, also show that a cognitive task with little or no overt motor activity may interfere asymmetrically with manual performance.

Hellige's and Longstreth's second experiment and several others summarized in Table 8-1, address the second issue, that is to say, whether it is possible to demonstrate selective disruption of left-hand performance. Hellige's and Longstreth's second experiment shows that the direction of interference asymmetries may be reversed, that is, an activity putatively lateralized to the right hemisphere interfered more with concurrent left-hand performance than with concurrent right-hand performance. Nevertheless, the Hellige and Longstreth Block Design task falls short of being an ideal nonverbal analogue for recititation. The use of different organs to interfere with the left and right hands (use of the left hand to interfere with the right and vice versa) introduces some complications into the picture. It is difficult to ascertain whether the task is equally difficult for both hands and whether attention is allocated to each hand in comparable ways across conditions. Moreover, there is evidence that the spread of motor activity and transfer of motor training from one hand to the other is greater from left to right than from right to left (Hicks, Frank, & Kinsbourne, 1982), and it is not clear how these factors might affect dual-task performance.

The ideal nonverbal analogue for speaking would entail non-verbal vocalization. If the cognitive rather than the motor component of speech generates lateralized interference with concurrent manual performance, one might expect to find reversed lateralization of interference with a nonverbal vocalic task, such as humming or "la-la-ing" a melody. Even if the motor act of vocalization generates some selective interference with the right hand

(Hellige & Longstreth, 1981), that asymmetry should be nullified or overridded by the right-hemispheric cognitive components of the nonverbal task. According to this argument, nonverbal vocalization should yield either equivalent levels of interference with left- and right-hand performance or selective interference with the left hand. Extant findings, however, fail to confirm this expectation. Of six experiments from Table 8-1 that entail nonverbal vocalization, none yielded a left-greater-than-right pattern of interference, and only one (Lomas & Kimura, 1976, Experiment 1) showed bilaterally equivalent levels of interference. In two experiments (Hicks, 1975, Experiment 4; Hicks, Bradshaw, Kinsbourne, & Feigin, 1978, Experiment 2), nonverbal vocalization interfered to a greater degree with right-hand than with left-hand performance, and in three other experiments (Johnson & Kozma, 1977; Lomas & Kimura, 1976, Experiments 2 & 3), nonverbal vocalization had no measurable effect on concurrent performance with either hand.

In his Experiment 4, Hicks (1975) compared the effects of humming with the effects of verbal recitation upon the dowel-rod balancing. Prior to each humming trial, the experimenter hummed a portion of a popular song from the 1950s, and the subject subsequently hummed that melodic segment while balancing a dowel rod. The verbal task entailed recitation of the lyrics corresponding to the tune, for example, "by the light of the silvery moon." Both vocalization tasks caused generalized and lateralized interference with rod balancing, and the respective effects of the two tasks could not be differentiated. Other investigators, using similar tasks, obtained different results. Lomas and Kimura (1976), in their first experiment, instructed subjects to "la-la" the tune of "Jingle Bells" while balancing a dowel rod. In this instance, interference was bilateral. The nonverbal vocalization disrupted the balancing performance of both hands about equally. Yet another outcome was reported by Johnson and Kozma (1977), whose subjects listened to a tape-recorded melody and then hummed it while balancing a dowel rod. These investigators selected short, simple melodies for which there were no lyrics. Statistical analyses revealed neither generalized nor lateralized interference in this study, that is, humming had no measurable effect on manual performance.

The situation is not clarified by the other three experiments, in which sequential finger or arm movement replaced dowel-rod balancing as the manual task. Hicks et al. (1978) instructed their subjects to "tra-la" the first stanza of "Reveille" while typing an eight-letter sequence with one hand or the other. As in the earlier experiment by Hicks (1975), verbalization and nonverbal vocalization had almost identical effects on manual performance and both disrupted right-hand performance more than left-hand performance. Nevertheless, Lomas and Kimura (1976, Experiments 2 & 3) reported that "la-la-ing" a tune had neither generalized nor lateralized effects on the ability of right-handers to tap telegraph keys in sequence with the index, middle, ring, and little finger, to tap telegraph keys in sequence with the clenched hand, or to tap a single key repetitively with the index finger. Comparison of the Hicks et al. study with the Lomas and Kimura study suggests that the discrepancy in outcomes might be attributable to differences in the difficulty of the manual task. Of the three levels of difficulty established by Hicks and his colleagues, only the easiest seems comparable in difficulty with the most difficult tapping task used by Lomas and Kimura. Since Hicks et al. found that the interfering effects of vocalization increased markedly as the manual task became more difficult, it seems plausible that Lomas and Kimura might also have found generalized and lateralized interference with their musical task, had the manual task been difficult. The nonverbal vocalization tasks used by the respective investigators seem also to differ in difficulty or at least in their disruptive properties. "Reveille" has a particularly compelling rhythm (presumable adapted to arousing soldiers from sleep). In fact, Hicks et al. found that the "tra-la-ing" of "Reveille" caused significantly more typing errors than did verbal recitation. This finding contrasts with Lomas's and Kimura's tendency to find generalized interference with verbal recitation but not with nonverbal vocalization.

A third theoretical issue has been raised by Lomas and Kimura (1976), who argue that speaking interferes selectively with right-hand activity only if the manual activity entails rapid sequential positioning with minimal visual guidance. The significance of this issue lies in its relevance to the view that the left cerebral hemisphere is specialized for the programming of manual sequences, irrespective of the hand with which they are executed (Kimura, 1976; Kimura & Archibald, 1974). Lomas's and Kimura's (1976) dual-task evidence, however, seems to run contrary to expectations. Their data suggest that speaking disrupts right-hand performance selectively for tasks requiring movement sequences but not for simple repetitive movement. Recitation of a nursery rhyme slowed sequential finger tapping only with the right hand and sequential arm tapping only with the right arm, but the same recitation task slowed repetitive finger tapping, bilaterally. If the left hemisphere controls sequential movement bilaterally and simple finger flexion contralaterally, then one would expect speaking to interfere with sequential movement bilaterally and with repetitive movement on the right side only. In other words, the results were exactly the opposite of what one would have expected. Lomas and Kimura (1976) recognize the paradoxical nature of their findings and suggest that the interference between speaking and sequential tapping must occur "at some point beyond the bilateral control exerted by the left hemisphere, i.e., at a point where the programme of movements has already been transmitted to the left hand" (p. 31). As the investigators acknowledge, that explanation cannot account for their failure to find lateralized interference with repetitive finger tapping.

TABLE 8-1.
Studies of Output–Output Interference in Adults

Study	Subjects	Manual Task	Concurrent Task(s)	Results
Kinsbourne & Cook, 1971	20 normal right-handed 19- and 20-year-olds	Balancing a dowel rod on the index finger	Continuous repetition of a sentence	Recitation decreased balancing duration with the right hand but increased balancing duration with the left hand.
Briggs, 1975	16 right-handed volunteers (8 males, 8 females)	Bimanual tracking on an NASA Complex Coordinator. Left and right hands were used concurrently in the performance of independent tracking tasks.	Continuous repetition of any memorized prose passage, with delayed (220 msec) auditory feedback	Recitation with delayed auditory feedback increased the number of right-hand errors and had no significant effect on the number of left-hand errors.
Hicks, 1975 Experiment 1	13 normal, right-handed males; 13 normal, left-handed males without familial sinistrality; 9 normal left-handed males with familial sinistrality	Balancing a dowel rod on the index finger	Continuous repetition of a phrase	Recitation decreased only right-hand balancing duration in right-handers, but it decreased balancing duration with both hands in left-handers. Recitation rate was faster with the right hand than with the left.

TABLE 8-1., Continued

Study	Subjects	Manual Task	Concurrent Task(s)	Results
Experiment 2	26 normal, right-handed males without familial sinistrality; 26 normal, right-handed males with familial sinistrality	Balancing a dowel rod on the index finger	Half of the subjects within each group repeated phonetically easy phrases, and half repeated phonetically difficult phrases ("tongue twisters").	Recitation decreased only right-hand balancing duration; the effect was greater with difficult phrases than with easy phrases. Verbal production did not differ in left- and right-hand conditions, but more errors were made when subjects were balancing with the right hand.
Experiment 3	39 normal, right-handed males without familial sinistrality; 18 normal, right-handed males with familial sinistrality	Balancing a dowel rod on the index finger; within each familial sinistrality group, one-third of the subjects were assigned to one of the following treatments: no practice in rod balancing, 2 practice trials with each hand, 6 practice trials with each hand.	Continuous repetition of a phrase	Recitation decreased only right-hand balancing duration in subjects without familial sinistrality; recitation decreased balancing duration with both hands in subjects with familial sinistrality. Practice in rod balancing did not affect either the magnitude or the asymmetry of interference. Verbal production did not differ in left- and right-hand conditions.

	Subjects	Manual task	Concurrent verbal task	Results
Experiment 4	12 normal, right-handed males without familial sinistrality; 12 normal, right-handed males with familial sinistrality	Balancing a dowel rod on the index finger	Continuous humming of a tune or continuous repetition of the lyrics corresponding to the tune	Both humming and recitation of lyrics decreased right-hand but not left-hand balancing duration.
Hicks, Provenzano, & Rybstein, 1975 Experiment 1	20 normal, right-handed university students (8 males, 12 females)	Repeated typing of a sequence requiring both hands; the left hand led the sequence on some trials, and the right hand led the sequence on other trials.	Vocal or silent rehearsal of letter strings with varying degrees of approximation to English	The concurrent tasks generated more interference with the right hand leading the sequence than with the left hand. Neither letter-string difficulty nor rehearsal mode altered the laterality of interference. Recall of letter strings did not differ between right-hand-leading and left-hand-leading conditions.
Experiment 2	24 normal, right-handed university students (9 males, 15 females)	Repeated typing of a sequence requiring 4 fingers of one hand	Vocal or silent rehearsal of letter strings with varying degrees of approximation to English	The concurrent tasks interfered more with right-hand performance than with left-hand performance. Neither letter-string difficulty nor rehearsal altered the laterality of interference.

TABLE 8-1., Continued

Study	Subjects	Manual Task	Concurrent Task(s)	Results
Majeres, 1975				
Experiment 1	20 right-handed male university students	Turning an activity wheel with the left or right hand	Naming colors at two levels of difficulty (The difficult task was a Stroop test.)	The hand used to turn the wheel had no effect on time required to name the colors. The effect on wheel turning was not assessed.
Experiment 2	24 subjects (details not specified in report)	Balancing a dowel rod on the index finger	Verbalizing (details not specified in report)	No significant asymmetry of interference
Lomas & Kimura, 1976				
Experiment 1	24 right-handed university students (12 males, 12 females)	Balancing a dowel rod on the index finger	Continuous repetition of a nursery rhyme; vocalization ("la-la") of a familiar tune	Overall and for females, the concurrent tasks had no lateralized effect on balancing duration. For males, nonspeech vocalization interfered with balancing bimanually, and speaking interfered only with right-hand balancing.
Experiment 2	48 university students (12 right-handed males; 12 right-handed females; 12 left-handed males; 12 left-handed females)	Sequential tapping of four telegraph keys with index, middle, ring, and little fingers of one hand	Continuous repetition of a nursery rhyme; vocalization ("la-la") of a familiar tune	For right-handers, recitation disrupted sequencing with the right hand but not with the left; nonspeech

				vocalization had no significant effect on performance with either hand. For left-handers, both vocal tasks disrupted performance with both hands.
Experiment 3	18 right-handed university students (9 males, 9 females)	1. Sequential tapping of four telegraph keys with the clenched hand 2. Repetitive tapping of a single telegraph key with the index finger of one hand	Continuous repetition of a nursery rhyme; vocalization ("la-la") of a familiar tune	Recitation disrupted arm-tapping performance with the right arm only; nonspeech vocalization had no significant effect on the performance of either arm. Recitation interfered with the finger tapping of both hands; nonspeech vocalization had no significant effect on the performance of either hand.

TABLE 8-1., Continued

Study	Subjects	Manual Task	Concurrent Task(s)	Results
Bowers, Heilman, Satz, & Altman, 1978 Experiment 1	24 right-handed university students (12 males, 12 females)	Repetitive tapping of a lever with the index finger of one hand	Reciting as many words as possible that begin with a specified letter	Recitation slowed tapping rate in both hands, but the right hand was affected more than the left. Tapping had no significant effect on verbal production.
Hicks, Bradshaw, Kinsbourne, & Feigin, 1978 Experiment 2	72 right-handed university students	Repeated typing of a sequence requiring the index, middle, ring, and little fingers; each subject performed the task at one of three levels of difficulty.	Continuous repetition of a sentence or continuous "tra-la-ing" of the first stanza of "Reveille"	Both vocalization tasks disrupted right-hand performance more than left-hand performance, and the asymmetry of interference increased linearly with the difficulty of the sequence to be typed.
Johnson & Kozma, 1977	18 right-handed university students (9 males, 9 females)	Balancing a dowel rod on the index finger	Continuous repetition of a sentence or continuous humming of a melody	For females, neither vocalization task had a significant effect on duration of rod balancing. For males,

274

Wolff & Cohen, 1980 Experiment 1	30 right-handed university graduates between the ages of 23 and 41 years (7 males and 7 females without familial sinistrality; 8 males and 8 females with familial sinistrality)	Tapping a key with the index finger in synchrony with a metronome; unimanual and alternating bimanual tasks were performed.	Continuous repetition of the first part of a nursery rhyme	sentence recitation disrupted right-hand performance only; humming had no effect on performance with either hand. In the unimanual conditions, recitation had no significant effect on the regularity of tapping with either hand; in the bimanual condition, recitation disrupted mainly right-hand performance in women.
Experiment 2	30 right-handed university graduates between the ages of 23 and 40 years (7 males and 8 females without familial sinistrality; 8 males and 7 females with familial sinistrality)	Tapping a key with the index finger in synchrony with a metronome; unimanual and alternating bimanual tasks were performed.	Reading aloud from unfamiliar text	In both unimanual and bimanual conditions, reading disrupted the regularity of tapping with the left and right hands; there was no significant lateralization of interference, even though 24 of the 30

TABLE 8-1., Continued

Study	Subjects	Manual Task	Concurrent Task(s)	Results
				subjects showed greater interference with the right hand than with the left on the unimanual task.
Dalby, 1980	30 right-handed university students (15 males, 15 females)	Repeated typing of a sequence requiring the index, middle, ring, and little finger of one hand	1. Continuous repetition of a sentence 2. Reading aloud from a word list	Both verbal tasks disrupted right-hand performance more than left-hand performance. For both verbal tasks, more words were produced during left-hand tapping than during right-hand tapping.
Lomas, 1980 Experiment 1	32 right-handers (16 males, 16 females)	1. Sequential tapping of four telegraph keys with the clenched hand 2. Sequential tapping of four telegraph keys with the index, middle, ring, and little finger of one hand On half of the	Continuous repetition of a nursery rhyme	When the arm was moved without opportunity for visual guidance, recitation disrupted tapping with the right arm only; when visual guidance was possible, recitation did not disrupt tapping with either arm. When the fingers were moved without

276

Study	Subjects	Task	Results
		trials in each condition, the subject's view of the keys was occluded.	opportunity for visual guidance, recitation disrupted tapping with the right hand only; when visual guidance was possible, recitation disrupted tapping with only the left hand.
Experiment 2	16 right-handers (8 males, 8 females)	Continuous repetition of a nursery rhyme / Sequential tapping of four telegraph keys with the index, middle, ring, and little finger of one hand	Irrespective of whether visual guidance of finger movements was possible, recitation disrupted tapping with the right hand only.
Hellige & Longstreth, 1981 Experiment 1	48 right-handed university students (26 males, 22 females)	Repetitive tapping of a telegraph key with the index finger of one hand / Reading aloud from unfamiliar text; reading silently from unfamiliar text; half of the subjects expected to be tested on the material, and the other subjects were told that the content of the material was irrelevant.	Reading aloud disrupted right-hand tapping more than left-hand tapping in both the test and no-test groups. Silent reading disrupted right-hand tapping more than left-hand tapping only in the test group. For both groups, the asymmetry of

TABLE 8-1., Continued

Study	Subjects	Manual Task	Concurrent Task(s)	Results
				interference was greater when subjects were reading aloud than when they were reading silently.
Experiment 2	48 right-handed university students (24 males, 24 females)	Repetitive tapping of a telegraph key with the index finger of one hand	Solving Wechsler Block Design problems of two difficulty levels, using the hand opposite to the tapping hand; each subject performed one of two motor-only control tasks, placing blocks into a box or continuously rotating a block.	Solving Block Design problems disrupted left-hand tapping more than right-hand tapping. The motor-only tasks also disrupted left-hand tapping more than right-hand tapping, but the asymmetry was less marked than in the Block Design conditions. Performance on Block Design problems did not differ between hands.

Lomas (1980) reiterated the argument that asymmetric interference is seen only with sequential tasks that require little or no visual guidance, and he attempted to demonstrate the importance of visual guidance. In his first experiment, Lomas duplicated the two conditions from the Lomas and Kimura study—sequential arm tapping and sequential finger tapping—that had yielded lateralized interference. On half of the trials, however, the screen occluding the keys was removed, and the subjects were encouraged "to view their arm and the keys to help performance" (Lomas, 1980, p. 142). Lomas speculated that sequential finger tapping would be guided by a nonvisual limb-positioning system, irrespective of whether visual guidance were available, but that arm tapping would become visually guided if the opportunity for such guidance were available. If lateralized interference depends upon involvement of a nonvisually guided system, lateralized interference should be found, Lomas reasoned, with finger tapping, irrespective of the availability of visual guidance and with arm tapping only when visual guidance is not available. These predictions were only partially supported. Speaking interfered only with right-arm performance on the arm-tapping task with occluded vision and with neither arm's performance on the same task with the occluding screen removed. Interference effects on the sequential finger-tapping task were anomalous; speaking interfered only with right-hand tapping when vision was occluded and only with left-hand tapping when the occluding screen was removed. Moreover, since subjects tapped faster when the screen was absent than when it was present, the data contradict Lomas's assumption that sequential finger tapping would be controlled via a nonvisual limb-positioning system even when visual guidance was available. Lomas repeated the sequential finger-tapping experiment and obtained entirely different results, that is to say, the availabilty of visual guidance did not improve performance significantly, and speaking interfered with right-hand but not left-hand tapping, irrespective of whether or not the hand was occluded. The reason for the striking disparity between the outcomes of Experiments 1 and 2 is not evident.

What can be concluded about the claim that lateralized interference is obtained only with sequential tasks and only when nonvisual control is involved? First, some investigators have found asymmetric interference, using repetitive finger tapping (Bowers et al., 1978; Hellige & Longstreth, 1981). In the child literature, to be reviewed subsequently, there are numerous examples in which speaking interferes asymmetrically with simple repetitive finger tapping. It has been shown repeatedly that speech has an asymmetrical effect on dowel-rod balancing (Hicks, 1975, Experiments 1–4; Kinsbourne & Cook, 1971). Although dowel-rod balancing does not entail repetitive movement in the same sense that finger tapping does, the movements required to balance a dowel rod are not sequential in the way that the movements required to tap a series of keys are sequential. Thus, apart from the Lomas and Kimura (1976) study, there is little evidence to suggest that a manual must require sequential movement if lateralized interference is to be obtained. The same might be said about the necessity to prevent visual guidance of the manual act; in most of the studies outlined in Table 8-1, the investigators obtained asymmetric interference effects without finding it necessary to occlude their subjects' view of their hands. Hicks et al. (1978) presumably accentuated the role of vision by color-coding the typewriter keys and instructing subjects to strike a key of a particular color with a particular finger. Although subjects must fixate on the rod rather than on the hand while balancing a dowel rod, the hand and arm movements are made in response to visual information. If other investigators have obtained asymmetric interference effects using nonrepetitive, visually guided tasks, one might ask why Lomas and Kimura (1976) and Lomas (1980) failed to find such effects under similar circumstances. A parsimonious explanation is that task difficulty exerts a strong influence on the outcome of dual-task studies. In Experiment 1 of Lomas's and Kimura's (1976) study, the expected results were obtained with males, that is, nonverbal vocalization disrupted dowel-rod balancing bilaterally, and recitation disrupted balancing with the right hand only. In contrast, neither vocalization task had a significant effect, either generalized or lateralized, on the balancing performance of females. Inspection of the mean balancing times reveals that, in the control conditions, females balanced the dowel rod less than half as long as did males, even though data for 9 of 21 females had been discarded because these women failed to meet the minimum balancing time criterion of 5 seconds. For some reason, dowel-rod balancing seems to be more difficult for females than for males (see Johnson & Kozma, 1977). In the Lomas and Kimura (1976) study, females performed so poorly on the task in the control conditions that balancing performance actually improved slightly when the recitation task was being performed concurrently (a nonsignificant average increase of 11% from 19.2 to 21.3 seconds, as compared with males' significant average decrease of 17% from 48.2 to 40.0 seconds). Clearly, there can be no lateralization of interference if there is no interference. One could argue that other tasks used by Lomas and Kimura (1976) and by Lomas (1980) were too easy to ensure the generation of stable interference effects. In Experiment 3 of the Lomas and Kimura study, subjects were required to combine the relatively easy speaking task of nursery rhyme recitation with the relatively easy manual task of tapping a telegraph key repetitively. Consequently, tapping rate in the dual-task condition, averaged across hands, decreased only 5.1% from the rate in the control conditions. Although this decrement was statistically significant, it constitutes a small range in which to detect an asymmetry. In comparison, sequential finger tapping and sequential arm tapping in the same study reduced mean tapping rate by 7.8% and 10.0%, respectively. Lomas (1980) failed to find asymmetric interference when subjects recited a nursery rhyme and engaged in sequential arm tapping with opportunity for visual guidance, but generalized interference in that condition was only 3.6%, as compared with 13.7% when vision was occluded (in which case a significant asymmetry of interference was found). Although it is possible to find statistically significant lateralization of interference with as little as 4% or 5% decrease in manual performance, relative to baseline conditions (Hellige & Longstreth, 1981, Experiment 1; Lomas, 1980, Experiment 2), it seems that asymmetric interference is more likely to be observed when the combination of tasks is sufficiently difficult to decrease manual performance by several percentage points. For example, Hicks et al. (1975) found a strongly lateralized interference effect under conditions in which verbal rehearsal decreased manual performance by 19.2%. In this case, the lateralization of interference was so marked that there was a crossover interaction between leading hand and condition; right-hand-leading performance was superior to left-hand-leading performance in the control condition, but the effect was reversed when concurrent rehearsal was required.

Within certain limits, task difficulty may be altered without radically altering the lateralization of interference (e.g., Hellige & Longstreth, 1981; Hicks, Provenzano, & Rybstein, 1975). Under some circumstances, however, increasing the difficulty of either the manual task (Hicks, Bradshaw, Kinsbourne, & Feigin, 1978) or the concurrent vocalic task (Hicks, 1975) increases the degree to which interference is lateralized. When one task or the other becomes excessively difficult, lateralization of interference might decrease again, although this has not been shown in a parametric study. The influence of task difficulty upon asymmetries of verbal-manual interference probably varies from task to task and probably is dependent upon the exact nature of the interaction between tasks. Unless two different tasks are equated for difficulty or for degree of generalized interference with a concurrent task, one cannot be sure that laterality differences are attributable to specific properties of the tasks—such as sequential or repetitive movement—or to differences in task difficulty.

Motor-Motor Interference in Children

The evidence for asymmetric vocal-manual interference in children is summarized in Table 8-2. These studies are similar to those outlined in Table 8-1, except that the difficulty of the tasks has been adjusted to make the tasks more appropriate for children. There are no studies that require dowel-rod balancing or tapping sequentially with four fingers; instead, the manual tasks consist of either repetitive tapping with the index finger or of alternate tapping of two keys. Usually the vocal task consists of recitation of a nursery rhyme or list of familiar words, but children also have hummed, recited "tongue twisters," and read a list of words while engaged in concurrent finger tapping.

Most of the studies with children were undertaken for the purpose of demonstrating the same kind of interference asymmetry as seen in adults. Since this asymmetry would be expected only if speech is lateralized, evidence from dual-task experiments with children could be used to infer the presence or absence of speech lateralization in children. Thus, the dual-task procedure constitutes a novel means of addressing the long-standing controversy over the developmental course of left-hemispheric specialization for speech (see Kinsbourne & Hiscock, 1977; Lenneberg, 1967; Porter & Berlin, 1975; Satz, Bakker, Teunissen et al., 1975). The results in this regard are remarkably consistent across studies; not a single study has failed to find asymmetric interference in normal, right-handed children. Moreover, a lateralized effect of speaking upon finger tapping has been found in the youngest children tested (3-year-olds), and the magnitude of the asymmetry appears to remain constant between the ages of 3 and 12 years (Hiscock & Kinsbourne, 1978, 1980; Kinsbourne & McMurray, 1975; Piazza, 1977; White & Kinsbourne, 1980). There are only two exceptions to the finding of constant interference asymmetry across childhood (Hiscock, 1982; Hiscock, Kinsbourne, Samuels, & Krause, 1982b). Both of these studies are cross-sectional; both study children across a limited age range; and the developmental trends observed are in opposite directions. In an experiment requiring children to recite a "tongue twister" while tapping two telegraph keys alternately (Hiscock, 1982), it was found that the asymmetry of interference increased from grade three to grade five. The opposite pattern was found with one of the dependent variables in a study in which children in grades one through four recited a list of animal names while tapping a telegraph key repetitively (Hiscock et al., 1982b). When interference was measured in terms of change in tap-to-tap variability from the control conditions to the dual-task conditions, the asymmetry of interference decreased with increasing age. However, when the usual measure of interference was used, that is, change in tapping rate from the control conditions to the dual-task conditions, the asymmetry of interference remained constant across the four-year age range. These two conflicting findings of developmental change in degree of asymmetry may reflect sampling error, or they may show valid age-related changes that may be found with particular tasks and particular measures of interference; nevertheless, in most cases, the degree to which interference is lateralized remains invariant across a wide span of childhood years.

Task difficulty was not varied systematically in any of the studies of verbal-manual interference in children, but one study suggested that children's proficiency in an activity influences the degree to which that activity exerts lateralized interference on a concurrent manual task (Hiscock, Antoniuk, & Prisciak, 1982). In this study children at two age levels were asked to read aloud from a word list while tapping with either the left or right index finger. Half of the children at each age level were slightly less proficient in reading than would be predicted on the basis of a group IQ test, and the other children were slightly more proficient. Although the selection criteria were not strong, assignment to poor- and good-reader groups was validated by the finding that good readers read significantly more words than did poor readers in dual-task competition. Moreover, the poor readers showed a significantly greater degree of lateralized interference than did the good readers. The laterality of the two groups did not differ when recititation and tapping were performed concurrently; only the reading task differentiated the groups. This finding is consistent with Hicks's (1975) report that the degree to which interference is lateralized increases as the nonmanual task becomes more difficult, although in the Hiscock et al. (1982a) study, it was group differences in proficiency rather than task differences that caused the task to be more difficult for one group than for the other. It is noteworthy that age did not have a similar effect on the lateralization of interference.

Apart from the laterality aspect of dual-task performance in children, it is useful to determine how overall performance changes with increasing age. The dual-task paradigm may be used to address the issue of changing mental capacity during development (see Pascual-Leone, 1970). Studies of verbal-manual time sharing (e.g., Hiscock & Kinsbourne, 1978, 1980) show that children's performance on each of the concurrent tasks increased between the ages of 3 and 12 years, but these increases need not be taken as evidence for increasing time-sharing capacity. It has been claimed by Case (1978) that older children perform better than younger children on these tasks because older children perform with greater "operational efficiency." In other words, if the tasks are held constant across age levels, then the older children are, in effect, performing easier tasks, and what appears to be greater ability to perform two such tasks concurrently is derived from the relatively lesser demands of the tasks. In fact, inspection of the data for children from 3 to 12 years of age reveals that the proportionate decrement in tapping rate, which is attributable to the addition of the verbal task, decreases linearly with increasing age. This developmental decrease in interference accompanies an increase in performance on each of the two tasks. Thus, it appears that children at all age levels are performing both tasks at the limits of their ability, but that older children can, in addition, time-share more effectively than younger children (Hiscock, Kinsbourne, Samuels, & Krause, 1982b).

Studies with children have been used to address another issue of theoretical significance: the transitivity of interference between concurrent tasks. Kinsbourne and Hicks (1978) state the "paradoxical proposition" that the functional distance between left- and right-hand areas in the cortex differs as a function of the direction in which activation is spreading. Studies of motor overflow and studies of transfer of training indicate that the functional distance from the cortical area for left-hand control to the cortical area for right-hand control is less than the distance between the same cortical areas in the reverse direction. Kinsbourne and Hicks (1978) suggest that this intransitivity may be attributable to a "species-specific preprogrammed rightward response bias" (p. 357). Several studies of dual-task performance reveal a directionality of a different kind, that is, speaking interferes asymmetrically with manual activity, but verbal output remains constant, irrespective of which hand is performing the manual task. This unidirectional effect frequently is found with adults as well as with children (e.g., Hicks, 1975, Experiments 2 and 3; Hicks, Provenzano, & Rybstein, 1975), although the results with adults are contradictory (see Dalby, 1980; Hicks, 1975, Experiment 1) and frequently obscured by differences between tasks, by failures to determine whether there is any generalized interference from manual activity to vocalization, and by failure even to measure performance on the vocalization task. Many of the studies with children are better designed for the assessment of trade-offs between tasks.

White and Kinsbourne (1980) reported that children verbalized more syllables of the nursery rhyme, "Jack and Jill," when tapping with the left hand than when tapping with the right hand. This seems to be the one exception to the rule in the studies of children. In the same study, children emitted about the same number of animal names, irrespective of whether they were tapping concurrently with the left or with the right hand, and in numerous other studies of concurrent speaking and finger tapping, verbal production was invariant across left- and right-hand tapping conditons (Dalby & Gibson, 1981; Hiscock, 1982; Hiscock et al., 1982a; Hiscock & Kisbourne, 1978, 1980; Hiscock et al., 1982b). Why should manual activity have no lateralized influence on speaking when speaking has so strongly lateralized an effect on manual activity? Hiscock (1982) proposed that children "protect" their speaking at the expense of degraded performance on the manual task (see Kahnemann, 1973). It was pointed out that, when speaking is performed concurrently with tapping, tapping rate—averaged across hands—decreases quite dramatically in comparison with single-task tapping rate, but the rate of verbal production changes relatively little in comparison with a condition in which only speaking is required. In a study by Hiscock and Kinsbourne (1980), in which the magnitude of interference in both directions can be compared, it was found that reciting a nursery rhyme decreased tapping rate by 19.1%, but tapping reduced the rate of production of words in the nursery rhyme by only 4.0%. The argument, then, is identical to that applied previously to some of the adult studies except that now it applies to the vocalization task rather than to the manual task; if the amount of generalized interference falls below a certain level, there is little likelihood of finding lateralized interference.

Hiscock (1982) attempted to test the "protection of speech" hypothesis by instructing children to emphasize either tapping or speaking on any particular dual-task trial. It was expected that any tendency to protect speaking would be overridden by instructions to emphasize tapping and that, under those circumstances, left- and right-hand tapping might interfere differentially with speaking. The results, in fact, did not conform to this expectation. Although instructions to emphasize tapping had the expected facilitative effect on tapping, children not only tapped faster in this condition but they also produced more words from a "tongue twister" than when told to emphasize speaking. Subsequent analysis of errors in the different task-priority conditions illuminated the paradoxical increase in verbal production with instructions to emphasize tapping. When children were told to emphasize tapping, they emitted more words, but they also made many more speech errors than when told to emphasize speaking. Nevertheless, even though the number of speech errors when tapping was emphasized increased by over 60% relative to a speaking-control condition, there was no tendency to commit more errors when tapping with the right hand than when tapping with the left. This outcome casts doubt on the "protection of speech" hypothesis and leaves unexplained the repeated failures to find any difference between the hands in their disruption of concurrent speech.

Finally, it should be noted that Piazza (1977) did what no one had been able to do, despite six attempts with adults, that is, she found that nonverbal vocalization interfered to a greater degree with left-hand finger tapping than with righ-hand finger tapping. Piazza's method was straightforward; preschool children were required to tap with the left or right index finger while reciting a familiar rhyme, while humming an unspecified tune, and while remaining silent. The results were exactly as predicted. Recitation disrupted right-hand tapping more than left-hand tapping, and humming had the opposite effect. There also was generalized interference associated with both vocalization tasks such that both hands were affected by both tasks. The reason for the predicted outcome in Piazza's study, in light of the very different findings for nonverbal vocalization tasks in the adult literature, is unknown.

TABLE 8-2.
Studies of Motor–Motor Interference in Children

Study	Subjects	Manual Task	Concurrent Task(s)	Results
Kinsbourne & McMurray, 1975	48 kindergarten students, mean age 5.7 years (24 males, 24 females; 41 right-handers, 7 left-handers)	Repetitive tapping on a table top with the index finger	Continuous repetition of a nursery rhyme or a list of animal names	Both recitation tasks reduced tapping rates for both hands. The reduction was asymmetric, as right-hand rate exceeded left-hand rate in the control conditions but not in the dual-task conditions.
Piazza, 1977	36 right-handed children; 3-, 4-, and 5-year-old groups (18 males, 18 females)	Repetitive tapping of a finger-tapping apparatus with the index finger	Continuous repetition of a familiar rhyme or humming; the experimenter recited and hummed along with the child.	Both vocalization tasks reduced tapping rates for both hands. Recitation reduced right-hand rate more than left-hand rate, and humming reduced left-hand rate more than right-hand rates. The asymmetries were additive across age levels.

Hiscock & Kinsbourne, 1978	151 right-handed children in 9 age groups from 3 to 12 years (79 males, 72 females)	Repetitive tapping of a telegraph key with the index finger	Continuous repetition of a nursery rhyme or a list of animal names	Both recitation tasks reduced right-hand tapping rate more than left-hand tapping rate, and the asymmetry was additive across age levels. Verbal production was equivalent with left- and right-hand tapping.
Hiscock & Kinsbourne, 1980	155 right-handed children in 9 age groups from 3 to 12 years (84 males, 71 females)	Repetitive tapping of a telegraph key with the index finger	Continuous repetition of a nursery rhyme or a list of animal names	Both recitation tasks reduced right-hand tapping rate more than left-hand tapping rate, and the asymmetry was additive across age levels. Longitudinal data for 115 children confirmed the findings of the cross-sectional analyses. Verbal production was equivalent with left- and right-hand tapping.

TABLE 8-2., Continued

Study	Subjects	Manual Task	Concurrent Task(s)	Results
Obrzut, Hynd, Obrzut, & Leitgeb, 1980	96 right-handed children in three age groups from 7 to 12 years (16 normal and 16 learning–disabled children at each age level)	Repetitive tapping of a telegraph key with the index finger	Continuous recitation of a list of animal names	Recitation reduced the right-hand tapping rate significantly more than the left-hand tapping rate for the entire sample of normal and learning–disabled children. Interference was significantly greater for learning–disabled children, but the difference was additive across hands.
White & Kinsbourne, 1980	105 right-handed children in 9 age groups from 3 to 12 years (53 males, 52 females)	Repetitive tapping of a metal key with the index finger	Continuous repetition of a nursery rhyme; naming as many animals as possible	Rhyme task: Recitation reduced right-hand tapping with more than left-hand tapping rate; the asymmetry was additive across age levels; children produced more syllables of the rhyme during left-hand tapping than during right-hand tapping.

Study	Subjects	Motor task	Verbal task	Results
				Naming task: The verbal task reduced right-hand tapping rate more than left-hand tapping rate; the asymmetry was additive across age levels; verbal production was equivalent with left- and right-hand tapping.
Dalby & Gibson, 1981	60 right-handed boys between the ages of 9 and 12 years (15 with nonspecific reading disability, 15 dysphonetic, 15 dyseidetic, 15 average readers)	Alternate tapping of the first and second fingers on a typewriter	Continuous recitation of a list of animal names	Recitation reduced right-hand tapping rate more than left-hand tapping rate for average readers and boys with nonspecific reading disability. Verbal production was equivalent with left- and right-hand tapping for all groups.
Hiscock, 1982	83 right-handed children in 3 age groups from 8 to 11 years (43 males, 40 females)	Alternate tapping of two telegraph keys with the index finger	Continuous repetition of a "tongue twister"; children were instructed to emphasize tapping on half of the dual-task trials and to emphasize speaking on the other half of the trials.	Recitation reduced right-hand tapping rate more than left-hand tapping rate, and the degree of asymmetry increased with increasing age but was additive across task priorities.

TABLE 8-2., Continued

Study	Subjects	Manual Task	Concurrent Task(s)	Results
				Verbal production and number of errors were equivalent with left- and right-hand tapping, irrespective of task priority.
Hiscock, Antoniuk, & Prisciak, 1982 Experiment 1	55 right-handed boys in 2 grade-level groups (grades 2 and 3 vs. grades 4 and 5); subjects in each group were divided into good and poor readers.	Repetitive tapping of a microswitch tapping apparatus with the index finger	Continuous repetition of a "tongue twister"; reading a list of words aloud	Recitation of the "tongue twister" slowed right-hand tapping more than left-hand tapping, and the asymmetry was additive across age and reading ability. Reading aloud slowed right-hand tapping more than left-hand tapping, and the asymmetry was additive across age levels. However, the asymmetry was more marked in poor readers than in good readers. Verbal

| Hiscock, Kinsbourne, Samuels, & Krause, 1982 | 73 right-handed children in 4 age groups from 6 to 10 years (39 males, 34 females) | Repetitive tapping of a telegraph key with the index finger | Continuous repetition of a nursery rhyme or a list of animal names | production in recitation and reading were equivalent with left- and right-hand tapping. Both recitation tasks reduced right-hand tapping rate more than left-hand tapping rate, and the asymmetry was additive across age levels. Recitation of animal names increased the variability of right-hand tapping more than that of left-hand tapping, and the asymmetry was additive across age levels. Recitation of the nursery rhyme increased the variability of right-hand tapping more than that of left-hand tapping for males but not females and for younger but not older children. Irrespective of vocalization task, verbal production was equivalent with left- and right-hand tapping. |

COMPETITION BETWEEN A COGNITIVE PROCESS AND A MOTOR PROCESS

Cognitive-Motor Interference in Adults

The next group of studies, which is described in Table 8-3, entails competition between unimanual activity and concurrent performance of a cognitive task. The line of demarcation between the motor-motor experiments summarized in Table 8-1 and the cognitive-motor experiments summarized in Table 8-3 is somewhat arbitrary, as there are a few experiments that could appear in either category. For example, Table 8-1 includes two experiments by Hicks, Provenzano, & Rybstein, (1975), in which subjects rehearsed letter strings silently while performing a sequential typing task. It also includes an experiment by Hellige and Longstreth (1981), in which subjects read silently while engaging in finger tapping. Even though silent rehearsal and silent reading do not require overt vocalization, these experiments were placed into the motor-motor category because the nonvocal tasks served as control tasks for other tasks in the same experiments that did require vocalization. The word fluency task used by Bowers et al. (1978) combines the cognitive process of generating words within a category with the motor act of articulating the words. This experiment was categorized as a study of motor-motor competition, even though the cognitive component seems greater than that involved in reciting a nursery rhyme, for example. However, a study involving repetition of digits in reverse sequence (Botkin, Schmaltz, & Lamb, 1977) was included in the cognitive-motor category on the assumption that the cognitive demands of the digit-span test are of primary importance. The arbitrary nature of these classificatory decisions serves to emphasize the continuity of the various dual-task studies. There is no clear-cut distinction between motor and cognitive tasks; all of the vocalization tasks mentioned in Table 8-1 require some cognitive programming, and all of the cognitive tasks outlined in Table 8-3 presumably involve some motor activity, such as visual scanning, subvocal verbalization, and response preparation. Nevertheless, for expository purposes at least, it seems useful to distinguish between dual-task studies in which both tasks require activity that is primarily motoric and studies in which one task is performed with little or no overt motor activity.

The manual tasks represented in this group of experiments include repetitive finger tapping, alternate tapping of two buttons with the index finger, sequential tapping with four fingers, and attempting to hold a stylus within a hole without allowing it to touch the sides. In most experiments involving tapping, subjects were instructed to tap as fast as possible, but in one instance (McFarland & Ashton, 1978b) subjects attempted to maintain a rate that had been established by a metronome. In the experiment with metronome cuing, the investigators assessed the effects of concurrent tasks by measuring the variability of tapping in different experimental conditions. The same authors, in a study of speeded finger tapping (McFarland & Ashton, 1978c), measured variability of tapping as well as rate of tapping, but other investigators measured manual performance in terms of only rate. Numerous cognitive tasks were used in these studies. They included perceptual tasks, such as embedded figures tests and closure tests; tasks requiring the encoding of verbal or nonverbal material for subsequent recognition or recall; silent reading; backward repetition of digit strings; tests of running memory span; and tests of nonverbal reasoning. In most instances, performance on the cognitive task was measured, thus, information about the effects of manual activity upon cognitive performance is available.

Each of the studies summarized in Table 8-3 yielded some evidence of generalized or lateralized interference, or both, between cognitive and manual performance. Consequently, the results confirm the findings of Hicks, Provenzano, & Rybstein, (1975) and of Hellige and Longstreth (1981), insofar as they establish that cognitive tasks without overt motor components may disrupt manual performance and may do so asymmetrically. The findings described in Table 8-3 leave little room for arguing that overt motor activity is necessary to generate asymmetric interference with concurrent manual activity. However, since none of the experiments compares a cognitive-plus-motor condition with a cognitive-only or a motor-only condition while holding other variables constant, these studies shed no additional light on the question of whether the effects of the cognitive and motor components upon left- and right-hand performance are additive or interactive.

As a means of measuring laterality, the cognitive-motor interference paradigm offers a great advantage over the motor-motor paradigm, that is to say, a much wider choice of nonverbal (putatively right-hemispheric) control tasks. As mentioned previously, the only satisfactory nonverbal counterpart to speaking is nonverbal vocalization, such as humming or "la-la-ing" a tune, and there is reason to doubt that such activity is controlled exclusively or even predominantly by the right hemisphere (see Gates & Bradshaw, 1977; Hicks, 1975). The use of verbal cognitive tasks potentially allows the investigator to find or design a nonverbal cognitive task that is well matched in all respects except the verbal or nonverbal nature of the required processing.

Unfortunately, investigators frequently have failed to take advantage of this opportunity to match verbal and nonverbal tasks. For example, McFarland and Ashton (1978a) required their subjects to vocalize while performing each of six verbal tasks but apparently not while performing most of the nonverbal tasks. Similarly, Dalby (1980) contrasted reading aloud and sentence repetition, on the one hand, with solving Raven's Matrices and Space Relations problems, on the other. Although it is reassuring to find that verbal and nonverbal tasks generated differentially lateralized interference with manual performance, the verbal and nonverbal tasks in these studies differ along so many dimensions that it would be imprudent to conclude that the verbal-nonverbal difference is responsible for the differential lateralization of interference. Perhaps differences in difficulty level, mode of responding (vocal vs. nonvocal), or some other uncontrolled factor accounts for these findings.

The strongest evidence for differential lateralization of cognitive processes comes from studies in which there are fewest differences between the verbal and nonverbal tasks being compared. One of the best tasks in this regard is the running memory span test (Shepard & Teghtsoonian, 1961), used by McFarland and Ashton in two of their studies (1978b, c). During this task, stimuli to be learned are presented visually at a rate that varies randomly between certain limits to prevent subjects from using presentation rate as a cue in timing their tapping. Each item in the list is presented twice, with a variable number of items between occurrences. The average span may be prescribed by the experimenter as a means of controlling the difficulty of the task. The subject's task is to classify each item as either an old or a new item. By changing the stimuli from words to random shapes (McFarland & Ashton, 1978b) or to photographs of faces (McFarland & Ashton, 1978c), it is possible to convert the task from a verbal task to a nonverbal task without changing other attributes of the task. Although the difficulty (average span) of the running memory span task and the spacing of the tapping buttons influenced the results, findings from both of McFarland's and Ashton's (1978b, c) experiments conformed quite well with the prediction that the verbal memory span task would interfere mainly with right-hand performance. Nevertheless, despite the investigator's effort to devise comparable verbal and nonverbal tasks, they found that the nonverbal task in both instances was more difficult than the verbal task. Even when the average span for random shapes was halved to compensate for subject's difficulty in recognizing these stimuli (McFarland & Ashton, 1978b), the error rate for this material was much higher than the error rate for words. Consequently, the conclusion that words and random shapes have differentially lateralized effects on manual perform-ance must be qualified because the tasks were unequal in difficulty.

None of the experiments summarized in Table 8-3 demonstrate unequiv-ocally that lateralization of interference depends only upon the verbal or nonverbal nature of the cognitive task. As a group, however, these studies show that the pattern of interference usually is quite different for verbal and nonverbal tasks. If the pattern of lateralization is not actually reversed (Dalby,

1980; McFarland & Ashton, 1975b, 1978b, c), the usual right-greater-than-left pattern is likely to be absent for a nonverbal cognitive task (Bowers et al., 1978; McFarland & Ashton, 1978a). The only exception to this general conclusion is found in the results of Summers and Sharp (1979), who obtained no differential interference effects among cognitive tasks classified as verbal, spatial, and verbal-spatial. The verbal task required retention of a string of eight visually presented letters; the spatial task required retention of the positions of eight circles within a matrix; and the verbal-spatial task required retention of eight letters, along with their positions, within a matrix. All three tasks had bilaterally equivalent effects on sequential key pressing, irrespective of whether the key pressing was unimanual or bimanual, and all three tasks disrupted right-hand performance but not left-hand performance on a test of repetitive finger tapping. As pointed out by the investigators, their cognitive tasks and their sequential manual tasks were difficult, and there is some reason to believe that bilateral interference becomes more likely as task difficulty increases (McFarland & Ashton, 1978b, c). The difficulty factor might account for the indistinguishable effects of the three tasks in the experiment involving repetitive tapping, that is, for the finding that all three tasks interfered only with right-hand performance. One might speculate that the spatial and verbal-spatial tasks were amenable to verbal strategies. However, there was one set of findings that did differentiate the three tasks in the third experiment; whereas recall in the verbal condition was not affected by tapping with either hand, recall in the spatial and verbal-spatial conditions was disrupted by left-hand tapping but not right-hand tapping. Interpretation of this pattern of results is obscured by the fact that left-hand tapping interfered with both verbal and nonverbal components of the verbal-spatial task, that is, with both the recall of letter names and with the positions in which the letters occurred.

In all but the first of the experiments summarized in Table 8-3, investigators assessed performance on both the manual and cognitive tasks. In one instance (McFarland & Ashton, 1978a), no errors were made on the cognitive tasks. The remaining studies provide some information about the transitivity of cognitive-manual interference and about the lateralization of interference in each direction. Unfortunately, the findings do not lead to a straightforward conclusion.

In some instances (Dalby, 1980; McFarland & Ashton, 1978b, c), left- and right-hand activity had differential effects on the performance of the cognitive tasks. Most notable is McFarland's and Ashton's (1978c) finding that right-hand tapping increased the error rate and decreased recognition sensitivity in the running memory span task for words only, and that left-hand tapping increased the error rate and decreased recognition sensitivity in only the faces task. Even this finding, however, was qualified by the effect of spacing between the button switches being tapped. The selective effect of right-hand tapping upon verbal performance was found only when the buttons were 12 cm apart. With 6-cm spacing between buttons, tapping caused only a criterion shift in word recognition, and this shift was associated with left-hand rather than right-hand tapping. Hand effects upon cognitive performance in another study by McFarland and Ashton (1978b) depended upon the length of the average span, Dalby (1980) found a hand difference only for males and only for one of two nonverbal tasks. From these findings, one may conclude that the two hands may have a differential effect on cognitive performance, depending upon the cognitive task, but that it is difficult to predict the circumstances under which this selective interference will materialize.

Other studies have failed to find any evidence that performance on the cognitive task differs, as a function of the hand being used to perform the manual task. The repeated failure of Bowers et al. (1978) to find any effect of repetitive finger tapping upon cognitive performance might be attributed to the low difficulty level of the manual task. However, as noted previously, Summers and Sharp (1979) found that repetitive finger tapping with the left hand interfered with subjects' performance on tasks classified as spatial and verbal-spatial. Thus, if difficulty is a critical factor, it appears that the difficulty of the manual and the cognitive task must be considered together. Increased difficulty, however, may not be sufficient to ensure finding asymmetric interference. Summers and Sharp (1979) found that their more difficult manual tasks, which required either unimanual or bimanual performance of an eight-step sequence, interfered about equally with spatial and verbal-spatial recall, irrespective of which hand was executing the sequence (or of which hand was leading the sequence, in the case of bimanual performance).

The data discussed thus far have yielded three distinct outcomes with respect to hand effects upon cognitive performance: neither left- nor right-hand activity interferes with cognitive performance (Bowers et al., 1978); left-hand activity and right-hand activity have equivalent effects on cognitive performance (Summers & Sharp, 1979, Experiments 1 & 2); and left-hand activity and right-hand activity have unequal effects on cognitive performance (Dalby, 1980; McFarland & Ashton, 1978b, c; Summers & Sharp, 1979, Experiment 3). As noted previously, the unequal effects have been obtained under some circumstances and not under others within the same study. The experiment by Botkin, Schmaltz, & Lamb (1977) does not fit well into any of these three categories, as the investigators failed to measure either manual performance or cognitive performance under control (single-task) conditions. Consequently, there is no direct means of measuring interference between tasks. Botkin et al. asked subjects to perform a hole steadiness task while engaged in the Digits Backward test from the Wechsler Adult Intelligence Scale (WAIS). Half of the subjects performed the steadiness task with the right arm, and half performed with the left arm. It was found that subjects who used the right arm repeated significantly fewer digits, but they also performed significantly better on the steadiness task. In the absence of information about performance on each task in isolation, it is difficult to interpret the results. An obvious possibility is that the subjects who performed with the right arm tended to emphasize manual performance at the expense of digit-span performance. However, subjects' self-reports concerning their strategy did not support this explanation that the left hemisphere was "overloaded" by simultaneous performance of the digit-span task and the steadiness task with the right arm.

Cognitive-Motor Interference in Children

The final group of studies is summarized in Table 8-4. In each of these studies, right-handed children performed a cognitive task while they tapped with one hand or the other. There was relatively little variation in the tapping task from one study to another. In all but two experiments, children engaged in speeded repetitive tapping with the index finger. Children in one experiment (Dalby & Gibson, 1981) alternately struck two typewriter keys with the index and middle fingers, and children in another experiment (Cermak, Drake, Cermak, & Kenney, 1978) grasped a metal stylus in one hand and used the stylus to alternately tap two metal plates. In most instances, tapping speed was the primary dependent variable, although McFarland and Ashton (1975a) and Hiscock, Kinsbourne, Samuels, and Krause (1982) analyzed variability of tapping as well as its rate. Cognitive tasks were more heterogenous; they included reading silently, finding hidden figures, finding missing letters, encoding nonsense shapes or faces for later recognition, solving items from Raven's Matrices, solving arithmetic problems, and encoding the orientation of line segments.

The Cermak et al. (1978) study combined tapping with performance of dichotic listening task. Although dichotic listening might be classified as a perceptual task rather than a cognitive task, the digit strings presented in the Cermak et al. experiment probably challenged children's memory and other higher level cognitive processes as much as they challenged perceptual ability (see Bryden & Allard, 1978; Porter & Berlin, 1975). Consequently, the Cermak et al. study seems to be related quite closely to the other studies summarized in Table 8-4.

The findings described in Table 8-4, taken collectively, confirm the major findings from studies of cognitive-manual interference in adults, that is to say, that cognitive tasks are capable of interfering significantly with the concurrent performance of a manual task and that the interference may be asymmetric under certain circumstances. As a rule, the interference asymmetries were consistent with those expected on the basis of current concepts of left- and right-hemispheric specialization. For example, if the spatial-verbal task of McFarland's and Ashton's (1975a) experiment is disregarded, the results are exactly as predicted: finding hidden figures had a selective effect on the speed and variability of left-hand tapping, and reading had a selective effect on the speed and variablility of right-hand tapping. When the spatial-verbal task was substituted for tapping alone as a control condition, the results were altered substantially. However, it is not clear what one should find when a task that is partially verbal and partially spatial is used as a control task. Hiscock et al. (1982) found that silent reading disrupted right-hand tapping more than left-hand tapping, but encoding the orientation of lines disrupted left-hand and right-hand tapping to approximately the same extent. Similarly, White and Kinsbourne (1980) found bilaterally equivalent interference when children finger-tapped and encoded nonsense shapes. Dalby and Gibson (1981) found that, when "dyseidetic" boys and their normal controls attempted to solve items from Raven's Matrices test, the left-hand tapping rate was affected more than the right-hand rate. No asymmetry of interference was found with "dysphonetic" boys or for boys with a nonspecific reading disability.

These findings make it clear that various nonverbal tasks affect concurrent finger tapping in children in a way that is quite different from the way in which verbal tasks affect their finger tapping. With children, as with adults, the asymmetry of interference is not always reversed, but it may merely be absent when nonverbal tasks are performed. This particular discrepancy among studies is of questionable significance; one could argue that all nonverbal tasks are likely to be amenable in some degree to verbal mediation and that the opportunity for verbal mediation decreases the likelihood of finding consistent left-greater-than-right asymmetries. Thus, irrespective of whether a cognitive task disrupts left-hand performance selectively or whether it disrupts the performance of both hands equally, the outcome might be taken as evidence that the right cerebral hemisphere is contributing substantially to the processing of the cognitive task. Alternatively, one might interpret the difference between unilateral and bilateral interference more literally and conclude that some nonverbal tasks, such as encoding nonsense shapes, require bilateral cerebral processing whereas other nonverbal tasks, such as solving Raven's Matrices problems, involve only the right hemisphere. However, literal interpretations of this kind probably are premature, as the lateralization of interference may be influenced by factors other than the lateralized or non-lateralized nature of the required cognitive processing. In particular, it should be noted that McFarland and Ashton (1978b) found that the processing of random shapes interfered selectively with left-hand tapping when the task was relatively easy (i.e., when the average memory span was relatively short) but that processing the same stimuli interfered about equally with left- and right-hand tapping when the task was made more difficult. Until the potentially confounding effects of difficulty and other factors are better understood and controlled, it is prudent to avoid concluding that one nonverbal task is processed in only the right hemisphere and another is processed bilaterally.

In addition to the expected findings, there are some anomalous findings in the literature on cognitive-motor interference in children. Hiscock et al. (1982a, b), in two different studies, found that the encoding of faces disrupted right-hand tapping more than left-hand tapping. In the second of these studies, the face-encoding task was matched closely with a number-encoding task. Although the average memory load was less with faces (two faces) than with numbers (three two-digit numbers) in order to compensate for inherent differences in the ease with which faces and numbers are recognized, all other aspects of the two tasks were identical. It found that number-encoding slowed finger tapping to a greater degree than did face-encoding, but the lateralization of interference was about the same in both instances. This outcome duplicated the results of another similar study with children (Hiscock, et al., 1978a), but both findings are contrary to the results of McFarland and Ashton's (1978c) study of face recognition and finger tapping in adults. In that study, a memory-for-faces task interfered selectively with left-hand tapping, and left-hand tapping but not right-hand tapping interfered with recognition of faces. There are at least three possible explanations for these differences among the studies. First, there is little resemblance between the running memory span methodology used by McFarland and Ashton and the study-test procedure used by Hiscock et al. For example, the former entailed sequential presentation of 50 stimuli for 800 msec each and the latter entailed presentation of one, two, or three faces for 5 seconds, followed by a 5-second retention interval. In view of the likelihood that both left- and right-hemisphere mechanisms are involved in facial recognition (see Benton, 1980; Sergent, 1982), laterality effects in face-recognition tasks may be especially susceptible to methodological alterations. A second possibility is that the processing of faces differs in some important way between children and adults (Carey & Diamond, 1977; Carey, Diamond & Woods, 1980). Yet another is that the Hiscock et al. results were influenced by carry-over effects. When nonverbal trials are interspersed randomly among verbal trials, perhaps subjects establish a verbal set that influences their laterality not only on the verbal trials but also on the interspersed nonverbal trials. Such an effect occurred in a visual laterality study (Hellige, 1978). Although McFarland and Ashton also presented both verbal and nonverbal stimuli to the same subjects within the same session, they gave the two sets of 50 stimuli in two separate blocks. Further research is required to account for the divergent findings from the studies using physiognomic stimuli.

TABLE 8-3.

Studies of Interference between Cognitive Processing and Motor Output in Adults

Study	Subjects	Manual Task	Concurrent Task(s)	Results
McFarland & Ashton, 1975b	12 right-handed university students (7 males, 5 females)	Alternate pressing of two microswitches, 2 inches apart, with the index finger of one hand.	1. Spatial; finding hidden figures in a design. 2. Verbal; performing simple arithmetic calculations 3. Spatioverbal; solving a geometric problem requiring use of letters and digits	Performing the spatial task slowed tapping with both hands, but the left hand was affected more than the right. Performing the verbal task slowed tapping with both hands, but the right hand was affected more than the left. Tapping rate in the spatial condition did not differ from that in the spatioverbal condition. Left-hand tapping rate, but not right-hand rate, in the verbal condition was greater than that in the spatioverbal condition.
Botkin, Schmaltz, & Lamb, 1977	102 right-handed university undergraduates (51 male, 51 female)	Performing a steadiness task, i.e., holding a stylus within a 1/4-inch hole and attempting to avoid	Repeating digit strings in reverse order (Digits Backwards test from the Wechsler Adult Intelligence Scale)	Subjects who performed the steadiness task with the left arm repeated more digits and had a higher error rate for.

		contact with the edge of the hole; half of the subjects held the stylus with the left hand, and half held the stylus with the right hand.		the steadiness task than did subjects who performed with the right arm.
Bowers, Heilman, Satz, & Altman, 1978				
Experiment 2	18 right-handed university students (9 males, 9 females)	Repetitive tapping of a lever with the index finger of one hand	Listening to a recorded story for about 30 sec, after having been told that recall would be tested upon termination of the story	Listening to stories slowed tapping in both hands, but the right was affected more than the left. Tapping had no significant effect on recall of the stories' content.
Experiment 3	18 right-handed university students (9 males, 9 females)	Repetitive tapping of a lever with the index finger of one hand	Reading a story for 30 sec, after having been told that recall would be tested upon completion of the story; the stories were the same as those used in Experiment 2. Presumably, the reading was done silently.	Reading stories slowed right-hand tapping but not left-hand tapping. Tapping had no significant effect on recall of the stories' content.

TABLE 8-3., Continued

Study	Subjects	Manual Task	Concurrent Task(s)	Results
Experiment 4	18 right-handed university students (9 males, 9 females)	Repetitive tapping of a lever with the index finger of one hand	Scanning a set of 12 photographs of faces for 30 sec., after having been told that subsequent recognition would be tested	Scanning faces slowed left-hand and right-hand tapping by equivalent amounts. Tapping had no significant effect on recognition performances.
McFarland & Ashton, 1978a	20 right-handed university students (number of males and females not specified)	Alternate pressing of two button switches, 5 cm apart, with the index finger of one hand	Verbal tasks (all of which required vocalization): 1. Reading a paragraph of abstract material 2. Reading a paragraph of concrete material 3. Identifying the words in a series of anagrams 4. Scanning a word list for 3 specified words 5. Incorporating words into a sentence	When data were pooled within each task category (i.e., verbal and non-verbal), it was found that verbal tasks slowed right-hand but not left-hand tapping and that nonverbal tasks slowed both right- and left-hand tapping. Results for each of the verbal tasks and for each of the nonverbal tasks conformed to the category pattern, except

302

Study	Subjects	Motor task	Cognitive tasks	Results
McFarland & Ashton, 1978b	40 right-handed university students (number of males and females not specified)	Alternate pressing of two button switches, 5 cm apart, with the index finger of one	6. Rehearsing the alphabet with the objective of detecting the missing letter Nonverbal tasks: 1. Scanning for 3 random shapes 2. Scanning for 3 geometric figures 3. Identifying a picture (closure task) 4. Identifying a printed word (closure task) 5. Solving an embedded figures task 6. Matching segments of a line drawing to parts of a completed picture Performing running-memory-span tasks at 2 levels of difficulty; the stimuli for one task	that the closure tasks had little effect on tapping rate. Subjects' ratings of task difficulty revealed no difference between verbal and nonverbal tasks. Performing the short-span words task disrupted right-hand but not left-hand tapping

303

TABLE 8-3., Continued

Study	Subjects	Manual Task	Concurrent Task(s)	Results
		hand; subjects attempted to maintain a pace (1 tap per 380 msec) set during an initial metronome-cued period.	consisted of words; the average memory span was either 10 or 20 items. The stimuli for the other task consisted of random shapes; the average memory span was either 5 or 10 items.	regularity. The long-span words task disrupted both right-hand and left-hand performance. Performing the short-span shapes task disrupted left-hand but not right-hand tapping regularity. The long-span shapes task disrupted both right- and left-hand performance. Only right-hand tapping increased the errors score on the words task, and the effect was obtained only in the short-span condition. Only left-hand tapping increased the error score on the shapes task, and the effect was obtained only in the long-span condition.

McFarland & Ashton, 1978c	16 right-handed university students (number of males and females not specified)	Alternate pressing of two button switches with the index finger of one hand; the distance between buttons was 6 cm for half of the subjects and 12 cm for the other half.	Performing running-memory-span tasks in which the items consisted either of words or of photographs of faces; the average memory span in each case was 15 items.	Performing the words task decreased right-hand but not left-hand rate, and performing the faces tasks decreased left-hand but not right-hand rate. Analysis of variability data yielded the same pattern of lateralized disruption, but only for subjects who pressed buttons that were 6 cm apart. For subjects in the 12-cm condition, both cognitive tasks disrupted tapping regularity in both hands. Right-hand tapping with 12-cm spacing increased errors and decreased sensitivity (d') during the words task. Left-hand tapping, irrespective of distance between buttons, increased errors and decreased d' during the faces task.

TABLE 8-3., Continued

Study	Subjects	Manual Task	Concurrent Task(s)	Results
Summers & Sharp, 1979				
Experiment 1	16 right-handers (7 males, 9 females)	Pressing 8 keys in a prescribed sequence with the index, middle, ring, and little fingers of both hands; one hand led the sequence on day 1, and the opposite hand led on day 2.	Retaining in memory, over a 30-sec interval, material classified as verbal (a random string of 8 letters), spatial (8 randomly positioned circles), or verbal-spatial (8 randomly positioned letters)	Each of the three concurrent tasks reduced the number of correct manual responses, and the effect was additive across right-hand leading and left-hand leading conditions. Bimanual sequencing decreased recall of spatial and verbal-spatial information. The interference was not lateralized.
Experiment 2	16 right-handers (7 males, 9 females)	Pressing 4 keys in a prescribed 8-part sequence with the index, middle, ring, and little finger of one hand; one hand performed the sequence on day 1, and the opposite	Retaining in memory, over a 30-sec interval, material classified as verbal (a random string of 8 letters), spatial (8 randomly positioned circles), or verbal-spatial (8 randomly positioned letters)	Each of the three concurrent tasks reduced the number of correct manual responses, and the effect was additive across hands. Unimanual sequencing decreased recall of spatial and and verbal-spatial

306

information, but not of verbal information. The interference was not lateralized.

hand performed on day 2.

Experiment 3

16 right-handers (7 males and 9 females)

Pressing 1 key as rapidly and as regularly as possible with the index finger of one hand

Retaining in memory, over a 15-sec interval, material classified as verbal (a random string of 8 letters), spatial (8 randomly positioned circles), or verbal-spatial (8 randomly positioned letters)

Each of the three concurrent tasks reduced the number of taps with the right hand but not with the left. Tapping did not affect verbal recall, regardless of which hand performed the tapping. Left-hand tapping but not right-hand tapping decreased recall of spatial and verbal-spatial information.

TABLE 8-3., Continued

Study	Subjects	Manual Task	Concurrent Task(s)	Results
Dalby, 1980	30 right-handed university students (15 males, 15 females)	Repeated typing of a sequence requiring the index, middle, ring, and little finger of one hand	Solving items from Raven's Progressive Matrices and from the Space Relations test of the Differential Aptitude Tests; a response (mode unspecified) was made at the end of a 15-sec trial.	Solving Raven's Matrices problems disrupted left-hand performance more than right-hand performance. Solving Space Relations problems disrupted left-hand performance more than right-hand performance for males only. For males, left-hand tapping but not right-hand tapping decreased performance on Raven's Matrices. For females, tapping had no effect on Raven's Matrices scores. Irrespective of the subject's sex, tapping had no effect on Space Relations scores.

TABLE 8-4.
Studies of Interference between Cognitive Processing and Motor Output in Children

Study	Subjects	Manual Task	Concurrent Task(s)	Results
McFarland & Ashton, 1975	16 right-handed children in 4 age groups from 9 to 12 years	Repetitive tapping of a button switch with one hand; tapping was scored for speed and regularity.	1. Spatial task: finding hidden figures 2. Verbal task: reading a section of a book 3. Spatial-verbal task: finding missing letters from a spatially random array	Performing the spatial task decreased left-hand tapping speed and increased left-hand variability, relative to a "no activity" control condition, but the spatial task had no effect on right-hand tapping. Performing the verbal task decreased right-hand tapping. Performing the verbal task decreased right-hand tapping speed and increased right-hand variability, relative to a "no activity" control condition, but the verbal task had no effect on left-hand tapping. Only the effect of the spatial task on left-hand variability was significant when the spatial-verbal task was used as a control task. An age ×

TABLE 8-4., Continued

Study	Subjects	Manual Task	Concurrent Task(s)	Results
				treatment × hand interaction suggests that the treatment × hand interaction was more marked at age 9 than at ages 10, 11, and 12.
Cermak, Drake, Cermak, & Kenney, 1978	61 right-handed boys between the ages of 8 and 14 years (14 normal boys, 47 learning-disabled boys; of the learning-disabled boys, 16 had higher performance IQ than verbal IQ, and 16 had less than a 5-point discrepancy between verbal and performance IQ.)	Alternate tapping of two metal plates with a metal stylus held in one hand	Listening to three dichotic pairs of digit names through stereophonic headphones	When right-hand tapping was performed, none of the groups showed a significant right-ear advantage for the dichotic stimuli; when left-hand tapping was performed, all groups except the high verbal, low performance IQ group showed a significant right-ear advantage. However, only the low verbal, high performance IQ group showed a significant change in ear asymmetry between the dichotic-listening-alone condition and a

Study	Sample	Task	Findings
White & Kinsbourne, 1980	105 right-handed children in 9 age groups, from 3 to 12 years (53 males, 52 females)	Repetitive tapping of a metal key with the index finger	listening-plus-tapping condition. This change occurred with left-hand tapping.
		Encoding nonsense shapes for subsequent recognition	Shape encoding reduced tapping rate, but the effect was not lateralized. Shape recognition was equivalent with left- and right-hand tapping.
Dalby & Gibson, 1981	60 right-handed boys between the ages of 9 and 12 years (15 with nonspecific reading disability, 15 dysphonetic, 15 dyseidetic, 15 average readers)	Alternate tapping of the first and second fingers on a typewriter	
		Solving an item from Raven's Colored Progressive Matrices; a pointing response was made at the end of the trial.	Solving Raven's Matrices problems reduced left-hand tapping rate more than right-hand rate for average readers and boys in the dyseidetic group. Both left- and right-hand tapping decreased scores on Raven's Matrices, but there was no significant difference between hands.

311

TABLE 8-4., Continued

Study	Subjects	Manual Task	Concurrent Task(s)	Results
Hiscock, Antoniuk & Prisciak, 1982 Experiment 1	55 right-handed boys in 2 grade-level groups (grades 2 and 3 vs. grades 4 and 5); subjects in each group were divided into good and poor readers.	Repetitive tapping of a microswitch tapping apparatus with the index finger	Encoding 4 pictures of boys' faces for subsequent recognition	Face encoding slowed right-hand tapping more than left-hand tapping. The effect was additive across grade level and reading ability. Recognition of faces did not vary as a function of the hand that had performed the tapping.
Experiment 2	64 right-handed children in grades 2-5 (8 males, 8 females at each grade level); all children were average readers; half were in the upper 1/3 of their class in mathematics, and half were in the lower 1/3.	Repetitive tapping of a microswitch tapping apparatus with the index finger	1. Silent reading of a word list; the number of words read was assessed at the end of each trial. 2. Encoding the orientation of a line; subsequent to each trial, the child tried to find a line of identical orientation within a set of 3 lines.	All three cognitive tasks slowed finger tapping. Silent reading affected the right hand more than the left, but interference from the line-orientation and arithmetic tasks was not lateralized.

Hiscock, Kinsbourne, Samuels, & Krause, 1982	73 right-handed children in 4 age groups from 6 to 10 years (39 males, 34 females)	Repetitive tapping of a telegraph key with the index finger	3. Solving a visually presented aritimetic problem; subsequent to each trial, the child tried to find the correct answer among 3 choices. Encoding a variable number of faces or numbers for subsequent recognition	Both memory-encoding tasks slowed right-hand tapping more than left-hand tapping; number-encoding was more disruptive than face-encoding; the amount of interference increased as a linear function of memory load; effects were additive across age levels. None of these effects were significant in the analysis of tapping variability. Performance on the recognition tasks was equivalent with left- and right-hand tapping.

It might also be considered unexpected that performing arithmetic calculations interfered equally with the left- and right-handed tapping (Hiscock et al. 1982a), insofar as left-hemisphere lesions seem to affect calculation ability more frequently and severely than do right-hemisphere lesions (Grafman, Passafiume, Faglioni, and Boller, 1982; Hécaen, 1962). However, McFarland and Ashton (1975b) found that a calculation task interfered more with right-hand tapping than with left-hand tapping in adults. But, McFarland and Ashton did find significant interference with left-hand tapping as well as with right hand tapping. In addition, in their study, the arithmetic problems were presented in the form of sentences to be read. Thus, the asymmetric interference might be due to reading of words rather than to calculation. Hiscock et al. presented their calculation problems in symbolic form, for example, $[75 + 8 = \underline{\quad}.]$

Only one study from Table 8-4 addresses the issue of task difficulty directly. Hiscock et al. (1982b) varied the memory load in their face-encoding and number-encoding tasks across three levels of difficulty. Irrespective of task, increasing the memory load caused a linear decrease in the rate of concurrent finger tapping. However, the decrease was additive across the hands; the degree of asymmetry remained constant as the concurrent task became more difficult. As stated previously, task difficulty may be manipulated in moderate degrees without changing the degree of asymmetry. This conclusion is further supported by evidence that the degree of asymmetry in children does not change with increasing age (Hiscock et al., 1982b; White & Kinsbourne, 1980). In these studies, the cognitive task was the same for children of different ages. Consequently, the task was more difficult for the younger children than for the older children. The differential difficulty was reflected in significant age effects in their performance on the cognitive tasks. Nevertheless, the degree to which interference between the cognitive task and finger tapping was lateralized did not change with age.

Among the studies summarized in Table 8-4, only the Cermak et al. (1978) study showed an asymmetry in the reverse direction, that is, from manual activity to cognitive activity. The Cermak et. al study differed from the others in many respects, but it does suggest that the left and right hand may have differential effects on concurrent cognitive (or perceptual) processing. Three groups of learning-disabled boys and a control group of normal boys accomplished a dichotic listening task while tapping with the right hand, and while performing no concurrent task. Although the condition X ear interaction failed to reach statistical significance, it was noted that three of the four groups showed a significant right-ear superiority in the left-hand tapping condition, as compared with one group in the single-task condition and no groups in the right-hand tapping condition. Direct comparison of ear scores among conditions revealed that only one group of learning-disabled boys showed significant changes as a result of the concurrent finger tapping. For boys in that group, left-hand tapping was associated with significant increase in recall of digit names from the right ear and with a significant decrease in recall of digit names from the left ear. Overall, the study provides preliminary evidence that manual activity may alter asymmetries of dichotic listening. Cermak et al. did not report the effects of dichotic listening upon left- and right-hand tapping rates.

The other studies—those designed primarily to measure interference in the cognitive-to-manual direction—failed to provide any evidence of asymmetry in the reverse direction. In one study (McFarland & Ashton, 1975a), performance on the cognitive task apparently was not measured. Cognitive performance was assessed in the other studies, but none of these four studies suggest that activity with one hand is more disruptive than the same activity performed with the other hand. To some extent, the negative findings may reflect a lack of generalized interference in the motor-to-cognitive direction. Hiscock et al. (1982a) found that children read as many words while tapping as when no concurrent task was being performed. This is reminiscent of the "protection" of speech that seemed to occur in studies of competition between speech and manual performance. Dalby and Gibson (1981), however, found that both left- and right-hand tapping disrupted performance on Raven's Matrices, but even then the effect of one hand was not greater than that of the other. In the other studies yielding no hand difference (Hiscock et al., 1982b; White & Kinsbourne, 1980), the generalized interference from manual activity could not be measured, as there was no control condition in which the cognitive tasks were performed without concurrent manual activity. Thus, apart from the qualified and preliminary findings of Cermak et al. (1978), there is no evidence from studies of children that the left and right hands have differential effects on cognitive performance.

Two of the studies of cognitive-motor interference in children raise the question of whether tapping variability provides information in addition to that provided by tapping rate. McFarland and Ashton (1975a) found that rate and variability measures were largely redundant, for example, when a concurrent task selectively slowed tapping in one hand, that task also selectively increased the variability of tapping in the same hand. In one of their studies with adults (McFarland & Ashton, 1978c), the same investigators measured both rate and variability of tapping and found similar effects for the two measures. However, the two measures diverged in the group that tapped buttons spaced 12 cm apart. For subjects in this group, the cognitive tasks had the predicted lateralized effects upon tapping speed, but the variability measure showed bilateral interference. A study by Hiscock et al. (1982b) reveals some marked differences between interference as measured by rate and interference as measured by variability. Most notably, rate data showed asymmetric interference between memory-encoding and tapping, but variability data did not. Variability has been defined differently by the different groups of investigators. McFarland and Ashton defined tapping variability as either the variance (McFarland & Ashton, 1975a) or the standard deviation (McFarland & Ashton, 1978c) of the mean intertap interval for each condition. Hiscock et al. (1982) defined tapping variability in terms of the coefficient of variation or the standard deviation of the average tap-to-tap rate for each condition, divided by the average tap-to-tap rate. In other words, McFarland and Ashton worked with intervals (in msec) and Hiscock et al. converted each interval into tap-to-tap rate (in taps/second). Moreover, Hiscock et al. chose the coefficient of variation as an estimate of tapping variability that would be largely independent of rate. Since the mean and standard deviation are more likely to be correlated than are the mean and coefficient of variation, one would expect that McFarland's and Ashton's approach would result in greater redundancy between measures of rate and variability.

DUAL-TASK RATIONALE: IMPLICATIONS FOR LATERALITY STUDIES

The dual-task experiment need not be complicated in the conceptualization, design, instrumentation, or data analysis. Some of the most important findings are derived from relatively simple studies in which the most elaborate piece of equipment was a stopwatch or an electromechanical counter. If the results were consistent from one study to the next and if the results did not vary with minor alterations in task or procedure, investigators might be justified in viewing the technique as a straightforward and convenient means for studying cerebral lateralization. Different combinations of subject and task variables could be explored in an effort to understand how the cerebral hemispheres interact under various controlled conditions. In fact, as this review has shown, the dual-task literature has become progressively less coherent as research reports have accumulated. While this incoherence may destroy any overly optimistic preconceptions about immediate usefulness of the technique as a means of measuring cerebral lateralization, it also serves more constructive purpose insofar as it alerts laterality researchers to the need for an understanding of basic principles. Only if these principles are understood and applied to the design of experiments will the inconsistencies and contradictions in the literature become interpretable.

The cognitive psychology literature on time-sharing delineates many of the basic issues that apply to all dual-task experiments, irrespective of whether laterality is a factor (Friedman & Polson, 1981; Kantowitz & Knight, 1976;

Navon & Gopher, 1979, 1980; Norman & Bobrow, 1975, 1976). In particular, this literature points out some of the assumptions inherent in the logic of the dual-task technique. Many of these assumptions are implicit in the design and interpretation of the dual-task laterality experiments discussed in this chapter. At least some of the assumptions, and perhaps all of them, are invalid under some circumstances. Violation of an assumption may invalidate the dual-task technique for the purpose of studying hemispheric functioning, or it may have little impact on the laterality aspects of the study. Navon and Gopher (1979) have discussed six assumptions underlying dual-task studies, all of which are problematic within the framework of single-channel theory and even more problematic from a perspective of multiple resources theory. Each of these assumptions can be related to the study of dual-task laterality.

The first assumption underlying what Navon and Gopher (1979) term "the strict central capacity interference model" is that performance on a task is sensitive to the amount of resources made available for the task. In the ideal dual-task situation, as more and more resources are transferred from one task to the other, performance on the first task declines at a fixed rate and performance on the second task improves at a fixed rate. However, there is no reason to suppose that the actual relationship between resources and performance must be consistent across a wide range of resource levels, or that it must be comparable for different tasks. Norman and Bobrow (1975) suggest that the performance-resource function may have a minimum threshold value of resource, below which there is no performance, and that other portions of the curve may be characterized by plateaus and changing slopes. In most dual-task laterality studies, nothing is known about the performance-resource function for either task or about the nature of performance trade-offs between tasks when two tasks are performed concurrently. It is only known that the subject is operating at a point that represents one of many possible combinations of performance on one task and performance on the other, that is, at one point of an uncharted performance operating characteristic (POC) curve. Transferring one unit of resource from one task to the other may have a dramatic effect or no effect at all upon the performance of either task, depending upon the shape of the subject's POC curve and the subject's current position on that curve.

Empirical determination of performance-resource functions may be an unattainable goal (see Norman & Bobrow, 1975, pp. 52–53), and plotting of POC curves has been accomplished only rarely (see Navon & Gopher, 1979, pp. 221–222). Nevertheless, the laterality researcher at least can ensure that performance on the manual task changes from the single-task to the dual-task condition as the difficulty of the concurrent task is varied. In this way, it is possible to infer that performance is being measured within what Norman and Bobrow (1975) termed the performance-limited portion of the performance-resource function, that is, that performance is sensitive to changes in resource allocation. However, if increasing the allocation of resources has no effect on performance, the task is said to be data limited. Presumably, most tasks are resource limited throughout some range of resource levels, above which further allocation of resources produces no further improvement in performance. If there is no improvement in performance from dual-task condition to single-task condition (e.g., the dowel-rod balancing performance of females in Lomas's and Kimura's Experiment 1; 1976), one could argue that performance of the task in question falls within its data-limited region; additional allocation of resources will not improve performance. When performance falls within this region, the dual-task method yields no useful data.

Second is the assumption that the processing demands of tasks are additive, that is, that the amount of resources required for concurrent performance of two tasks is the sum of the resources required to perform each task in isolation. This assumed additivity of resources is vital in dual-task studies whose purpose is to evaluate the relative resource demands imposed by two different tasks. For example, in a traditional dual-task experiment, the relative demands of tasks A and B might be evaluated by requiring subjects to perform each task, in turn, concurrently, with task X. If task X is performed less well in conjunction with A than in conjunction with B, the investigator might conclude that A demands more resources than does B. Such a conclusion overlooks the "concurrence" effects (Navon & Gopher, 1979) that may be created by the combination of tasks. Perhaps task A demands no more resources than task B, but more resources are required to prevent maladaptive cross talk between A and X than between B and X. In terms of the functional distance model, a larger inhibitory barrier is needed to keep the respective neural circuits for A and X isolated from each other. Depending upon the precise nature of the tasks, nonadditivity of resources may be beneficial rather than deleterious. Performance would benefit when certain task components are identical, thus allowing duplicate utilization of common resources.

How is resource additivity relevant to studies of dual-task laterality? The basic premise of such studies is that resources are *not* additive. The presumed reason that a task disrupts concurrent performance with one hand more than with the other hand is that one combination of tasks (e.g., speaking and right-hand tapping) tends to produce more cross talk than another combination (e.g., speaking and left-hand tapping). Consequently, more resources must be devoted to the third task, that is to say, that of maintaining isolation between the two overt tasks. The greater the amount of resources devoted to this third task, the smaller the amount of resources available for control of the two overt tasks.

Nonadditivity of resources becomes a source of ambiguity in dual-task laterality experiments only when two different tasks (rather than two hands) are being compared. Even though the two tasks may be of comparable difficulty, as assessed from single-task performance, one may disrupt manual performance to a greater degree than the other (Hiscock et al., 1982b). The disparity might reflect differences between tasks in resource demands, or it might reflect differences in degree of nonadditivity when the tasks are combined with the manual task. In either case, differences between the tasks along a verbal-nonverbal dimension, for example, would be confounded with other differences. This potential confound is not likely to be a problem when one task interferes predominantly with the right hand and the other with the left hand. The problematic outcome is that in which the task producing the greater generalized interference also produces the greater amount of lateralized interference. One could then argue that any differences in the lateralization of interference are secondary to differences in generalized interference, that is, asymmetry of interference cannot be demonstrated in the absence of interference. The same kind of confound might exist if the tasks differed in difficulty when performed alone. The main point, however, is that differences in additivity of resources may affect task differences in dual-task laterality even if the tasks are equated with respect to difficulty in the single-task situation.

A third assumption is that the two tasks remain independent when being performed concurrently. From the prior discussion of additivity of resources, one might suspect that the integrity of the tasks is not always preserved in the dual-task situation. The concept of concurrence benefits (Navon & Gopher, 1979), in particular, implies that one task may be altered to make use of "by-products" of the other task or to eliminate components that are redundant with those of the other task. Probably the independence of tasks is compromised further with practice; proficiency in dual-task performance may be achieved largely by learning to amalgamate the two separate tasks into one more complex task (Gopher & North, 1977; LaBerge, 1973). Violation of the assumption of independence between tasks can affect laterality studies in two ways. First, if the two tasks are consolidated to an increasing degree with practice and if there are carry-over effects from one hand to the other, the degree to which interference is lateralized may depend upon the order in which the hands are tested (see Hiscock & Kinsbourne, 1978, 1980). Normally, order effects might be eliminated or minimized by training each hand to asymptotic performance. In the case of dual-task performance, however, it may require an unusually great amount of practice to obtain asymptotic performance (LaBerge, 1973; Norman & Bobrow, 1975), and dual-task performance at asymptote may be such that both tasks are performed as well as either task separately (Spelke, Hirst, & Neisser, 1976). In that event, there would be no measurable interference and thus no opportunity to demonstrate lateralized interference. The second potential effect of nonindependence upon laterality concerns comparisons between different tasks. The problem is the same as that discussed with respect to nonadditivity: even though two cognitive tasks, for example, are matched for difficulty in the single-task situation, one of them may be more readily amalgamated with the manual task in the dual-task situation. Consequently, one task might yield little evidence of generalized or lateralized interference because it is easily combined with the manual task.

The fourth problematic assumption discussed by Navon and Gopher holds that the general pool of capacity is constant across situations. This conflicts with Kahneman's (1973) claim, based in part on evidence of correlation between task demands and physiological responses, that capacity varies with arousal. No one would assert that capacity is unlimited, but any substantial variability in the limit of capacity is sufficient to undermine the logic of the dual-task experiment. Particularly if capacity increases to meet increased demands, one might question the interpretation of comparisons between performance of a task in isolation and performance of the same task within a dual-task situation. If the heavier demands of the dual-task situation cause an increase in arousal and thus in available resources, performance in the dual-task condition might equal or even surpass that in the single-task condition. In any event, the resource demand of the added task would be underestimated. If the problem of elastic capacity is added to those of nonadditivity of resources and nonindependence of tasks, it becomes clear that single-task versus dual-task comparisons may not yield meaningful estimates of a task's resource demands. Again, however, laterality investigators are in the relatively favorable position of attempting to assess differential effects on left- and right-hand performance rather than to calculate the amount of processing resource required by different tasks. Variable capacity would not confound the interpretation of lateralized interference effects unless there were some reason to suspect that arousal would be increased differentially, as a function of the hand performing the manual task. If arousal level did vary as a function of hand, one would expect that the greater effect would occur with the hand that is more affected by the concurrent task, that is, the more difficult combination of tasks. Consequently, any left versus right differences in arousal would be expected to counteract asymmetries of interference rather than to create artifactual aymmetries. Nevertheless, whenever two different tasks are being compared in dual-task laterality studies, it is possible that they will differ in their tendencies to heighten arousal and that conclusions about task differences might be confounded by arousal differences.

The fifth point made by Navon and Gopher is that humans cannot always achieve complete control over the allocation of their processing resources. Navon and Gopher argue that some stimuli or stimulus dimensions are so compelling that they cannot be ignored. This lack of total control violates the assumption that the system can select any combination of performance levels that does not overtax its capacity (Navon & Gopher, 1979).

As a consequence, there may be a lower limit of demand imposed by a task. Despite the subject's intention to withdraw resources from that and apply those resources to the concurrent task, those resources cannot be freed. A major implication of this contingency is that the upper limit of performance on a second task will differ, depending upon whether the second task is performed in isolation or in the presence of the stimuli associated with the first task. In other words, the mere presence of stimuli associated with the first task may impair performance on the second task. Navon and Gopher assert that violation of the controllability assumption is important, primarily in studies of perception; if so, it may have little relevance to the literature discussed here. Nevertheless, it might be informative in some instances to use not only a no-concurrent-task control condition but also a control condition in which stimuli from a second task are present but not processed (i.e., what Navon and Gopher refer to as a dual-task focused-attention situation).

The final assumption in Navon's and Gopher's analysis of the strict central capacity model is labeled "complementarity of supplies." It assumes that the resources allocated to one task plus the resources allocated to the other task always sum to the total resources available. It follows, of course, that the amount of the resource allocated to one task at any moment is the total amount of resource minus the amount allocated to the other task. Navon and Gopher describe several hypothetical situations in which the principle of complementarity would be violated: (a) when the performance-resource function consists of discrete levels (Norman & Bobrow, 1975) (performance will not improve with increasing resource allocation until a threshold amount is available); (b) when performance is coordinated such that performance on one task cannot improve if performance on the other task deteriorates; (c) when the tasks are totally incompatible and must be performed alternately (the performance of either task alone at any instant may not consume all the available resources); and (d) when the joint resource demand of both tasks is comfortably within the capacity of the system. Violation of complementarity may occur in dual-task laterality studies, but it probably has no specific effect on the degree to which interference is lateralized. Contingency (b) above, which Navon and Gopher discuss under the heading of "substitutability of outputs," may occur in studies involving concurrent recitation and speeded finger tapping. The present authors have observed that, in children, there is a substantial positive correlation between verbal production and speed of tapping. It appears that the respective rhythms are coordinated to some extent so that the pace of one activity determines the pace of the other. Hiscock (1982) found that instructions to emphasize tapping not only increased the tapping rate but also increased the rate of speaking (with a corresponding rise in the number of speech errors). The asymmetry of interference was unaffected by manipulation of task priority. Perhaps this partial synchronization of tapping and speaking accounts for the intransitivity of interference between tapping and speaking. Despite the greater right-than-left effect of speaking on tapping, right-hand tapping rate in the dual-task situation usually equals or exceeds left-hand rate. In other words, concurrent speaking usually fails to reduce right-hand rate below the level of left-hand rate. If tapping rate tends to set the pace for speaking, then the relatively high right-hand rate might offset any tendency for speaking rate to diminish during right-hand activity. This analysis implies that speech errors should increase during right-hand tapping (see Hicks, 1975). As was the case with other assumptions, violation of the complementarity principle is more likely to affect between-task comparisons than between-hand comparisons, with the task held constant. For example, it may not be feasible to compare performance on a continuously measured task (e.g., speaking) with performance on a discretely measured task (e.g., solving an item from Raven's Matrices test). Since the Raven's Matrices performance can only assume values of zero and one, it quite likely would fall under contingency (a) above: a change in the amount of resources made available would have no effect until a certain threshold level was crossed.

This brief review of concepts from cognitive psychology accentuates two characteristics, one negative and one positive, of the dual-task laterality literature. First, on the negative side, it shows clearly that tasks and task parameters often have been chosen in an arbitrary, "hit-or-miss" fashion. With no regard for POC curves, resource-limited versus data-limited regions of performance, or any of the other theoretical accoutrements from cognitive psychology, investigators have combined pairs of tasks and measured changes in performance relative to single-task conditions. In many instances, the experiments yielded results as expected. When they did not, the investigators often resorted to post hoc explanations in terms of hemispheric specialization when, in all probability, the results reflected the experimenters' particular choice of task and task parameters. The more favorable implication of the cognitive psychology literature is that comparisons of left- and right-hand performance, with the concurrent task held constant, are relatively free of the problems that stem from violations of the assumptions underlying the dual-task technique. Irrespective of whether single-channel theory is tenable as a model of dual-task performance (Friedman & Polson, 1981; Kinsbourne, 1981; Navon & Gopher, 1979) and irrespective of whether the dual-task method can be used to measure the resources demanded by a particular task, it is possible to derive useful neuropsychological information from well-designed dual-task experiments.

What are the methodological attributes of a well-designed experiment? There are several attributes, although probably all of them cannot be incorporated into a single experiment. First, it is highly desirable that performance on both the manual and nonmanual tasks be measured. In addition, performance on each task should be measured in a single-task condition, as this allows the investigator to determine the pattern of performance trade-offs, that is, whether there was interference in both directions (nonmanual task to manual task and vice versa) and whether the interference in each direction was lateralized. Both tasks should be sensitive to changes in resource allocation, that is, performance should be within the resource-limited region of the performance-resource function. For the reason discussed previously, tasks characterized by discrete levels of performance should be avoided. If two different manual tasks are to be contrasted, the tasks should be as similar to each other as possible. Violations of Navon's and Gopher's (1979) various assumptions appear to become more damaging as the tasks become divergent. In addition, it is impossible to know why two tasks produce differentially lateralized interference with manual performance if the tasks differ along several dimensions. When analyzing the dual-task data, it is important to assess generalized interference as well as lateralized interference so that failures to find asymmetries may be evaluated more adequately. In some cases, the absence of lateralized interference may be attributable to experimental conditions that result in no generalized interference between tasks. Although it would be unrealistic to suggest that laterality researchers generate families of POC curves for their tasks before they attempt to find interference asymmetries, the interpretability of findings would increase if some effort were made to assess the generality of outcomes across different conditions of performance. To date, some investigators (e.g., Hellige & Longstreth, 1981: Hicks et al., 1975, 1978; Hiscock et al. 1982b; McFarland & Ashton, 1978b, c) have manipulated the difficulty of one or the other task in dual-task laterality study, but task priority was manipulated in only one study (Hiscock, 1982). The latter manipulation may be more informative, as it produces a change in position along a POC curve rather than two points on separate POC curves. However, either manipulation constitutes an improvement over the usual practice of assessing performance at one arbitrary point on an arbitrarily selected POC curve.

CONCLUSIONS

As studies of dual-task laterality accumulate, the literature begins to resemble a set of simulateneous equations with a greater number of variables than equations. Just as the equations cannot be solved without more information, the dual-task data cannot be reduced to a few conclusions without more information. Perhaps the greatest asset and greatest liability of the technique are the same: its potential for exploring a vast number of diverse behaviors. With other laterality measures, such as dichotic listening and visual half-field (tachistoscopic) presentation, the technique imposes fairly rigid limits on the phenomena that may be investigated. For example, only auditory phenomena may be studied using dichotic listening, and only briefly exposed visual stimuli may be used in tachistoscopic studies. In contrast, the dual-task method allows the investigation of an almost unlimited range of vocal and cognitive tasks. Researchers have sampled rather promiscuously from this universe of possible tasks; the literature lacks focused, systematic attention to a few tasks and a few task parameters. Consequently, apparent discrepancies among findings are not easily explained. If two different investigators, for example, use two completely different nonverbal tasks in combination with somewhat different manual tasks, it may be impossible to explain why one investigator finds bilateral interference and the other finds selective interference with the left hand. In the absence of detailed knowledge about the characteristics of the various tasks and the characteristics of pairs of tasks in combination—the extent of their resource-limited regions, the additivity of their resources—discrepant results will remain enigmatic.

Despite the unsystematic nature of the facts thus far assembled, a few findings appear quite consistently. First and most fundamental is the pervasiveness of dual-task interference. Nearly all of the studies reviewed in this chapter provide some evidence that either speaking or performing a cognitive task may disrupt the performance of a concurrent manual task. There is very little evidence of intertask facilitation. Second, it is equally clear that certain verbal tasks—recitation, reading aloud, reading silently, and probably several other activities— disrupt right-hand performance more than left-hand performance. Although it is difficult to specify the conditions under which the performance of a nonverbal task will disrupt left-hand activity more than right-hand activity, it is clear that the performance of many putatively nonverbal tasks generates interference that is either bilaterally equivalent or greater on the left side than on the right. Thus, the third general conclusion is that nonverbal tasks, considered collectively, yield a pattern of manual interference that is distinct from the pattern associated with verbal tasks. This conclusion is not as strong as might be desired, as it implies that little has been learned about the cerebral lateralization of specific nonverbal processes. Nonetheless, it is crucial to show that at least one category of task does not produce a right-greater-than-left pattern on interference. Only then can one be confident that the consistent asymmetry of interference achieved with verbal tasks is not an invariant property of dual-task performance in humans, for example, an artifact of the disparity between the hands in single-task performance. A fourth conclusion from the extant literature is that dual-task performance in children closely resembles that in adults, although overall capacity for dual-task performance seems to increase developmentally.

Children show patterns of asymmetric interference that are similar to those observed in adults.

The basic criteria can be applied to the dual-task method for studying cerebral organization—its usefulness for determining the extent to which each hemisphere subserves a particular process (e.g., solving Raven's Matrices) and its ability to elucidate general principles of brain organization. As concluded previously, there already has been partial success in meeting the first criterion. Dual-task studies confirm other evidence that certain verbal functions are performed asymmetrically in the brain, but the literature thus far provides little consistent information regarding the lateralization of nonverbal processes. The second objective is the ultimate one, and it is not likely to be achieved easily. At present, one can only speculate as to what the available dual-task data imply about cerebral organization in general. However, it is possible to identify some important issues that must be clarified if dual-task experiments are to facilitate the understanding of the brain.

One of the most important general questions concerns the existence of discontinuous channels, or resource pools, in the brain. As the limitations of the strict single-channel model become more evident, it is necessary to find a more satisfactory theory to explain how processing resources are allocated (Kinsbourne, 1981; Navon & Gopher, 1979). There are arguments for abandoning single-channel theory in favor of multiple-resources models (Navon & Gopher, 1979; Wickens, 1980) or models incorporating both central attention and multiple resources (Posner, 1978). It has even been proposed that each cerebral hemisphere constitutes an independent pool of resources (Friedman & Polson, 1981; Hellige, Cox, and Litvac, 1979). Both kinds of models—single-channel and multiple resources—give a good account for subjects' performance in some situations but not in others (Kinsbourne, 1981). The critical question is whether the machine-based concept of discrete channels is at all applicable to the human brain. In many of the experiments discussed in this chapter, interference did not vary between hands in a binary fashion; instead, the concurrent task merely had a greater effect on one hand than on the other hand. In other words, there was a left-right gradient of interference, as predicted by the functional distance model. Although discrete-channel formulations may be able to account for this common outcome, their explanations are post hoc. For example, it could be argued from a two-resource-pools perspective that optimal control of either hand involves mechanisms from both channels (hemispheres) and that the mechanisms required for performance of the concurrent task overlap to some extent with the hand-control mechanisms in both channels. It is more parsimonious to dispense with the assumption that the brain contains discontinuous channels.

A second related question concerns the reason that performance of a secondary task causes a decline in performance of the first. This is the most basic question of dual-task research, but it never has been answered satisfactorily. Usually it is assumed that a person's ability to perform two tasks concurrently is limited by a finite endowment of some resource, which is referred to as attention, effort, processing capacity, and so forth. Research has been focused on task demands for that resource as well as on the manner in which people allocate their resources to meet the task demands as effectively as possible. Task difficulty and allocation policy have been manipulated, but little attention has been paid to task similarity as a factor that also influences the success of dual-task performance. In the lexicon of cognitive psychology, structural interference (cross talk between, or competition for, specific mechanisms) has been regarded as less interesting than capacity interference (diversion of attention from one task to another). The current disillusionment with single-channel theory represents a reaction to this overemphasis on capacity. It is now clear that the kind of resources required by a task is as important as the amount of resources. The dual-task laterality literature thus far has failed to distinguish between capacity interference and structural interference. Findings that asymmetries of interference are invariant with changes in task difficulty (Hellige & Longstreth, 1981; Hicks, Provenzano, & Rybstein, 1975; Hiscock et al., 1982b) suggest that lateralized interference effects may reflect structural rather than capacity interference, although there are other findings that do not lend themselves to this interpretation (Hicks, 1975; Hicks et al., 1978; McFarland & Ashton, 1978b, c; Summers & Sharp, 1979). From the functional distance model, one would predict that changes in task difficulty would produce changes in interference that are largely generalized but that changes in the degree of similarity between tasks would be more likely to affect the lateralization of interference.

Finally, the principles to be extracted from dual-task studies must be validated across a wider range of phenomena. What are the explanatory powers of single-channel theory, multiple capacity models, and the functional distance model with respect to facilitative interactions between tasks, to interactions among limbs, to perceptual phenomena, to turning tendencies, to interference effects in learning and memory? Ultimately, the value of dual-task studies will lie not in the facts accumulated about performance of people on artificially conjoined tasks but in the insight gained of the organization of the brain.

REFERENCES

Allard, F., & Bryden M.P. The effect of concurrent activity on hemispheric asymmetries. *Cortex*, 1979 *15*, 5–17.

Allport, D.A. Attention and performance. In G. Claxton (Ed.), *Cognitive psychology: New directions*. London: Routledge & Kegan Paul, 1980.

Ammons, R.B., & Ammons, C.H. Decremental and related processes in skilled performance. In L.E. Smith (Ed.), *Psychology of motor learning*. Proceedings of C.I.C. Symposium on Psychology of Motor Learning, University of Iowa, 1970.

Anrep, G.V. The irradiation of conditioned reflexes. *Proceedings of the Royal Society*, 1923, *96B*, 604–626.

Bahrick, H.P., Noble, M., & Fitts, P.M. Extra-task performance as a measure of learning a primary task. *Journal of Experimental Psychology*, 1954, *48*, 298–302.

Bahrick, H.P., & Shelley, C. Time sharing as an index of automatization. *Journal of Experimental Psychology*, 1958, *56*, 288–293.

Benton, A.L. The neuropsychology of facial recognition. *American Psychologist*, 1980, *35*, 176–186.

Berlin, C.I., Porter, R.J., Jr., Lowe-Bell, S.S., et al. Dichotic signs of the recognition of speech elements in normals, temporal lobectomees, and hemispherectomees. *IEEE Transactions on Audio and Electroacoustics*, 1973, *AU-21*, 189–197.

Blyth, K.W., Experiments on choice reactions with the hands and feet. Unpublished doctoral dissertation, University of Cambridge, 1962.

Boles, D.B. Laterally biased attention with concurrent verbal load: Multiple failures to replicate. *Neuropsychologia*, 1979, *17*, 353–361.

Botkin, A.L., Schmaltz, L.W., & Lamb, D.H. "Overloading" the left hemisphere in right-handed subjects with verbal and motor tasks. *Neuropsychologia*, 1977, *15*, 591–596.

Bowers, D., & Heilman, K. Material specific hemispheric arousal. *Neuropsychologia*, 1976, *14*, 123–128.

Bowers, D., Heilman, K.M., Satz, P., & Altman, A. Simultaneous performance on verbal, nonverbal, and motor tasks by right-handed adults. *Cortex*, 1978, *14*, 540–556.

Briggs, G.G. A comparison of attentional and control shift models of the performance of concurrent tasks. *Acta Psychologica*, 1975, *39*, 183–191.

Broadbent, D.E. The role of auditory localization in attention and memory span. *Journal of Experimental Psychology*, 1954, *47*, 191–196.

Bryden, M.P., & Allard, F. Dichotic listening and the development of linguistic processes. In M. Kinsbourne (Ed.), *Assymmetrical function of the brain*. New York: Cambridge University Press, 1978.

Carey, S., & Diamond, R. From piecemeal to configurational representation of faces. *Science*, 1977, *195*, 312–314.

Carey S., Diamond R., & Woods, B. Development of face recognition—A maturational component? *Developmental Psychology*, 1980, *16*, 257–269.

Case, R. Intellectual development from birth to adulthood: A neo-Piagetian interpretation. In R. Siegler (Ed.), *Children's thinking: What develops?* Hillsdale, N.J.: Erlbaum, 1978.

Cermak, S.A., Drake, C., Cermak, L.S., & Kenney, R. The effect of concurrent manual activity on the dichotic listening performance of boys with learning disabilities. *The American Journal of Occupational Therapy*. 1978, *32*, 493–499.

Cernacek, J. Contralateral motor irradiation—cerebral dominance: Its changes in hemiparesis. *Archives of Neurology*, 1961, *4*, 165–172.

Clare, M.H., & Bishop, G.H. Electromyographic analysis of the physiologic component of tremor. *Archives of Physical Medicine*, 1949, *30*, 559–566.

Cook, T.W. Studies in cross education. 1. Mirror tracing the star-shaped maze. *Journal of Experimental Psychology*, 1933a, *16*, 144–160.

Cook, T.W. Studies in cross education. 2. Further experiments in mirror tracing the star-shaped maze. *Journal of Experimental Psychology*, 1933b, *16*, 679–700.

Cook, T.W. Studies in cross eductaion. 3. Kinesthetic learning of an irregular pattern. *Journal of Experimental Psychology*, 1934, *17*, 749–762.

Cullen, J.K., Jr., Thompson, C.L., Hughes, L.F. et al. The effects of varied acoustic parameters on performance in dichotic speech perception tasks. *Brain and Language*, 1974, *1*, 307–322.

Dalby, J.T. Hemispheric timesharing: Verbal and spatial loading with concurrent unimanual activity. *Cortex*, 1980, *16*, 567–573.

Dalby, J.T., & Gibson, D. Functional cerebral lateralization in subtypes of disabled readers. *Brain and Language*, 1981, *14*, 34–48.

Davis, R.C. The pattern of response in a tendon reflex. *Journal of Experimental Psychology*, 1942a, *30*, 452–463.

Davis, R.C. The pattern of muscular action in simple voluntary movements. *Journal of Experimental Psychology*, 1942b, *31*, 347–366.

Dawson, G.D., Investigations on a patient subject to myoclonic seizures after sensory stimulation. *Journal of Neurology, Neurosurgery and Psychiatry*, 1947, *10*, 141–162.

Dawson, G.D. A summation technique for detection of small evoked potentials, *Electroencephalography and Clinical Neurophysiology*, 1954, *6*, 65–84.

Deatherage, B.H., & Evans, T.R. Binaural masking: Backward, forward, and simulataneous effects. *Journal of the Acoustical Society of America*, 1969, *46*, 362–371.

Duncan, J. Divided attention: The whole is more than the sum of its parts. *Journal of Experimental Psychology: Human Perception and Performance*, 1979, *5*, 216–228.

Fitts, P.M., & Posner, M.I. *Human performance*. Belmont, Calif.: Brooks/Cole, 1967.

Friedman, A., & Polson, M.C. Hemispheres as independent resource systems: Limited-capacity processing and cerebral specialization. *Journal of Experimental Psychology: Human Perception and Performance*, 1981, *7*, 1031–1058.

Gardner, E.B., & Branski, D.H. Unilateral cerebral activation and perception of gaps: A signal detection analysis. *Neuropsychologia*, 1976, *14*, 43–53.

Gardner, E.B., Eagan, M.J., & Branski, D.M. Attentional bias in gap-detection: An investigation of "the Kinsbourne effect." Paper presented to the American Psychological Association, Montreal, 1973.

Gates, A., & Bradshaw, J.L. The role of the cerebral hemispheres in music. *Brain and Language*, 1977, *4*, 403–431.

Gibson, E.J. Sensory generalization with voluntary reactions. *Journal of Experimental Psychology*, 1939, *24*, 237–253.

Goodglass, H. Shai, A., Rosen, W., & Berman, M. New observations on right-left differences in tachistoscopic recognition of verbal and non-verbal stimuli. Paper presented at the International Neuropsychological Society meeting, Washington, D.C., 1971.

Gopher, D., & North, R.A. Manipulating the conditions of training in time-sharing performance. *Human Factors*, 1977, *19*, 583–593.

Grafman, J., Passafiume, D., Faglioni, P., & Boller, F. Calculation disturbances in adults with focal hemispheric damage. *Cortex*, 1982, *18*, 37–50.

Hécaen, H. Clinical symptomatology in right and left hemispheric lesions. In D.B. Mountcastle (Ed.), *Interhemispheric relations and cerebral dominance*. Baltimore: Johns Hopkins Press, 1962.

Hellige, J.B., Visual laterality patterns for pure- versus mixed-list presentation. *Journal of Experimental Psychology: Human Perception and Performance*, 1978, *4*, 121–131.

Hellige, J.B., & Cox, P.J. Effects of concurrent verbal memory on recognition of stimuli from the left and right visual fields. *Journal of Experimental Psychology: Human Perception and Performance*, 1976, *2*, 210–221.

Hellige, J.B., Cox, P.J., & Litvac, L. Information processing in the cerebral hemispheres: Selective hemispheric activation and capacity limitations. *Journal of Experimental Psychology: General*, 1979, *108*, 251–279.

Hellige, J.B, & Longstreth, L.E. Effects of concurrent hemisphere-specific activity on unimanual tapping rate. *Neuropsychologia*, 1981, *19*, 1–10.

Hicks, R.E. Intrahemispheric response competition between vocal and unimanual performance in normal adult human males. *Journal of Comparative and Physiological Psychology*, 1975, *89*, 50–60.

Hicks, R.E., Bradshaw, G.J., Kinsbourne, M., & Feigin, D.S. Vocal-manual trade-offs in hemispheric sharing of human performance control. *Journal of Motor Behavior*, 1978, *10*, 1–6.

Hicks, R.E., Frank, J.M., & Kinsbourne, M. The locus of bimanual skill transfer. *Journal of General Psychology*, 1982, *107*, 277–281.

Hicks, R.E., Provenzano, F.J., & Rybstein, E.D. Generalized and lateralized effects of concurrent verbal rehearsal upon performance of sequential movements of the fingers by the left and right hands. *Acta Psychologica*, 1975, *39*, 119–130.

Hiscock, M. Verbal-manual time sharing in children as a function of task priority. *Brain and Cognition*, 1982, *1*, 119–131.

Hiscock, M., & Kinsbourne, M. Ontogeny of cerebral dominance: Evidence from time-sharing asymmetry in children. *Developmental Psychology*, 1978, *14*, 321–329.

Hiscock, M., & Kinsbourne, M. Asymmetry of verbal-manual time sharing in children: A follow-up study. *Neuropsychologia*, 1980, *18*, 151–162.

Hiscock, M., Antoniuk, D., & Prisciak, K. Dual-task performance as a function of children's age and academic skill level. Manuscript in preparation, 1982a.

Hiscock, M., Kinsbourne, M., Samuels, M., & Krause, A.E. The development of dual-task performance: Effects of speaking and memory-encoding upon the rate and variability of children's finger tapping. Manuscript in preparation, 1982b.

Johnson, O., & Kozma, A. Effects of concurrent verbal and musical tasks on a unimanual skill. *Cortex*, 1977, *13*, 11–16.

Johnston, W.A., Greenberg, S.N., Fisher, R.P., & Martin, D.W. Divided attention: A vehicle for monitoring memory processes. *Journal of Experimental Psychology*, 1970, *83*, 164–171.

Kahneman, D. *Attention and effort*. Englewood Cliffs, N.J.: Prentice-Hall, 1973.

Kantowitz, B.H., & Knight, J.L., Jr. On experimenter-limited processes. *Psychological Review*, 1976, *83*, 502–507.

Keele, S.W. *Attention and human performance*. Pacific Palisades, Calif: Goodyear, 1973.

Kerr, B. Processing demands during mental operations. *Memory and Cognition*, 1973, *1*, 401–412.

Kimura, D. Cerebral dominance and the perception of verbal stimuli. *Canadian Journal of Psychology*, 1961, *15*, 166–171.

Kimura, D. The neural basis of language qua gesture. In H. Whitaker and H. Whitaker (Eds.), *Studies in neurolinguistics, Vol. 2*. New York: Academic Press, 1976.

Kimura, D., & Archibald, Y. Motor functions of the left hemisphere. *Brain*, 1974, *97*, 337–350.

Kinsbourne, M. The cerebral basis of lateral asymmetries in attention. In A.F. Sanders (Ed.), *Attention and performance III*. Amsterdam: North-Holland, 1970.

Kinsbourne, M. The control of attention by interaction between the cerebral hemispheres. In S. Kornblum (Ed.), *Attention and performance IV*. New York Academic Press, 1973.

Kinsbourne, M. The mechanisms of hemispheric control of the lateral gradient of attention. In P.M.A. Rabbitt & S. Dornic (Eds.), *Attention and performance V*. New York: Academic Press, 1975.

Kinsbourne, M. Single channel theory. In D.H. Holding (Ed.), *Human skills*. Chichester, Sussex: Wiley, 1981.

Kinsbourne, M. Hemispheric specialization and the growth of human understanding. *American Psychologist*, 1982, *37*, 411–420.

Kinsbourne, M., & Cook, J. Generalized and lateralized effects of concurrent verbalization on a unimanual skill. *Quarterly Journal of Experimental Psychology*, 1971, *23*, 341–345.

Kinsbourne, M., & Hicks, R.E. Functional cerebral space: A model for overflow, transfer and interference effects in human performance. In J. Requin (Ed.), *Attention and performance VII*. Hillsdale, N.J.: Erlbaum, 1978.

Kinsbourne, M., & McMurray, J. The effect of cerebral dominance on time sharing between speaking and tapping by preschool children. *Child Development*, 1975, *46*, 240–242.

Klapp, S.T. Doing two things at once: The role of temporal compatibility. *Memory and Cognition*, 1979, *5*, 375–381.

LaBerge, D. Attention and the measurement of perceptual learning. *Memory and Cognition*, 1973, *1*, 268–276.

LeDoux, J.E., Wilson, D.H., & Gazzaniga, M.S. Manipulo-spatial aspects of cerebral lateralization: Clues to the origin of lateralization. *Neuropsychologia*, 1977, *15*, 743–750.

Lenneberg, E.H. *Biological foundations of language*. New York: Wiley, 1967.

Lomas, J. Competition within the left hemisphere between speaking and unimanual tasks performed without visual guidance. *Neuropsychologia*, 1980, *18*, 141–149.

Lomas, J., & Kimura, D. Intrahemispheric interaction between speaking and sequential manual activity. *Neuropsychologia*, 1976, *14*, 23–33.

Lundervold, A. Electromyographic investigations during sedentary work, especially typewriting. *British Journal of Physical Medicine*, 1951, *14*, 32–36.

Luria, A.R. *Higher cortical functions in man*. New York: Basic Books, 1966.

Majeres, R.L. The effect of unimanual performance on speed of verbalization. *Journal of Motor Behavior*, 1975, *7*, 57–58.

McFarland, K., & Ashton, R. A developmental study of the influence of cognitive activity on an ongoing manual task, *Acta Psychologica*, 1975a, *39*, 447–456.

McFarland, K.A., & Ashton, R. The lateralized effects of concurrent cognitive activity on a unimanual skill. *Cortex*, 1975b, *11*, 283–290.

McFarland, K.A., & Ashton, R. The influence of brain lateralization of function on a manual skill. *Cortex*, 1978a, *14*, 102–111.

McFarland, K.A., & Ashton, R. The influence of concurrent task difficulty on manual performance. *Neuropsychologia*, 1978b, *16*, 735–741.

McFarland, K.A., & Ashton, R. The lateralized effects of concurrent cognitive and motor performance. *Perception and Psychophysics*, 1978c, *23*, 344–349.

Michon, J.A. A note on the measurement of perceptual motor load. *Ergonomics*, 1964, *7*, 461–463.

Michon, J.A. Tapping regularity as a measure of perceptual motor load. *Ergonomics*, 1966, *9*, 401–412.

Moray, M. Where is a capacity limited? A survey and a model. *Acta Psychologica*, 1967, *27*, 84–92.

Navon, D., & Gopher, D. On the economy of the human information processing system: A model of multiple capacity. *Psychological Review*, 1979, *86*, 214–225.

Navon, D., & Gopher, D. Task difficulty, resources and dual task performance. In R.S. Nickerson (Ed.), *Attention and performance VIII*. Hillsdale, N.J.: Erlbaum, 1980.

Noble, M., Trumbo, D.A., & Fowler, F. Further evidence of secondary task interference in tracking. *Journal of Experimental Psychology*, 1967, *73*, 146–149.

Norman, D.A., & Bobrow, D.G. On data-limited and resource-limited processes. *Cognitive Psychology*, 1975, *7*, 44–64.

Norman, D.A., & Bobrow, D.G. On the analysis of performance operating characteristics. *Psychological Review*, 1976, *83*, 508–510.

Obrzut, J.E., Hynd, G.W., Obrzut, A., & Leitgeb, J.L. Time sharing and dichotic listening asymmetry in normal and learning-disabled children. *Brain and Language*, 1980, *11*, 181–194.

Pascual-Leone, J. A mathematical model for the transition role in Piaget's developmental stages. *Acta Psychologica*, 1970, *63*, 301–345.

Peters, A. Why the preferred hand taps more quickly than the non-preferred hand: Three experiments on handedness. *Canadian Journal of Psychology*, 1980, *34*, 62–71.

Piazza, D.M. Cerebral lateralization in young children as measured by dichotic listening and finger tapping tasks. *Neuropsychologia*, 1977, *15*, 417–425.

Porter, R.J., & Berlin, C.I. On interpreting developmental changes in the dichotic right ear advantage. *Brain and Language*, 1975, *2*, 186–200.

Posner, M.I. *Chronometric explorations of mind: The third Paul M. Fitts lectures*. Hillsdale, N.J.: Erlbaum, 1978.

Posner, M.I. Cumulative development of attentional theory. *American Psychologist*, 1982, *37*, 168–179.

Posner, M.I., & Boies, S.J. Components of attention. *Psychological Review*, 1971, *78*, 391–408.

Purpura, D. Comparative physiology of dendrites. In G.C. Quarton, T. Melnechuk, & F.O. Schmitt (Eds.), *The neurosciences*. New York: Rockefeller University Press, 1967.

Satz, P., Bakker, D.J., Teunisson, J. et al. Developmental parameters of the ear asymmetry: A multivariate approach. *Brain and Language*, 1975, *2*, 171–185.

Searleman, A. A review of right hemisphere linguistic capabilities. *Psychological Bulletin*, 1977, *84*, 503–528.

Sergent, J. About face: Left-hemisphere involvement in processing physiognomies *Journal of Experimental Psychology: Human Perception and Performance*, 1982, *8*, 1–14.

Shepard, R.N., & Teghtsoonian, M. Retention of information under conditions approaching a steady state. *Journal of Experimental Psychology*, 1961, *62*, 302–309.

Sherrington, C.S. *The integrative action of the nervous system*. New Haven, Conn.: Yale University Press, 1906.

Spelke, E., Hirst, W., & Neisser, U. Skills of divided attention. *Cognition*, 1976, *4*, 215–230.

Summers, J.J., & Sharp, C.A. Bilateral effects of concurrent verbal and spatial rehearsal on complex motor sequencing. *Neuropsychologia*, 1979, *17*, 331–343.

Trumbo, D.A., & Noble, M.E. Secondary task effects on serial verbal learning. *Journal of Experimental Psychology*, 1970, *85*, 418–424.

Trumbo, D.A., Noble, M.E., & Swink, J. Secondary task interference in the performance of tracking tasks. *Journal of Experimental Psychology*, 1967, *73*, 232-240.

Tukey, J.W. One degree of freedom for nonadditivity. *Biometrics*, 1949. *5*, 232-242.

Welford, A.T. The "psychological refractory period" and the timing of high speed performance: A review and a theory. *British Journal of Psychology*, 1952, *43*, 2-19.

Welford, A.T. Evidence of a single-channel decision mechanism limiting performance in a serial reaction task. *Quarterly Journal of Experimental Psychology*, 1959, *11*, 193-210.

Welford, A.T *Fundamentals of skill.* London: Methuen, 1968.

White, N., & Kinsbourne, M. Does speech output control lateralization over time? Evidence from verbal-manual time-sharing tasks. *Brain and Language*, 1980, *10*, 215-223.

Wickens, C. The structure of attentional resources. In R. Nickerson (Ed.), *Attention and performance VIII*. Hillsdale, N.J.: Erlbaum, 1980.

Witelson, S.F. Hemispheric specialization for linguistic and nonlinguistic tactual perception using a dichotomous stimulation technique. *Cortex*, 1974, *10*, 3-17.

Wolff, P.H., & Cohen, C. Dual task performance during bimanual coordination. *Cortex*, 1980, *16*, 119-133.

9

Brain Potential (BP) Evidence for Lateralization of Higher Cognitive Functions

Alan S. Gevins

INTRODUCTION

In the last few years, many studies have reported human brain potential (BP) evidence for cerebral lateralization of cognitive functions. Most of these studies have seemingly supported the idea that the left cortical hemisphere of right-handers mediates language processing and other sequential cognitive processes, while the right hemisphere mediates spatial, "gestalt," and even affective aspects of cognition. Recently, this entire body of BP research has been called into question on methodological grounds. Essentially, there seems to have been a preoccupation with finding left-right differences to the exclusion of more basic issues, including the mechanisms of mass neural processing, the representation of higher cognitive functions in the mass electrical activity of the brain, and requisite experimental controls. This chapter will briefly review methods for recording and analyzing BP, their origin and transmission to the scalp, the implicit brain model in BP studies, and methodologic requirements for associating a BP with a cognitive function. This will be followed by a detailed critical review of EEG and evoked potential studies of lateralization of cognition. Finally, a summary of our latest research will be presented, in which we have found that even simple numerical and spatial judgments are associated with complex and rapidly changing BP patterns in many areas of both hemispheres. Lateralized patterns can develop and fade in successive fractions of a second.

METHODS OF STUDYING BP

There are two popular methods of studying brain potentials—electroencephalogram (EEG), or continuous recording, and averaged evoked potential (EP), or recording that is time registered to a stimulus or response. EEGs are recorded for tens of seconds to minutes, while EPs last about a second. EEGs may be recorded while a person performs complex problem-solving tasks while EPs are usually obtained during simple judgment tasks. (A hybrid paradigm, called "probe EP," computes EPs to irrelevant stimuli while a person performs a complex task; physiological interpretation is difficult.) Since EPs are synchronized to an external event, it is possible to obtain a clear picture of the sequence of brain electrical events (peaks and valleys) associated with a simple judgment by averaging the potentials over many repetitions of the judgment. Most BP studies of cognition presently use the EP method because its superior temporal resolution allows the association of a change in averaged BP peaks with a particular cognitive process. Changes in the amplitude or timing of these peaks have been associated with successive stages of the brain's stimulus processing over a 500 or so millisecond epoch, including expectation (prestimulus), encoding of stimulus properties, selective attention, detection of a novel or relevant stimulus, context updating, concept formation, and preparation for response.

The most well-known cognitive EP component is the "P3" or "P300." First discovered by Samuel Sutton, Roy John, and their associates in New York in 1965, this very prominent and reliable component is sometimes even visible on the unaveraged EEG polygraph. It is an endogenous component that does not necessarily covary with the physical properties of a stimulus but rather with some aspect of the stimulus' significance to the participant. There has been much discussion about the number of different types of P3 components and their psychological significance (Donchin, Ritter, & Cheyne, 1978; Roth, 1978; Sutton, Tueting, & Hammer, 1978; Teuting, 1978). Most interpretations of P3 associate it with updating of "subjective probabilities" (Donchin et al., 1978), stimulus set selection (Duncan-Johnson & Donchin, 1979), go/no-go judgments (Simpson, Vaughn, & Ritter, 1977), and other manipulations that seem to relate to the novelty or relevance of a stimulus (or its absence) to the participant. The latency of an earlier, sense modality dependent potential, N2, has been found to have a higher correlation with reaction time than P3 (Simpson et al., 1977). Additionally, a "P3-like" component has been found in the human hippocampus, with about the same latency and which reacts to the same experimental manipulations as the scalp P3 (Halgren et al., 1980). A hippocampal origin of the P3 would be consistent with its putative psychological significance as a sign of the detection of a novel stimulus. P3s have not often been reported to vary in lateralization, as a function of experimental manipulation.

There has been little support for lateralization of higher cognitive functions from EP studies. This may be due to the automization of the repeated simple judgments that are usually used in the EP paradigm. Alternatively, it may be that the commonly studied EP peaks are not cortical in origin. Finally, the insufficient spatial sampling of each hemisphere in most EP studies may be a contributing factor to negative results. Most positive reports of lateralization have been based on the EEG method. These reports may reflect the existence of linguistic and spatial "cognitive modes" in the brain, lasting tens of seconds or more, or they may be due to the confounding of the cognitive manipulation with uncontrolled differences in stimulus, performance-related factors, and efferent factors of complex problem-solving tasks.

Another basic point is that the recording equipment and analytical tools used in BP reseach are currently inadequate for actually measuring the very complex spatiotemporal electrical events that must be associated with higher brain functions. With even the most advanced technology, the best we can hope for at this time is to see some signs of where and when mass neural processing is specifically related to different types of cognitive tasks. This is very remote from measuring the brain's hypothesized mass electrical code for higher cognitive functions, for which a deeper understanding of the origin and significance of BP would seem to be necessary. Likewise, more powerful computerized analyses are needed for extracting the small BP signals related to higher cognitive functions from the vast sea of electrical "noise" unrelated to these functions. But even with current limitations, useful information may be gleaned from EEGs and EPs. Further, the noninvasive nature of BP recording and the very fine temporal resolution possible with BP motivate the further development of BP recording and analysis technologies.

Considering current technological limitations, it is apparent that BP has been too often used in a simplistic search for direct parallels between the mass electrical activity of the human brain and abstract psychological constructs. Often forgotten are the conclusions of the eminent neuropsychologist, A.R. Luria (1973, 1977), that abstract mental functions seem to involve complex interactions of many areas of the brain.

METHODS OF RECORDING BP

Electroencephalography measures summated neuronal electrical activity. Unaveraged scalp-recorded BPs normally range from 10 to 200 uV, but may rise to 1 mV during epileptic seizures (Figure 9-1). Between 3 and 20 electrodes are applied to the scalp in research studies, and the voltage changes over time in each electrode are recorded. When multiple electrodes are used, they are usually placed over each of the major lobes of the cerebral cortex of the brain. The electrodes are arranged in symmetrical patterns of connections called montages, and different montages can highlight or concentrate on particular electrode connections. Each electrode is connected with an electrically relatively "neutral" lead attached to the ear lobes, mastoids, chest, chin, nose, or the average of all other electrodes. This is called a "reference" montage. Each electrode can be connected with another "active" lead located over a different scalp area. This is called a "bipolar" montage. The type of reference can alter the magnitude of BP asymmetries. Unilateral references are especially problematical, since an asymmetry can result from potentials in the reference rather than the active electrode. EEGs are conventionally described as patterns of activity in five frequency ranges: delta (less than 4 Hz), theta (4 to 7 Hz), alpha (8 to 12 Hz), beta (13 to 30 Hz), and gamma (more than 30 Hz). The harmonic composition of BP is usually complex and only occasionally approaches a sinusoidal form. BP amplitude at the scalp generally decreases with increasing frequency, largely due to blur distortion from transmission through the cerebral spinal fluid, the skull, and the scalp. The origin of the low-voltage, scalp-recorded potentials above about 25 to 35 Hz can be ambiguous, possibly arising from a mixture of cortical activity and muscle action potentials. In EEG recordings the 3dB bandpass points of the amplifiers are typically set to 1 and 70 Hz, while in EP studies they may be set to 0.01 and 15 Hz.

Electrodes are also attached near the eye to record potentials produced by eye movements, to the arm to record muscle potentials if a finger or hand movement is required in the experiment, and sometimes to the throat to measure subvocalization. These signals are recorded because BP can be contaminated by artifacts originating from muscles and other physiological and instrumental sources, including sweating and loose or moving electrodes (Kooi, Tucker, & Marshall, 1978). In EEG polygraph tracings from clinically normal people, some of the characteristics of artifacts include fuzziness or thickness of the trace, sudden large changes in voltage, or repetitive sharp or saw-toothed waveforms. It is essential to delete portions of the tracings contaminated by such artifacts if one is to have the certainty that only BPs are being measured. Such editing is best done manually, as current automated editing is far from perfect. Machines or programs that compute summated BP indexes on-line (eg., EEG spectral intensities or averaged EPs) usually preclude careful manual editing. There is little reason to accept the results of a BP study that did not eliminate every segment of contaminated data.

A typical research recording session lasts about one to four hours and usually consists of repetitions of tasks such as signal detection, spatial rotation, block design, linguistic processing, arithmetic, and so forth. These tasks can require a switch press as a response or more complex efferent activity. As noted, a response is required to make strong inferences about the existence of a cognitive function.

SIGNAL PROCESSING OF BP

The importance of signal processing in studying the BP of higher cognitive functions cannot be overly stressed. Signal processing is our microscope, but unfortunately there are as yet few, if any, adequate standard products. Researchers must, therefore, make their own instruments. This section will only outline BP signal-processing techniques in order to organize the discussion below. Numerous detailed reviews and examples may be found in the published literature (Dolce & Kunkel, 1975; Gevins, 1980; Gevins et al., 1975; Glaser & Runchkin, 1976; John, Ruchkin, & Vidal, 1978; John 1977; Matejcek & Schenk 1975; Remond, 1977).

Five major steps are necessary for a complete BP analysis (Table 9-1): signal conditioning and digitization, primary analysis, feature extraction, classification and/or decision, and validation. Our computer system, ADIEEG, which performs these five steps, has been previously described (Gevins et al., 1975; Gevins, Zeitlin, Yingling et al., 1979; Gevins, 1980).

THE ORIGIN AND POSSIBLE SIGNIFICANCE OF BP

Unaveraged, spontaneous BPs, recorded by an electrode on the surface of the cortex, are thought to be largely a function of postsynaptic potentials of perhaps hundreds of thousands to millions of vertically oriented, columnarly organized, pyramidal cells in cortical layers three and five (Creutzfeldt, 1974; Elul, 1972a, 1972b). A number of studies have demonstrated that the probability of action potentials in neurons is highly correlated with the amplitude and phase of low-frequency extracellular macropotentials, although the exact phase relation varies with the type of neural tissue and the recording

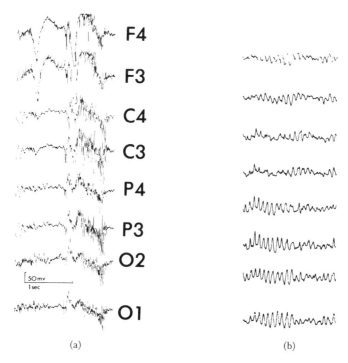

(a)

(b)

Figure 9-1, a-e. *EEG polygraph excerpts. Anatomic placements are the same in all excerpts except (c) (refer to outline of head in (c) to associate a symbolic designation with its anatomic location). The same amplitude and time scales have been used in (a) - (e). In (d) they are slightly expanded as shown. (a) Eye movement potential contamination evident as large V-shaped waves in frontal (F4 and F3) electrodes. Movement and muscle action potential contamination evident at right as large amplitude, high and low frequency components in all channels. (b) Relaxation (eyes closed) is associated with rhythmic waveforms of approximately 9 Hz (alpha rhythm) most prominent in the posterior (parietal-P, and occipital-O) channels. (c) Onset of drowsiness at about the "o" in the word "drowsy" is associated with a reduction in the alpha rhythm and an increase in low frequency (below approximately 8 Hz) components. (d) Valium, a commonly used tranquilizer, produces high frequency (above about 20 Hz) activity in all electrodes. (e) Variation of BEP's during visual fixation by three persons. (From Gevins, A.S.,* IEEE Trans. on Patt. Analys. and Intell. *PAMI*-2:5:383-404, 1980. © *1980 IEEE.*

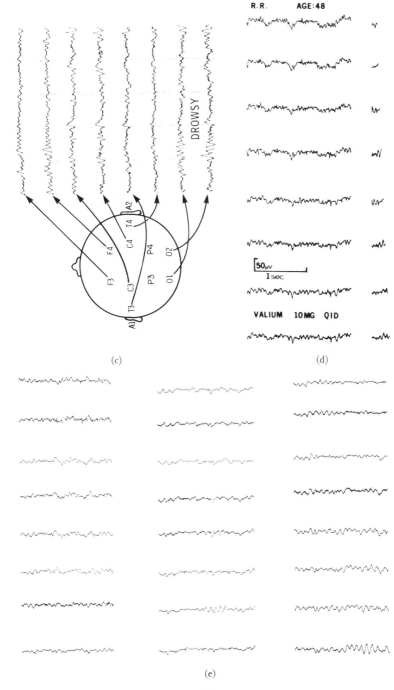

TABLE 9-1.
Complete BP Analysis

Step	Explanation	Example
Signal conditioning and digitization	Prepare BP for analysis; read into computer.	Filter out low- and high-frequency components.
Primary analysis	Compute important properties of the signal.	EEG frequency analysis; Averaged evoked potentials (EP)
Feature extraction	Summarize important properties.	EEG: amount of energy in delta, theta, alpha, and beta bands; EP: location and size of peaks or principal components analysis.
Classification	Decide how the BP analysis relates to the cognitive manipulation.	Classify BP patterns with their cognitive tasks.
Validation	Determine that the results apply in general.	Determine if the same BP pattern is associated with a particular cognitive task when performed by a new group of people.

site (Creutzfeldt, Watanabe, & Lux, 1966a, 1966b; Fox, 1970; Freeman, 1975; Purpura et al., 1966; Verzeano & Calma, 1954; Verzeano et al., 1970). The functional significance of mass BP is not known. Some neuroscientists think that these macropotentials are a useful epiphenomenon that may be likened to the smoke from a factory that may indicate when a factory is busy without signifying exactly what the factory is doing. An important minority of neuroscientists think that, under proper conditions, macropotentials may be found to contain more specific signs of neural information processing (Freeman, 1975, 1979a, 1979b, 1979c, 1980; Freeman & Schneider, 1982).

There is a gross correspondence between Broadman's cortical areas and some major functional systems of the human brain, particularly for sensory input and motor output, and for some elements of language and spatial processing. However, the knowledge of this localization has not been primarily based on scalp-recorded BP, but rather from the study of patients with localized brain lesions or with commissurotomies, from focally stimulated neurosurgery patients, and from radiologic studies, including regional cerebral blood flow and positron emission tomography (Ingvar, 1978; Ingvar & Lassen, 1975; Ingvar, Sjoland, & Ardo; 1976; Mazziotta & Phelps, in press; Mazziotta et al., 1980, 1981a, 1981b; Metter, 1981; Phelps, 1981; Phelps et al., 1981). Some supporting evidence also comes from averaged sensory and motor EP studies. While there is gross localization of some aspects of sensory, motor, linguistic, and spatial processing, no simple correspondence has been found between Broadman areas and abstract mental functions, such as different types of reasoning per se. Inferences from patients with focal brain lesions can be misleading in this regard since, as the nineteenth century British neurologist, John Hughlings Jackson, stressed, localization of a lesion that interferes with a mental function does not mean that the function itself has been localized. The plasticity of the brain following lesions must also be considered in this regard (Bach-y-Rita, 1972, 1980). It seems that, as our source of data shifts from behavioral or structural observations of brain-lesioned patients to direct imaging of healthy brain functioning, the emphasis in our modeling is shifting toward a more dynamic, mosaic model of higher brain functions (Gevins, 1981).

BRAIN MODELS IMPLICIT IN BP STUDIES

When studying the brain's mass electrical potentials during higher cognitive functions, it is useful to make explicit the underlying model of the brain as an information-processing system. In EEG spectral analysis studies, it is implicitly assumed that the brain consists of compartments corresponding in number to the scalp electrodes. The energy emitted by these compartments in several low-frequency bands is thought to be related to the number of neurons engaged in "cooperative processes" (Elul, 1969, 1972a, 1972b). In practice, the EEG is recorded for periods from several seconds to a minute while people perform arithmetic, geometric figure rotations, or other complex problem-solving tasks. These tasks consist of the concatenation of many more basic operations (e.g., arithmetic consists of operators, carries, stores, etc.). In this type of study it is implicity assumed that there are task-specific cognitive brain states that have characteristics spectral intensity patterns (Gevins & Schaffer, 1980). In fact, it has never been demonstrated that this assumption is true under conditions in which the type of mental task is varied while perceptual, performance-related, and efferent factors are controlled (Gevins et al., 1979a, 1979b, 1979c, 1980). On the contrary, the remarkable similarity of the EEG spatial distribution for different types of controlled mental tasks suggests that complex problem solving is widely distributed in the brain.

A more process-oriented model underlies averaged evoked potential studies of cognition. The average EP paradigm generally treats the brain as a black box that, on the average, emits voltage peaks at characteristic delays after a stimulus. Changes in the time, amplitude, and anatomic distribution of these voltage peaks are used to characterize stimulus and response properties as well as variations in the type of cognition. While the EP paradigm has been, and continued to be, very fruitful, the problem with this research model is that the relations between cognitive and neural processes are not actually as direct or as simple as they are assumed to be. For example, the recent work of Rohrbaugh, Lindsley, and associates (1980) demonstrated that a contingent negative variation (CNV) synthesized from unrelated stimuli and responses is indistinguishable from the "real" CNV discovered by the late British psychiatrist, Grey Walter (Walter et al., 1964). Consider another example of the nonunique association between EPs and cognitive functions. In 1973 Hillyard, at the University of California, San Diego, reported increased voltage of an EP peak, called N1, with selective attention. This phenomenon was thought to represent early stimulus set selection prior to full cognition of the meaning of the stimulus. However, recently Naatanen and Michie (1979) and Naatanen, Gaillard, and Mantysalo (1978) at Helsinki and Parasuraman and Beatty (1980) at UCLA have shown that the psychological manipulation of selective attention does not necessarily result in an enhancement of N1 component amplitude. Naatanen and Michie did this merely by lengthening the interstimulus interval to about 800 msec instead of 500 msec and by using many stimuli to make the average. Although much useful knowledge can be obtained from the EP, if the same EP effect can be produced under a variety of psychological circumstances and if the same psychological manipulations do not produce the same EP effects, the EP effects have no intrinsic existence outside the context of a particular experiment and are, therefore, not related to the specific content of cognitive processes. This is the upper bounds on their specificity.

Thus, while they continue to produce useful results, both currently popular paradigms, EEG and EP, are based upon very simplified models of the brain and cognition. The former has insufficient temporal resolution and lumps together too many cognitive processes, while the latter performs an excessive data reduction of the brain's electrical activity, resulting in too few parameters to characterize the content of cognitive processing. A somewhat more realistic research model may be to consider the brain as a local distributed computational network (outlined in Gevins, 1981).

COGNITIVE CONSIDERATIONS AND METHODOLOGICAL CRITERIA

It is not possible, in principle, to relate a BP pattern to a cognitive process. One cannot measure cognitive processes themselves; one can only measure the products of cognition, namely, the behavioral responses following performance of tasks requiring different cognitive processes. In psychological studies, statistical evaluation of behavioral measures (e.g., reaction time or solution accuracy) is used to infer that certain cognitive processes were performed. BP studies attempt to find correlates of this inferred activity. Yet experimental tasks usually require performance of a variety of afferent, efferent, and cognitive processes. For example, in addition to recall of an item, a "memory" task can involve watching or listening to a stimulus and activating a response switch. The clarity of a BP study thus depends upon the effectiveness of methodological controls designed to isolate and manipulate specific cognitive processes while eliminating or holding constant other task-related activities. When controls are inadequate, the error can be made of associating a BP pattern with a certain abstract psychological construct, such as " spatial imagery," when, in fact, it might actually be associated with a variety of other cognitive processes or with more mundane processes, such as finger movements. Even when other factors are controlled, it is difficult to deduce the characteristics (order, time of onset, and duration) of the component operations of any given complex problem-solving task. Such tasks are obviously heterogeneous composites of parallel and sequential cognitive operations, for example, mental multiplication consists of a series of "multiply," "store," "add," and "carry" operations; and mental rotation of geometric forms is composed of a series of "search," "transformation," "comparison," and "confirmation" operations, each lasting between 100 and 500 msec (Just & Carpenter, 1976). Thus, sampling several seconds of BP for analysis is based upon the supposition that the component operations together constitute a distinguishable neurophysiological state. In most instances, there is no strong evidence from healthy persons to support this supposition. This situation is improved in the EP paradigm by analysis procedures utilizing shorter samples that are time-locked to an event, but, as noted, there is the likelihood that simple judgment will become "automated" when repeated dozens of times to form an average EP.

It is difficult to isolate BP patterns during a task that may reflect the degree of metabolic activity of the cerebral cortex and subcortical structures from those that may characterize the specific information processing of a task. In fact, these two types of patterns are not distinct but reflect two hierarchically different levels of description of the same phenomenon. It is obviously even more difficult to measure the fine degree of spatial and temporal patterning specifically associated with different types of information processing. The overall cortical activity level is largely controlled by the reticular formation of the thalamus (Anderson & Anderson, 1968; Moruzzi & Magoun, 1949) which itself receives inputs from many cortical and subcortical areas. The ascending reticular activating system receives primary sensory signals, integrates them, and transmits signals that regulate the activity level of the cortex. In concert with areas of frontal cortex, specific thalamic nuclei gate sensory signals to local cortical areas (Skinner & Yingling, 1977). Since they are simpler to interpret, indexes of the activation of the autonomic nervous system, such as pupil size or heart rate, have been used as indirect measures of phasic activation of the central nervous system (CNS) during the execution of cognitive tasks (Kahneman, 1973). Yet automatic changes are systemic responses accompanying CNS changes. Direct measures of CNS activation, such as banded EEG spectral intensity, have so far only been used to differentiate gross differences along the sleep-walking continuum (Loomis et al., 1938; Rechtschaffen & Kales, 1973). While only limited attempts have been made to differentiate gradations of the walking state (Daniel, 1966; Simon, Schultz, & Rassman, 1977), there does not seem to be any fundamental obstacle to deriving such an EEG index (Gevins et al., 1977, 1979a).

The methodologic requirements for studies correlating BP with cognitive functions are discussed in recent books and review articles (Donchin, Kutas, & McCarthy, 1977; Gevins, 1980; Gevins & Schaffer, 1980; Thatcher & John, 1977). Table 9-2 summarizes the essential points. The first prerequisite is the control of irrelevant variables. BPs vary markedly as a function of age, state of arousal, handedness, and recent intake of common substances including coffee, cigarettes, alcohol, and tranquilizers. Unless one is explicitly studying these variables, they must be controlled to be as homogeneous as possible within the sample of persons studied. As noted, the elimination of contaminating nonneuroelectric artifacts is also prerequisite to any study using BP.

It is necessary to measure behavior during task performance to know that the participants are doing what the experimenter assumes that they are doing. In this regard, tasks that require a person to imagine something are not suitable. Only trials known to be performed correctly may, strictly speaking, be used for the BP analysis, unless one is studying errors. Tasks should be as short as possible, consistent with reasonable statistical stability of the BP measurements in order to reduce opportunities for behavioral variation within a task. Since BP characteristics, such as absolute amplitude in microvolts, vary greatly among individuals, it is useful to compare BP measurements among two or more tasks. If a "baseline" or "resting" task is to be used for comparison, it is important to carefully specify the participant's behavior, such as fixation on a dot and counting breaths. Even so, the sort of mental activity

TABLE 9-2.
Methodological Criteria for Studies of Brain Potentials and Cognition

1. *Neurophysiological Basis.* On the basis of animal research or human clinical data, are there good reasons to suppose that distinct BP patterns might be associated with the chosen cognitive processes?

2. *Sample Population*

   A. Restrictively define selection criteria for participants to maximize homogeneity among persons. Selection criteria should include: narrow age and educational level range, same handedness and sex, no neuroactive medications, etc.

   B. Select the minimal sample size using statistical power analysis or by estimating the variation within each class using behavorial data. Increase by about one-third to allow for data attrition due to contamination by nonneuroelectric artifacts, to poor recording conditions, or to behaviorally ambiguous data. Increase sample size to allow for an independent data set for validation of the classifier. Reconcile with the estimate of sample size obtained from the number of independent BP variables (see 3,F) by taking the maximum of the two estimates.

3. *Experimental Design*

   A. Select tasks for participants that can be behaviorally verified (e.g., count the number of flashes, estimate the passage of 5 seconds, etc.); account for learning effects.

   B. Include adequate controls to isolate the cognitive functions being investigated.

   C. Equate stimulus properties, efferent activities, and performance-related factors (behavioral measures of an individual's ability and effort) between tasks and between participants.

   D. Randomize or counterbalance order of presentation of tasks within and between persons.

   E. Retest several participants to assess retest reliability of both behavioral and BP measures.

   F. Include an adequate number of observations of each class from each participant so that (allowing for data attrition of about one-third) the number of observations per class will be at least 10 to 40 times the number of independent BP variables (depending upon the type of classifier). Allow for extra data if required by the type of cross-validation chosen.

4. *Recording Conditions*

   A. Unless studying variations in arousal, maintain uniformity in overall state of arousal; require a normal amount of sleep the prior night and record a fixed amount of time from waking and several hours from the last meal and coffee, etc.

TABLE 9-2., Continued

B. Maintain uniformity in state of arousal during each trial by requiring performance of a task to a behaviorally verifiable criterion level.

C. Apply an adequate number of electrodes to sample BP spatial variability.

D. Obtain data over an interval adequate to characterize BP temporal variability.

5. *Data Selection*

A. Unless studying variation in arousal, eliminate data from participants if analysis of their behavioral and BP data indicates a significant shift in level of arousal during the recording session.

B. If not studying variations in performance, eliminate data from participants if analysis of their behavioral responses indicates a significantly lower or higher level of task performance than the mean of all participants.

C. For the remaining participants, eliminate all trials with incorrect answers, unless studying BP patterns associated with correct vs. incorrect responses.

D. Eliminate all data segments contaminated by nonneuroelectric artifacts.

6. *Data Standardization.* In order to reduce the obscuring effect of irrelevant anatomical and physiological variables, standardize BP measures within persons and between classes, e.g., transform measures into standard scores by subtracting the mean and dividing by the standard deviation of the pooled (across classes) data.

---

accompanying a "baseline" is unknown and can be assumed to be quite variable.

Most BP studies of cognition have used 1 to 8 scalp channels. In contrast, several montages of 16 to 20 channels are used in routine clinical EEGs, the purpose of which is to find signs of gross pathology. This sparse spatial sampling has been justified by the observation that "not much difference" is seen in the components of the averaged EP for more closely spaced electrodes. The lack of a between-channels effect sometimes reported in analyses of variance of averaged EP has also been similarly interpreted. However, these conclusions cannot be correct in general. In a sense, they are circular in that a negative conclusion must follow from paradigmatic and analytic limitations of the studies in question and not from an inherent lack of spatial patterning of BP. To the contrary, much physical evidence suggests the presence of a very fine degree of spatial patterning, including the approximate 0.5 to 1 mm diameter of cortical macrocolumns, empirical measurements of the relative independence of cortical potentials at distances greater than 1 to 2 mm

(Cooper et al., 1965), and, at a larger scale, the known functional differentiation of the major cortical regions. Finer spatial sampling is required to measure such patterning, in conjunction with experimental paradigms and signal-processing techniques designed to modulate and quantify more localized processes. Since the intervening tissue acts as a spatial low-pass filter, about 2.5 cm is the closest that electrodes can usefully be placed on the scalp. About 60 channels are needed to cover the scalp with this spacing (Picton et al., 1978).

EEG STUDIES OF LATERALIZATION OF COGNITION

A popular procedure for detecting evidence of hemispheric specialization of cognition in normals has been the comparison of EEG alpha power measures recorded from bilateral, symmetrically placed electrodes. Typically, a set of tasks assumed a priori to be either "verbal-analytic" or "spatial-appositional" is presented to subjects while their EEGs are recorded for up to several minutes. Alpha band spectral intensities of the EEG from each task are transformed into a relative index that represents the difference or ratio between the two hemispheres. In the pioneering EEG study of its type, David Galin and Robert Ornstein (1972) at the Langley Porter Institute, San Franscisco, reported the existence of different lateralized EEG patterns during performance of spatial and language tasks. During block design, the EEG from the right hemisphere of dextrals had a reduced amplitude as compared with the left side, while during the writing task the opposite pattern predominated in that left hemisphere EEG was reduced compared with that of the right (Figure 9-2, A). This lateralized amplitude reduction was presumed to be a sign of the formation of cooperative mass neural processes in the underlying tissue, implying that the neural population was engaged in task-associated processing. Many experiments have been performed since this report that seem to confirm the finding of anatomically localized EEG differences corresponding to these two different classes of mental functions, but the patterns are not always so clear-cut (Figure 9-2 B). Donchin et al. (1977) focus on several crucial shortcomings of these results, including:

1. Failure to demonstrate that the cognitive manipulations were the major distinctions among the tasks selected. Usually the tasks are chosen to represent a certain type of cognitive activity for which the presumption of an anatomical locus is based either upon previously noted performance deficits in neurologically impaired populations or upon intuitive similarity to other activities "localized" in this fashion. But, as noted above, tasks usually also differ in difficulty and on

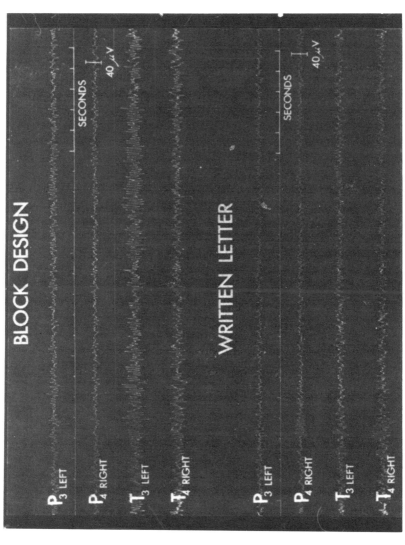

Figure 9-2A. *EEG excerpt showing asymmetry during Koh's block design and writing tasks. Note smaller voltage of right parietal (P4 electrode) during block design task.*

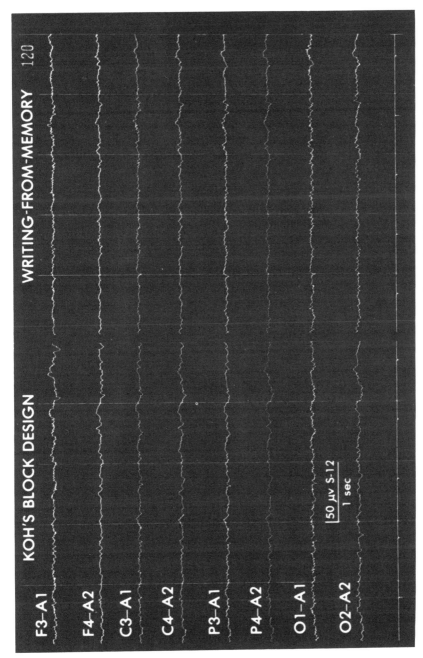

Figure 9-2B. *EEG excerpt in which asymmetry of the Koh's block design and writing-from-memory tasks is not obvious.*

stimulus and response-related factors. In addition, tasks are rarely composed of a set of homogeneous iterative operations; thus, the notion of a specific type of cognitive activity is often vague.

In a series of studies, we found no evidence of lateralization or other spatial EEG spectral intensity differences associated with different cognitive functions during performance of several (5 to 15) tasks, which differed in type of mental operations but which were otherwise controlled for perceptual, efferent, and performance-related factors (Gevins et al., 1979a, b, c; Gevins, Doyle, Schaffer et al., 1980) (Figure 9-3). We concluded that previous studies were unable to prove that the EEG patterns noted were strictly due to the cognitive aspects of task performance.

2. Failure to validate that the tasks were actually performed. For example, many studies utilized tasks such as imagining scenes (Doyle Ornstein, & Galin, 1974; Morgan et al., 1971) for which subject performance could not be validated. Also, rarely has performance assessment been used to eliminate data from trials with wrong answers.

3. Neglect in proving that a demonstrated EEG asymmetry is attributable to the experimental tasks and not to a combination of irrelevant factors, such as handedness, asymmetric skull thickness (Leissner, Lindholm, & Petersen, 1970), or improperly balanced electrode placements. Since EEG asymmetries have been reported during the "neutral baseline" task (Doyle et al., 1974; Rebert, 1978; Galin et al., 1978), if a task-associated modulation of baseline EEG asymmetry cannot be demonstrated, it has not been proved that lateralized cortical activity patterns are related to the task.

4. Using a between-person design to infer within-person differences. Furst (1976) and Glass and Butler (1977) rank-order-correlated each volunteer's mean solution time over all trials with mean relative occipital alpha activity and demonstrated an overall relationship between relative hemispheric activation and performance. However, it would not be correct to conclude that the significant correlations found were evidence that each person's reaction time was a function of the relative amount of occipital alpha activity during task performance.

5. Relying on measures that are ambiguous with respect to the actual locus of, or difference between, right and left hemisphere EEG activities. In our study, differences in alpha band intensity during the "spatial" Koh's block design task, as compared with the writing-from-memory task, were significant only for left hemisphere locations and right hemisphere sites showing little intertask differences (Gevins et al., 1979a) (Figure 9-4 A). Converting the spectral intensities into right/left ratios could produce data that could be misinterpreted as demonstrating right hemisphere activation during the former task (Gevins & Schaffer, 1980) (Table 9-3). In fact, only left-sided changes were found in most EEG studies (see below for possible exceptions). For example, McKee (McKee, Humphrey, & McAdam, 1973) demonstrated relative left hemisphere voltage reductions for three linguistic tasks and one musical task but did not find a task that reduced right hemisphere alpha voltage.

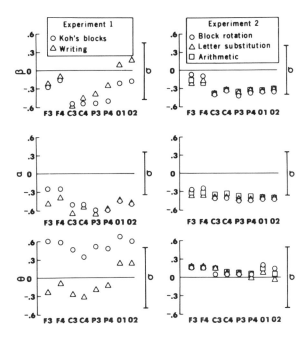

Figure 9-3. *Results of two experiments designed to assess EEG correlates of higher cognitive functions. Tasks of Experiment 1 (left) were one minute long and involved limb movements and uncontrolled differences in stimulus characteristics and performance-related factors. Tasks of Experiment 2 (right) were less than 15 seconds long and required no motion of the limbs: stimulus characteristics and performance-related factors were also relatively controlled. The graphs display means over all subjects of standard scores of EEG spectral intensities (expressed as changes from visual fixation values) recorded during performance of these tasks. Upper, middle, and lower sets of graphs are for spectral intensities in the beta (β, 14 to 20 Hz), alpha (α, 8 to 13 Hz), and theta (θ, 4 to 7 Hz) bands. The abscissa shows scalp electrode placements: left frontal (F3), right frontal (F4), left central (C3), right central (C4), left parietal (P3), right parietal (P4), left occipital (O1), and right occipital (O2). Thus these plots compare how EEG spectral intensities measured during the tasks differed from those during visual fixation. Standard deviations, which differed but slightly between electrode placements, are indicated at right of each plot. While there are prominent EEF differences between the uncontrolled tasks of Experiment 1, EEG differences between the relatively controlled tasks of Experiment 2 are lacking. Each of the controlled tasks is, however, associated with a remarkably similar bilateral reduction in alpha and beta band spectral intensity over occipital, parietal, and central regions. There is no evidence in these results that "logical" and "spatial" cognitive processes are associated with differentially lateralized EEG patterns. (From Gevins, A., et al., Science, 203, 665, 1979. © 1979 by the American Association for the Advancement of Science.)*

TABLE 9-3.
Ratios of Right Parietal to Left Parietal Average EEG
Spectral Intensity (P4/P3) for each Volunteer on a
"Spatial" and "Verbal" Task

Subject number	Ratios	
	Spatial task: Koh's block design	Verbal task: writing from memory
1	1.06	1.68
2	.93	1.04
3	.83	1.16
4	1.18	1.11
5	.95	1.52
6	.74	.93
7	1.61	1.15
8	.98	1.22
9	.92	1.17
10	.94	1.10
11	1.14	1.03
12	1.09	1.00
13	1.24	1.98
14	1.03	1.23
15	.77	.96
16	1.36	1.14
17	1.09	1.31
18	.73	1.01
19	.68	.89
20	1.02	1.56
21	.79	.86
22	.99	1.22
23	.86	.96
x =	1.00^{a}	1.18^{a}

Significant difference (p < .01), Wilcoxon matched-pair signed ranks test (2-tailed). (Reprinted from Gevins, A. & Schaffer, R. *CRC Critical Reviews in Bioengineering,* Oct. 1980, *pp.* 113–164. © The Chemical Rubber Co., CRC Press, Inc.)

Since one or more of these five methodological inadequacies characterize almost all recent research in this field, the existence of EEG indexes of differential hemispheric activation for different types of cognition remains

NORMALIZED THETA BAND SPECTRAL INTENSITY
(average of 23 subjects)

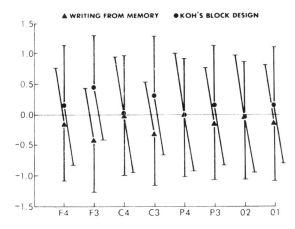

Figure 9-4a. *Spectral analysis of alpha band spectral patterns during a "language" and a "spatial" task. Standard ("z") scores were computed over two tasks for each volunteer, and then the mean and standard deviation for each task over volunteers were computed to produce the figure. Abscissa: electrode placements. Ordinate: average and standard deviation (for the 23 volunteers in the study) of the alpha band z-scores. Note that the only obvious changes are at left-sided (odd-numbered) placements except for FU.*

unsettled. The remainder of this section will consider some of the representative studies purporting to have verified this phenomenon. Table 9-4 lists methodological weaknesses in a number of frequently cited studies.

Doyle, Ornstein, and Galin (1974) noted changes of EEG asymmetry, especially among tasks with limb movements. In one of the most comprehensive studies to date, the investigators compared spectrally analyzed EEGs from four spatial or musical and four language or arithmetic tasks (Figure 9-5). Of the task comparisons, only one, tonal memory versus verbal listening, did not involve limb movement or presentation of stimuli to different sensory modalities, and tasks were not controlled for subject performance or for differences in difficulty. For each task-pair comparison, nonparametric tests for significant differences were performed (ratios of R/L delta, theta, alpha, and beta spectral intensity in the temporal and parietal regions). Only ratios of

NORMALIZED ALPHA BAND SPECTRTAL INTENSITY
(average of 23 subjects)

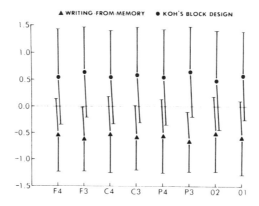

Figure 9-4b. *Standard theta band spectral intensities during performance of KB and WR by 23 subjects. Note the relatively large separation between the tasks. (Reprinted from Gevins, A. et al.* Electroencephalogr Clin Neurophysiol, *1979, 47:693–703.)*

parietal delta and high-frequency beta were significantly different between this pair of tasks.

Beaumont and associates (Beaumont, Mayes, & Rugg, 1978) compared interhemispheric ratios of alpha band spectral intensity and alpha band coherence from the final minute of each task while 16 volunteers each performed two "verbal-analytic" and two "spatial-appositional" tasks. The authors reported that coherence was more sensitive to asymmetries in hemispheric activity than in spectral intensity. While both the spectral intensity and coherence ratios revealed significant task-related changes, these measures were so labile that their standard deviations were sometimes larger than their mean values by a factor of 100. In addition, since no overt responses were made, task performance could not be validated.

Davidson et al. (1976) have noted sex differences in EEG asymmetry patterns during tasks involving either singing, whistling, or reciting the lyrics to familiar tunes for one-minute periods. Left and right occipital alpha bursts were counted with logic modules, and ratios of the difference in alpha bursts $(R - L/R + L)$ were computed for each of the 14 individuals in each condition and were subjected to a repeated measures analysis of variance. There was

TABLE 9-4.
Critique of Studies Reporting EEG Patterns
Related to "Lateralization of Cognitive
Mode"

Study	Fails to meet guidelines[a,d]
Beaumont, Mayes, and Rugg (1978)	c, d
Bennett and Trinder (1977)	a, b, c, d, e, f
Butler and Glass (1974)	c, d, f
Davidson and Schwartz (1977)	b, c, e, f?[b]
Dumas and Morgan (1975)	a, b, c, d, e, f
Doyle, Ornstein, and Gallin (1974)	a, b, c, d, e
Ehrlichmann and Wiener (1979)	a, b, c, d, e, f?[b]
Hirshkowitz, Earle, and Paley (1978)	c, d, e, f
McKee, Humphrey, and McAdam[c] (1973)	c, e, d?,[b] f
McLeod and Peacock (1977)	a, c, d, e
Morgan, McDonald, and MacDonald (1971)	b, c, d, e, f
Morgan, MacDonald, and Hilgard (1974)	b, c, d
Ornstein, Johnstone, Herron, and Swencians (1979)	a, b, c, d, f
Osborne and Gale (1976)	a, c, d, f
Robbins and McAdam (1974)	c, d, f
Schwartz, Davidson, and Pugash (1976)	d, e, f
Warren, Peltz, and Hanetas (1976)	c, d, f

[a] Guidelines for experiments on EEG correlates of cognition: (a) minimal or no differences between tasks in stimuli, (b) minimal or no differences between tasks in efferent activities, (c) minimal or no differences in performance-related factors (e.g., amount of time to solve and percentage of trials correct) between tasks or volunteers, (d) use of behavioral validation of continuous task performance to select EEG data for analysis, (e) present data on each electrode separately, (f) complete elimination of EEG data contaminated by extracerebral artifact.

[b] Items with question mark (?) denote insufficient evidence in report to evaluate guideline.

[c] Sample size was 4.

[d] a, b, d, e from Donchin et al., 1977.

Source: Reprinted from Gevins, A. & Schaffer, R. *CRC Critical Reviews in Bioengineering,* Oct. 1980, pp. 113–164. © The Chemical Rubber Co., CRC Press, Inc.

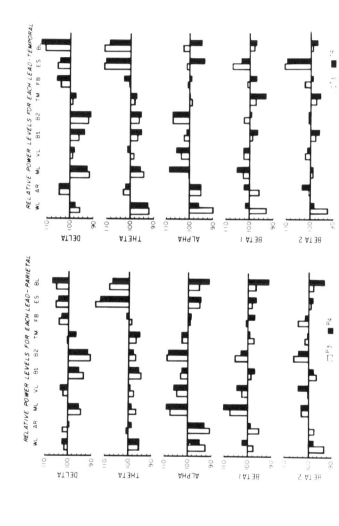

Figure 9-5. *EEG spectral analysis during "verbal and arithmetic" and "spatial and musical" tasks. Each graph displays the "average relative power levels" for each task averaged across subjects. "B₁" and "B₂" are baseline "resting" conditions, tasks listed to the left of these are "verbal" or "arithmetic," and those to the right are "spatial" or "musical." P3 and T3 represent left parietal and temporal activity, respectively; P4 and T4 represent right parietal and temporal activity. The magnitude of the asymmetries is greater at the temporal leads. (From Doyle, J., Ornstein, R., & Galin, D., Psychophysiology, 11, 567, 1974. With permission.*

358

significantly greater relative left hemisphere activation for talking, compared with whistling. Further analysis revealed this effect to be restricted to four right-handed females who had no familial left-handedness. An attempt was made to replicate this study by calculating parietal alpha ratios from ten males and ten females. The whistle versus talk comparison was not significant, nor was there any effect of sex. Since the EEG pattern of the intended "words plus music" (singing) condition was in one study intermediate but in the replication significantly extreme (compared with the values for the whistle and talk conditions), the a priori continuum of the musical-verbal cognitive dimension was not reflected in the pattern of relative hemispheric EEG activation.

Gale et al. (1978) also noted sex differences in total EEG asymmetry recorded during both "resting" and performance of "verbal-logical" and "spatial-appositional" tasks. Both sexes had greater left than right hemisphere integrated EEG voltage during tasks requiring volunteers to describe a real or imagined trajectory. However, for all other task and "rest" conditions, females had relatively greater left hemisphere integrated voltage, contrary to interhemispheric integrated voltage comparisons in males. While these results seem to provide an instance of right hemisphere EEG changes during performance of a "spatial" task, when a verbal component was added, relative right-sided suppression was increased for females, contrary to expectations.

Recently, Ornstein et al. (1980) compared integrated central and parietal alpha activity from ten males and ten females, each performing six "spatial" and one "verbal" task for three minutes each. While between-task differences in gross motor activity and stimulus characteristics were roughly controlled, differences in oculomotor activity and problem difficulty remained. Most importantly, the level of effort applied to the task during the course of the three-minute trials was not assessed. The authors reported that right hemisphere changes accounted for most of the significant task-associated differences in EEG. They concluded that performing a modified version of Shepard's and Metzler's spatial rotation task required an "analytic" cognitive strategy that engaged the volunteer's left hemispheres more than all the other "spatial" tasks except one. However, bilateral parietal intensities during this task were relatively large, indicating relatively less overall cortical activation. This result, coupled with the negative correlation between mental rotation performance level and associated right/left hemisphere alpha intensity ratios, suggests that not all of the volunteers were expending as much effort to perform this task as they were for some of the other tasks. If mental rotation performance was associated with relatively decreased left hemisphere alpha intensity, improved performance (more items correctly solved) would be expected to be associated with larger right/left alpha ratios and a positive, not a negative, correlation. While the authors demonstrated right hemisphere EEG changes accompanying performance of different "spatial" tasks and concluded that the volunteers' cognitive strategies determined the task-associated relative hemispheric activation, intertask differences in performance-related factors sensitive to task difficulty, effort and skill, and perceptual and efferent activities contributed to their results to an unknown extent.

At the EEG Systems Laboratory, we utilized the analysis methodology described above for evaluating EEG spectral changes associated with performance of various tasks, including reading, writing from memory, Koh's blocks design, mental paper folding (mentally reconstituting an unfolded cube to determine if two specified edges would be continuous), and several control tasks (Gevins et al., 1979a, 1979b). For each of the 23 right-handed volunteers, spectral features from nonartifacted EEG (as determined by two independent raters) from pairs of tasks were converted to standard scores so that the observations presented to the mathematical pattern classifier represented deviations from the mean of that spectral feature in that task pair of each person. The spectral features included theta (Figure 9-4, B), alpha (Figure 9-4, A), beta (14 to 20 Hz), and beta 2 (21 to 28 Hz) banded intensity, and four intra- and interhemispheric ratios of spectral intensity. Classification functions were generated and then validated on separate sets of data. Important features were extracted from significant functions according to an objective procedure (Table 9-5 and Figure 9-6). Consistent EEG patterns that distinguished pairs of tasks were uncovered, yet the task-specific EEG features created a complex spatial pattern of changes that could not be related to any particular perceptual, cognitive, or efferent aspect of the task. Most importantly, writing from memory could not be distinguished from merely scribbling.

We then performed a second study using simpler tasks (Gevins et al, 1979b, 1979c). "Other-than-cognitive" factors of task performance were contolled by utilizing tasks that were solvable within shorter (5- to 15-sec) trial periods, by eliminating limb movements, by reducing the magnitude of eye movements, by discarding the initial and final second of each trial to eliminate most sensory evoked and premotor potentials, and by analyzing only correct trials from volunteers whose overall performance ruled out guessing with 99% certainty. In addition, the tasks were made equally difficult for each participant by selecting sets of tasks following pretesting so that each person would be expected to correctly solve an average of 80% of the task items in an average of 7 seconds. The three tasks were serial addition, letter substitution, and mental block rotation. Based on factor analysis of psychometric batteries, the former two were considered to require primarily "analytic" processes and the latter, "spatial" cognitive processes. EEG data from 21 volunteers were analyzed, using the same methods as in the experiment described above, but the EEG spectra from the different cognitive tasks could not be distinguished (Figure 9-3 and Table 9-6). However, each of the tasks was about equally

TABLE 9-5.
Summary of EEG Pattern Recognition Analyses

Task-pair discrimination	Classification accuracy ($\bar{x}$ ± S.E., in %)	Spectral feature				
		θ	α	β_1	β_2	$\hat{f}$
Koh's block design (KB) vs. writing-from-memory (WR)	85 ± 1	F3↓C4↑P3↑O1↑		C↓	C↑P4↑	P4↓O1↓
Koh's block design (KB) vs. reading (RE)	85 ± 8	F↑P3↑O1↓	F3↑P3↓	F↓C3↓P↓O1↓	O↑	F3↓C↓P↓O↓
Reading (RE) vs. writing-from-memory (WR)*	84 ± 11	P4↑O↑	C↑P3↑	C↑P4↑		
Mental-paper-folding (FO) vs. reading (RE)*	81 ± 18	F↑O↓	P↓	C↓P3↓O↓	O2↑	F4↓O1↓
Mental-paper-folding (FO) vs. Koh's block design (KB)*	74 ± 3	F3↓C3↓O1↓		P↑O1↑	C3↑	C3↑

*Includes at least one non-significant classification accuracy (<74%).
Features from non-significant classifications are not included.

Note: The mean and standard error percentage correct pairwise classification accuracy of the cross-validation data is listed. Classification accuracies are the average of 8 analyses, one for each anatomic constraint. Location and type of spectral features distinguishing the pairs of tasks are shown. Each spectral feature entry indicates the derivation(s) for which the given feature discriminated the pair of tasks. A derivation without a subscript (e.g., C) indicates both channels of the homologous pair. The arrow indicates the direction of the change associated with the first-named task of the pair. For example, greater theta band spectral intensity at F3, C4, P3, and O1 associated with KB was important in distinguishing KB from WR.

Source: Reprinted from Gevins, A. et al. *Electroencephalogr Clin Neurophysiol,* 1979, 47:693–703.

KOH'S BLOCK DESIGN
DISTINGUISHED FROM WRITING-FROM-MEMORY

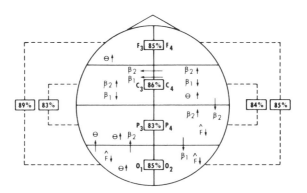

Figure 9-6a. *Topographic display of the major features distinguishing KB from WR as determined by the anatomically-constrained multivariate pattern recognition algorithm. In these displays, percentages denote classification accuracies achieved using testing (cross-validation) data from the two regions connected by boxes. Any classification accuracy enclosed by parentheses is not significant. Features from nonsignificant classifications are not included. Within a region, an arrow pointing up or down indicates the direction of change of the feature associated with performance of the first task. Here, increased theta and beta $_2$ band intensities and reduced $_f$ (characteristic frequency) distinguish KB from WR. An arrow connecting two regions points toward the region in which the feature increased relative to the other region in the first-named task. For example, theta and beta $_2$ intensity increased in P3 relative to O1 during KB.*

different from a visual fixation (passive) "task" (Figure 9-3). These results offered no evidence that EEG spectral intensity patterns over 5- and 15-second periods are sensitive to possible differences in mass neural processing between clearly different, relatively controlled cognitive tasks. This casts doubt as to whether previous EEG studies were actually measuring cognitive processes and not certain other-than-cognitive aspects of task performance (Gevins et al, 1980) (Table 9-4). The approximately uniform 10% reductions in alpha and beta band spectral intensity during task performance compared with visual fixation values might represent an equal level of electrocortical activation,

MENTAL PAPER-FOLDING
DISTINGUISHED FROM READING

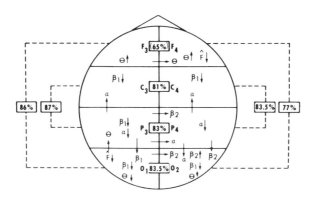

Figure 9-6b. *Topographic display of the major EEG features distinguishing FO from RE. (Reprinted from Gevins, A. et al. Electroencephalogr Clin Neurophysiol, 1979, 47:693–703.)*

attendant with performing different cognitive tasks to the same specified level of performance. Weaknesses of our study included the relatively long duration (5 to 15 sec) and internal heterogeneity of the tasks, the averaging of data within each trial to produce observations of arithmetic, block rotation or letter substitution "states," sole reliance on spectral analysis, and the inadequate sampling of the scalp topography with only eight electrodes.

Thus, although there are scores of studies of this phenomenon, because of their flaws, the existence of a background EEG index of lateralization of a background cognitive mode has not yet been proven.

With regard to lateralization as an index of performance, a study by Furst (1976) found a significant positive correlation betwen participants' R/L integrated voltage of occipital alpha and speed of performing any of three visuospatial problems. However, a significant correlation was also obtained between response speed and asymmetry during the "resting" condition. Furst assumed that these correlations resulted from a tonic asymmetry, rather than from a task-specific activation pattern. Again, the between-individual design weakens interpretation of the results. The significant correlation between performance and "resting" asymmetry highlights the criticism by Donchin et al. (1977) that task-related BP effects should be modulated by different types of tasks; if not, the influence of nontask-related factors cannot be distinguished—in this case, variation among people in tonic state of arousal,

TABLE 9-6.

Classification of Tasks in Experiment 2 (Controlled Tasks) by Means of the EEG. Each Entry is the Percentage of Correct Test-set Classifications of the Two Indicated Tasks.

Task	Serial arith- metic	Block rota- tion	Letter sub- stitu- tion
Visual fixation	75	76	75
Block rotation	62*		
Letter substitution		61*	
Serial arithmetic			59*

*Not significant

Source: Reprinted from Gevins, A. Doyle, Cutillo, et al. *Science,* 1981, *213*:918–922. © 1981 by the American Association for the Advancement of Science.

differences in BP attenuation due to asymmetries in skull thickness and conductance, and so forth.

Glass and Butler (1977) assessed the relation between alpha asymmetry and response time for 33 volunteers performing mental multiplications. A left/right ratio of integrated voltage for parietal alpha during the first five seconds of calculations was computed. This measure correlated significantly to the average response time but not to percent correct. Left hemisphere alpha voltage during an eyes-open "resting" condition also displayed a significant negative relationship to subsequent performance speed. As this was a replication of Furst's (1976) study using a task assumed to engage the "analytic" hemisphere, this study suffers from the same weaknesses as the former study.

In 16 volunteers, Galin, Johnstone, and Herron (1978) correlated integrated voltage of central and parietal alpha intensity with speed in solving Koh's blocks design, a "spatial" task. Integrated alpha intensities at the right parietal and both central derivations related to time to solve. Alpha in either the left, right, or both hemispheres increased for 10 of the 16 volunteers as they performed more difficult task items. To account for these mixed findings, the investigators emphasized individual variations in EEG changes during performance of tasks of unequal difficulty. Other weaknesses of this study include: only considering EEG activity in the alpha range (performance of this particular task is associated with dramatic theta band increases) (Doyle et al., 1974; Gevins et al., 1979a—Figure 9-4 B); using tasks that lasted several minutes without assessing moment-by-moment changes in performance; and adopting editing procedures that eliminated 40% of the participants tested, due to insufficient data (possibly eliminating the fast solvers). The remaining nonartifacted data might represent periods when subjects were not applying themselves to the task. In addition, the raw intensity values were normalized against the average intensity for each person, including not only the Koh's blocks task but also data from reading and writing sentences tasks. Normalizing the EEG with data from two "analytic" tasks that differed in difficulty and that had differing amounts of eye and hand movements had an unknown effect on the derived EEG patterns of task difficulty.

Rebert (1978b) and associates (Rebert & Low, 1978) (1978a) conducted four studies of the relation between EEG asymmetry and performance. In three of these studies about ten volunteers pressed a telegraph key in response to verbal or nonverbal target material. Alpha spectral intensities from bilateral occipital, parietal, temporal, and central locations were simultaneously recorded. The fourth study compared EEG spectra during listening to text and during performance of two "spatial" tasks: block rotation and viewing or playing "Pong" (an electronic table tennis game). For the first three studies, the authors noted individual differences in the relation between alpha lateralization and reaction time, but they did not find evidence that relatively higher alpha power in a hemisphere was associated with less efficient processing of a task presumably governed by that hemisphere. In the fourth study, the authors emphasized that task-related asymmetries occurred in the context of larger bilateral EEG changes.

EP STUDIES OF LINGUISTIC PROCESSING

As compared with the EEG, averaged EP studies have been very productive over the last 15 years in studying the BP correlates of "expectation," "selective attention," "orienting," "context updating," "conception formation," and so forth. While the existence of EP components is not in question, the above psychological interpretations given to them should be questioned since, as noted above, similar changes in the same components may be produced under a variety of psychological circumstances, and different EP effects may be produced with the same psychological manipulations. While lateralized EP patterns have not consistently been reported for simple judgments, one would expect them for linguistic tasks. However, study of EP patterns during linguistic processing is methodologically more complex than study of simple perceptual judgments. Not suprisingly, most previous studies have been less than satisfactory paradigmatically and analytically. This section will only discuss a few of the major ones in detail; similar criticisms could be properly directed at most other studies.

In their discussion of the implications of an important experiment, Friedman et al. (1975) presented a critique of prior EEG and EP studies of language. They ascribed previous reports of lateralization during linguistic tasks to: design or recording flaws, such as failure to use a nonlanguage control task, use of nonequivalent stimuli, and use of two unlinked lateral reference electrodes; and inadequate or inappropriate statistical analysis, such as failure to raise the significance criteria to adjust for multiple univariate comparisons. Friedman's 1975 study reported a significant left hemispheric lateralization of N1 amplitude evoked by signal words and of P3 amplitude evoked by nonsignal sounds. The P3 effect was attributed to a novelty manipulation, but the N1 effect may have been linguistically related. If so, this would be earlier than might be expected. Unfortunately, the spatial sampling was insufficient to resolve whether the N1 lateralization was maximal occipitally or more anteriorly—an obviously important neurolinguistic consideration. Another weakness of the study was that the task design required the identification of target words or sounds from only five highly familiar possibilities. After so many presentations, the stimuli might not have elicited the full hierarchy of linguistic processes for task performance. In order to have a strong inference that a particular linguistic process was actually performed, there must be a variety of examples of the task with behavioral validation of correct perform- ance in each trail.

Wood (1975) presented a study differentiating auditory and phonetic levels of processing in speech perception. Here the methodology was precise: auditory and phonetic judgments were made on identical stimuli, with the required distinctions adjusted to equal difficulty by pretest; control conditions and three nonphonetic experiments provided a pattern of inference specifically pointing to speech processing as the salient feature producing the effects; and convergent evidence from reaction times and EP support the proposed interpretation. The chief limitations were sparse spatial sampling and use of repeated univariate tests. Nevertheless, this study provided suggestive evidence that left hemisphere differences between auditory and phonetic processes may be measurable with EPs.

Other previous studies attempted to isolate BP patterns of grammatical or semantic functions. In a precedent-setting series of "homonym" studies, Marsh, Brown, and associates (Brown, Marsh, & Smith 1973, 1976, 1979; Marsh & Brown, 1977) took great care to control between-task differences in stimuli. Considered en masse, these studies seem to have demonstrated unequivocally BP differences between noun and verb forms of the same word.

However the possibility remains that the results are not actually related to the linguistic distinction, since no single study meets all the necessary methodological requirements. For example, since the 1976 and 1977 studies did not require the participant's response, there was no verification that the stimulus was perceived or processed as noun or verb. (Use of a nonlanguage control task would clarify this point.) Thus, the reported differences could be due to affect or arousal, among other factors. Since most studies used only one or two homonym pairs, as the investigators noted, there was the strong possibility of habituation to stimulus presentation. When they repeated the experiment on four consecutive days, the EP differences were attenuated on the second and disappeared by the third and fourth sessions (Marsh & Brown, 1977). Finally, the finding of a hemispheric asymmetry for "semantic stimuli" between Broca's area and its homologue and the absence of a finding over Wernicke's area seem to be at odds with neurolinguistic findings implicating posterior lesions for semantic receptive disorders. In addition, distinct "noun" and "verb" EP topographic distributions are findings that stand in isolation from other investigative procedures. In particular, studies of aphasics have not indicated separate component linguistic processes for nouns and verbs per se.

These investigators' current ingenious elaborations of their basic paradigm (Brown & Lehmann, 1979; Brown et al., 1979) support their previous conclusions. A noun/verb homonym was embedded in a phrase and presented in blocks to English-speaking ("rose/rows") and German-speaking ("fluege") participants. The German phrase was degraded with noise to produce an unintelligible utterance that was judged equally likely to be the original German noun or verb phrase, depending upon precue. Different scalp voltage field distributions were evoked by noun and verb stimuli, which seemed consistent across languages. Otherwise elegant, these studies contain some of the weaknesses noted above: use of only one noun/verb pair per study, presentation of the stimuli in blocks of 30 trials with precuing as to word type (thus possibly confounding expectancy, habituation, and linguistic processing), and the emphasis on the noun/verb distinction rather than on the other connotative or affective dimensions distinguishing the stimuli.

A study by Chapman (in Begleiter, 1979) used multivariate statistical methods to investigate connotative (affective) aspects of semantic meaning. Affective variations normally are associated with anatomically diffuse, "arousal"-related changes in electrocortical activity (e.g., "alpha blocking"). These diffuse changes would seem only indirectly related to component linguistic processes that are inferred to have a localized electrocortical representation. Since only one channel was analyzed, the Chapman studies were unable to distinguish diffuse from anatomically localized BP related to linguistic processing.

A series of studies by Molfese and associates (1979); and Molfese et al. (1979) have uncovered auditory EP factors sensitive to semantic and articulatory differences in stimuli matched by voicing and articulation. In the first study (Molfese, 1979), BP responses were measured from CVC nonsense syllables and words matched for articulatory features. Ten orthogonal factors for 160 EPs recorded from 10 participants were subjected to an analysis of variance. Certain factors varied as a function of meaning or voicing, but use of a 0.05 significance level without correction for multiple comparisons (i.e., the 10 factors) raises the possibility of Type I error. One factor, peaking at 6 to 60 msec poststimulus, was sensitive to the "meaning" manipulation. In noting that activity in this latency range is usually attributed to subcortical structures, the investigators concluded that some semantic processing (coarticulation) must occur subcortically. It is possible that the coarticulation effect might have the requisite degree of specificity to assess stimulus meaningfulness well before the final consonant at about 240 to 280 msec (e.g., meaningful-"peak"; nonsense -"paeb"). Alternatively, small but unmeasured differences in the acoustic properties of the stimuli or differences in task-associated effort between recognizing a word or nonword could be responsible for the early and later results, respectively. In a second experiment (Molfese, 1979), more specific semantic processes were studied. Participants were repeatedly presented with the word "ball" in two contexts by cuing the participant to think "baseball" or "dance" by means of verbal instructions or pictures. As noted, verification of imagining was difficult.

Thatcher (Thatcher, 1977; Thatcher & Maisel, 1979) performed several elegant studies that controlled for stimulus and response factors and measured behavior for each trial. The 1977 study demonstrated EP waveform asymmetries over temporal areas. The unknown neural and cognitive effects of the use of random dot stimuli as "baseline probes" before, between, and after stimuli (every 0.67 sec) complicates the interpretation of this otherwise exemplary study.

In other recent studies, Grabow et al. (1980a) unsuccessfully attempted to replicate the early study of Morrell and Salamy (1971), which reported N1 and P2 EP amplitude differences between spoken phonemes and other sounds. In a second study by the same authors (Grabow, Aronson, Offord et al. 1980b), an unsuccessful attempt was made to replicate the study of Wood et al. (1971). Stimuli were three computer-generated phonemes, two of which were the same but shifted in fundamental frequency. Although stimuli were adequately controlled, remaining methodological deficiencies (lack of control of performance-related factors and uncorrected multiple univariate significance tests) weakened the contrary result that EP amplitude to phonemes was reduced over the dominant temporal electrode.

In recent studies, improved in many respects over previous ones of their type, Neville (1981) used difficult tasks that produced behavioral asymmetries in reaction time studies. Visual examination of averaged EPs showed increased N1-P2 amplitude over the left parietal electrode in a visual word-pair recall task, an effect that was not present when the words were out of focus. Increased right central EP amplitudes were found for a line-drawing-recognition task. However, the tasks were not controlled for equality of stimulus and performance-related factors, and the conclusions were also weakened by use of an ipsilateral ear reference and sparse spatial sampling. In a new and further improved study (Neville, 1981), identity of stimuli between tasks was achieved by using a letter-maze stimulus and requiring a judgment either about letter identity or about position. Asymmetries in the averaged EP included greater left-sided positivity at about 200 msec for letter identity and greater right-sided (frontotemporal) positivity from about 300 msec to 1 sec for the position judgment. To specify this effect, the tasks must be even further controlled for difficulty, possible expectancy differences (CNV resolution), and possible small eye movement differences.

The lack of clear and consistent demonstrations of a lateralized BP pattern during linguistic processing may at first seem suprising, in light of the strong neurological evidence concerning the role of the dominant hemisphere in linguistic competence. Aside from methodological imprecision and analytical weakness, there may be neurophysiological reasons for this; Lassen, Ingvar, and Skinhoj (1978) have shown that nondominant hemisphere areas homologous to the dominant hemispere "language centers" show similar overall increases of regional blood flow during silent reading but with less spatial articulation than on the dominant side. This points to the necessity of finer BP spatial sampling to resolve potentially different spatiotemporal patterns associated with linguistic and nonlinguistic processing. (See also Wood, this volume.)

DYNAMIC SPATIAL BP PATTERN OF COGNITION

In this section, we will briefly summarize two new experiments. The first was designed to measure dynamic spatiotemporal BP patterns during simple numeric and spatial judgments (Gevins et al., 1981). The results from this study suggest that the brain's processing of even simple judgments is more dynamic and complex than can be accounted for by simple left/right theories of brain function. While lateralized patterns were found, they were sometimes simultaneously opposite in anterior and posterior areas, and shifted over split-second intervals.

As noted elsewhere (Gevins et al, 1981), there is evidence that increasing functional interrelation between neural areas may be reflected in increasing correlation of their low-frequency BP. To investigate this idea, a challenging, brief (about 1.2 sec) visuomotor task was developed that presumably established functional relations between visual, parietal, motor, and other neural areas. Two and one-half seconds following a task cue, a simple visual stimulus (an arrow, a target, and a number) was presented and required a judgment of magnitude. The response was to exert a force on an isometric transducer with a ballistic contraction of the right index finger, either proportional to the distance the target would have to move to intersect the arrow's projection, or proportional to the number (on a scale of 1 to 100). Arrow and number stimuli were always presented together, and the participant was cued as to task in randomly ordered blocks of 13 trials. Performance-related factors were equalized between tasks by computer-controlled on-line adjustment of the target size (arrow task) and the accuracy tolerance (number task) according to a moving average of recent performance. Thus, stimulus, response, and performance-related factors were held constant, while the type of judgment was varied between number decoding and spatial extrapolation.

Five clinically normal, right-handed adults each performed about 420 trials of each task. Sixteen electrodes were placed according to standard skull landmarks in positions covering the cranium. Vertical and horizontal eye movements were also recorded, as well as flexor muscle activity of the right index finger and the resultant output of the isometric force transducer. For each person, sets of trials of each task were selected so that there were no significant between-task differences in stimulus, response and performance-related factors. Stimulus-registered and response-registered averaged EP's were computed for each person and examined for consistent changes across tasks in peak latency or amplitude of the N1(N170), P2 (P240), P3a (P340), P3b (P450), P4 (P620), and RP ("readiness potential") peaks. No consistent, task-related amplitude or latency shifts were observed across persons, except for the P340 peak, which was always larger ($p < .05$) for the number task at all parietal electrodes (Figure 9-7). Thus the average EPs provided only limited information about the different types of judgments.

Since the peaks of the averaged EP signify the occurrence of neural processes that are consistently related in time to the stimulus, time intervals of 175 or 300 msec were centered on the peak time of the N1–P2, P3a, P3b, and P4 peaks of each person's averaged EPs, as well as a 300-msec prestimulus and a 175-msec preresponse interval. Single-trial, cross-correlation functions were computed between 44 pairwise combinations of 15 electrodes for each of these six latency windows. The raw correlations for each channel pair increased in magnitude with decreasing interelectrode distance. Mean correlation values for each latency interval were: prestimulus = .74, N1-P2 = .81,

P3a = .79, P3b = .75, P4 = .75, preresponse = .76. Analysis of variance was performed for each of the six intervals. The only significant task-related effect was a task × channel-pair interaction in three intervals. T-tests were performed between tasks on all single-trial values for each of the 44 correlations in each of the six intervals. Only 4 of the 264 tests were significant (p < .05, corrected for multiple comparisons).

Since these linear statistical methods were not informative, nonlinear, distribution-independent, multivariate pattern recognition was applied to determine how the correlation patterns of each task changed between sequential latency intervals, and how the two tasks differed in correlation within each latency interval (Gevins et al., 1979a, 1979b, 1979c; Gevins, 1980). In each analysis, functions were derived for each of nine cortical areas. A function consisted of a nonlinear combination of the correlations of the particular areas with 10 or 11 other areas (7 for the occipital area). Each classification function was developed on 788 trials and cross-validated on 400 previously unanalyzed trials. The correlations of a particular area were deemed to have changed with time or to have differed between tasks if the cross-validation classification accuracy was significantly better than chance at p < .005 or better. (Forty-nine attempted classifications with the data randomly assigned to the arrow or number categories did not produce significant cross-validation classifications at p < .005.) For each significant classification, correlations contributing most prominently to the classification function were identified. Diagrams of the contrasting areas and their most prominent correlations were drawn.

The within-task, interval-by-interval, analysis revealed similarities to as well as differences between tasks in the anatomic distribution of sequential changes in correlation. From the prestimulus to the N1–P2 interval, almost all areas changed, with most correlations increasing. From the N1–P2 through the P3b intervals, complex spatial patterns differed between tasks. From the P3b to the P4 interval, the areas showing change were identical for both tasks. From the P4 to the response interval, changes in midline-bilateral areas predominated in the arrow task, while all areas changed in the number task. In brief, the tasks evolved similarly following the stimulus and preceding the response, while they differed in the middle intervals.

When the pattern recognition analysis was applied to determine how the tasks differed from each other within each latency interval (Figure 9-8), significant differences were found in all but the preresponse interval, revealing a complex, rapidly shifting picture of lateralization. In the N1–P2 interval, correlations with the right parietal area were higher for the arrow task, while a more mixed pattern was seen over the left parietal area. In the P3a interval, a left-sided lateralization of differences was evident. During the P3b interval, a midline pattern was seen, while during the P4 interval, it was posterior right sided. No contrast was seen in the preresponse interval.

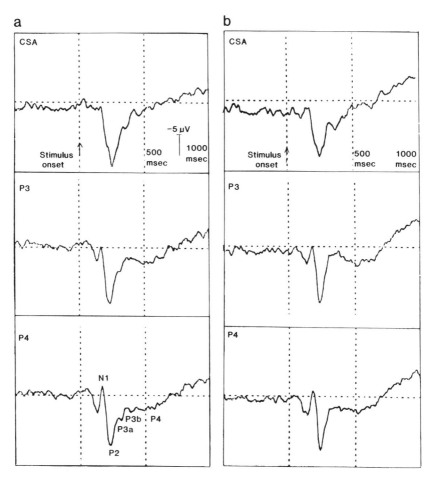

Figure 9-7. *Composites (average of averages) of five participants' stimulus-registered averaged evoked potentials for (a) number and (b) arrow tasks. Each composite is made up of about 55 trials from each of the five participants [277 trials in (a), 279 trials in (b)]. There were no consistent differences between tasks in the peak amplitudes or latencies of the individual averages forming the composite, except for the P3a (P340) component, which had a slightly larger amplitude parietally in the number task. (Reprinted from Gevins, A. et al.* Science, *1981, 213:918–922. c1981 by the American Association for the Advancement of Science.)*

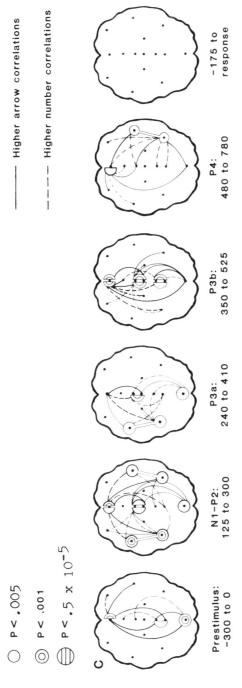

Key
○ P < .005
◎ P < .001
▦ P < .5 × 10⁻⁵

Key
——— Higher arrow correlations
- - - Higher number correlations

C

| Prestimulus: | N1-P2: | P3a: | P3b: | P4: | -175 to |
| -300 to 0 | 125 to 300 | 240 to 410 | 350 to 525 | 480 to 780 | response |

Figure 9-8. *Between-task pattern recognition analysis for each interval: areas outlined differed significantly in their correlation with other areas: a solid line connecting two areas indicates that the areas were more highly correlated for the arrow task. Note the contrasts between the arrow and number tasks in the prestimulus interval, a finding which might be interpreted as evidence of a "preparatory set." Also the lack of contrast on the prerespose interval may be interpreted as the completion of task-specific perceptual processing. (Reprinted from Gevins, A. et al. Science, 1981, 213: 918–922. © 1981 by the American Association for the Advancement of Science.)*

These between-task contrasts may be attributed to the difference in type of mental judgment, since there were no differences in stimuli, in magnitude, duration, velocity, or acceleration of response, in accuracy or response time, or in measures of "arousal," eye movements or EMG. The presence of frontal, parietal, and occipital contrasts during the cued prestimulus interval may be a sign of task-specific preparatory "set." The lack of contrast among tasks in the preresponse interval suggests that task-specific perceptual processing was completed by this time, and motor control commands common to both tasks were presumably being executed. These findings indicate that many areas in both hemispheres are involved in a complex manner even in simple judgments.

In a second study (Gevins, Schaffer, Doyle, Cutillo, Tannehill, & Bressler, 1982), an attempt was made to demonstrate simpler lateralized patterns more clearly related to established neuropsychological, radiological, and chronometric EP observations. This was done by employing a "move/no-move" version of the arrow task, in which the major effects of the difference between the move/no-move decision and between movement and nonmovement would be large and involve specific temporal intervals (the P300 and readiness potential intervals) and local neural areas whose function in such tasks has been well established (right parietal and left central, respectively).

Nine right-handed adults performed from 70 to 350 trials of the arrow task of the previous study. On a random 20 percent of the trials the stimulus number "0" was presented, indicating that no response was to be made (no-move trials). The recording and data screening procedure was the same as in the previous study, and about 1600 move and no-move trials formed the data set for analysis.

Analysis of EP peak amplitude and latencies revealed significant between-task differences only in the P350 and readiness potential intervals. The P350 peak was enhanced in the no-move trials, the greatest difference being at the anterior parietal electrode (Ps). No lateralization was observed. This agrees with previous reports of the behavior and topography of the P300 component in move/no-move paradigms (Simpson et al., 1977). In the readiness potential interval, centered 135 msec later, the expected left-lateralized negative shift was observed at the lateral central electrodes.

A more refined version of the pattern recognition analysis and a high significance level ($p < 5 \times 10^{-5}$) resulted in clear, simple patterns of between-task correlation contrasts that confirmed and elaborated the EP effects. In the P350 interval a single focus of difference between move and no-move tasks was observed at the right parietal electrode (P4), overlying an area of cortex known to be important for similar spatial judgments. It involved prominent correlation differences between the right parietal and the midline occipital, midline precentral, and right central electrodes. In the readiness potential interval 135 msec later the distinguishing focus shifted to the left central electrode (C3), involving correlation differences between that electrode and midline frontal, parietal, and occipital electrodes.

The right-parietal focus in the P350 interval provides a new type of evidence for the localization and lateralization of the processing of spatial judgments that was not evident in the average evoked potential. The left-central focus in the readiness potential interval may reflect the preparation and initiation of the right-hand finger movement. The rapid (135 msec) shift of locus from side to side may exemplify one reason why consistent brain potential lateralizations have been difficult to observe with previous methods that lack this degree of experimental control, sensitivity of analysis, and temporal resolution.

Although these results are clear and intuitively pleasing, it must be remembered that at a lower significance level ($p < .01$) a complex pattern of between-task differences in correlation is present in every interval.

It is not yet known whether or how these patterns of correlation are related to the participation of local neural areas in cognitive and motor processes, but their anatomic and temporal specificity in this study suggest that significant aspects of localized neural processing are being measured.

CONCLUSIONS

BPs are the measure of choice for directly assessing dynamic brain processes associated with higher cognitive functions. They may be recorded noninvasively, and their temporal resolution of small fractions of a second is sufficiently fine to measure the instant-by-instant fluctuations of mental activity. However, there have been few clear-cut and consistent BP confirmations of such seemingly incontrovertible findings as the involvement of Wernicke's and Broca's areas in linguistic comprehension and expression. The reasons for this are apparent when one considers the stringent experimental controls required to record BP and to allow a strong inference that they are associated with cognition, the excessively coarse spatial sampling of regional brain activity in most studies, and the immense technical complexity of the signal processing and pattern recognition analyses required to extract small BP signals related to cognition from the vast amount of unrelated brain electrical activity. These obstacles are currently being overcome.

ACKNOWLEDGMENTS

Supported by grants and contracts from the National Institutes of Mental Health, the Office of Naval Research, the Air Force Office of Scientific Research, the Air Force School of Aerospace Medicine, the John Fetzer Foundation, and Marilyn Brachman-Hoffman.

REFERENCES

Anderson, P., & Anderson, S.A. *Phsysiological basis of the Alpha rhythm* New York: Appleton, 1968.

Aunon, J.I., & McGillem, C.D. Signal processing in evoked potential research: Averaging and modeling. *CRC Critical Reviews in Bioengineering*, 1981, *3*(4):323-367.

Bach-y-Rita, P. *Brain mechanisms in sensory substitution*. New York: Academic Press, 1972.

Bach-y-Rita, P. (Ed.). *Recovery of function: Theoretical considerations for brain injury rehabilitation*. Baltimore: University Park Press, 1980.

Beaumont, J., Mayes, A., & Rugg, M. Asymmetry in EEG alpha coherence and power: Effects of task and sex. *Electroencephalography and Clinical Neurophysiology*, 1978, *45*:393.

Begleiter, H. *Evoked brain potentials and behavior*. New York: Plenum Press, 1979.

Brown, W., & Lehmann, D. Linguistic meaning-related differences in ERP scalp topography. In D. Lehmann & E. Callaway (Eds.), *Human evoked potentials*. New York: Plenum Press, 1979, pp. 31-42.

Brown, W., Marsh, J., & Smith, J. Contextual meaning effects on speech evoked potentials. *Behavioral Biology*, 1973, *9*:755-761.

Brown, W., Marsh, J., & Smith, J. Evoked potential waveform differences produced by the perception of different meanings of an ambiguous phrase. *Electroencephalography and Clinical Neurophysiology*, 1976, *41*: 113-123.

Brown, W., Marsh, J., & Smith, J. Principal components analysis of ERP differences related to the meaning of an ambiguous word. *Electroencephalography and Clinical Neurophysiology*, 1979, *46*: 709-714.

Chapman, R.M. Conative meaning and averaged evoked potentials. In H. Childers, E. (Ed.), *Modern spectrum analysis*. New York: IEEE Press, 1978.

Cooper, R. et al. Comparison of subcortical, cortical and scalp activity using chronically indwelling electrodes in man. *Electroencephalography and Clinical Neurophysiology*, 1965, *18*:217.

Creutzfeldt, O. The neuronal generation of the EEG. In A. Remond (Ed.), *Handbook of electroencehalography*. Part C, 2. Amsterdam: Elsevier, 1974.

Creutzfeldt, O., Watanabe, S., & Lux, H. Relations between EEG phenomena and potentials of single cortical cells. I. Evoked responses after thalamic and epicortical stimulation. *Electroencephalography and Clinical Neurophysiology*, 1966a, *20*:1-18.

Creutzfelt, O., Watanabe, S., & Lux, H. Relations between EEG phenomena and potentials of single cortical cells. II. Spontaneous and convulsoid activity. *Electroencephalography and Clinical Neurophysiology*, 1966b, *20*:19-37.

Daniel, R. Electroencephalographic pattern quantification and arousal continuum. *Psychophysiology*, 1966, *2*:146.

Davidson, R. et al. Sex differences in patterns of EEG asymmetry. *Biological Psychology*, 1976, *4*:119.

Dolce, G., & Kunkel, H. (Eds.). *CEAN, computerized EEG analysis*. Stuttgart: Verlag, 1975.

Donchin, E., Kutas, M., & McCarthy, G. Electrocortical indices of hemispheric utilization. In S. Harnard, R. Doty, L. Goldstein, J. Jaynes, & G. Krauthamer (Eds.), *Lateralization in the nervous system*. New York: Academic Press, 1977, pp. 339–384.

Donchin, E., Ritter, W., & Cheyne, W. Cognitive psychophysiology: The endogenous components of the ERP. In E. Callaway, P. Tueting, & S. Koslow (Eds.), *Event-related brain potentials in man*. New York: Academic Press, 1978, pp. 349–412.

Doyle, J., Ornstein, R., & Gallin, D. Lateral specialization of cognitive mode: II, EEG frequency analysis. *Psychophysiology*, 1974, *11*(5):567–578.

Duncan-Johnson, C.C., & Donchin, E. The relation of P300 latency to reaction time as a function of expectancy. 5th International Symposium on Electrical Potentials Related to Motivation, Motor and Sensory Processes of the Brain, Preliminary Papers. Ulm-Reisensburg, May, 1979, G1.

Elul, R. The physiological interpretation of amplitude histograms of the EEG. *Electroencephalography and Clinical Neurophysiology*, 1969, *27*:703.

Elul, R. Randomness and synchrony in the generation of the electroencephalogram. In H. Petsche & M. Brazier (Eds.), *Synchronization of EEG activity in epileptics*. New York: Springer-Verlag, 1972a, pp. 59–77.

Elul, R. Genesis of the EEG. *International Review of Neurobiology*, 1972b, *15*:227–272.

Fox, S. Evoked potentials, coding and behavior. In F. Schmitt (Ed.), *The neurosciences, second study program*. New York: Rockefeller University Press, 1970, p. 243.

Freeman, W.J. *Mass action in the nervous system*. New York: Academic Press, 1975.

Freeman, W.J. Nonlinear dynamics of paleocortex manifested in the olfactory EEG. *Biological Cybernetics*, 1979a, *35*:21–37.

Freeman, W.J. Nonlinear gain mediating cortical stimulus-response relations. *Biological Cybernetics*, 1979b, *33*:237–247.

Freeman, W.J. EEG anlaysis gives model of neuronal template-matching mechanisim for sensory search with olfactory bulb. *Biological Cybernetics*, 1979c, *35*:221–234.

Freeman, W.J. Analysis of spatial patterns of olfactory bulb EEG with the aid of a software lens. *IEEE Transactions, on Biomedical Engineering*, 1980, 27, 421–429.

Freeman, W.J., & Schneider, W. Changes in spatial patterns of rabbit olfactory EEG with conditioning to odors. *Psychophysiology*, 1982, *19*(1):44–56.

Friedman, D. et al. The late positive component (P-300) and information processing in sentences. *Electroencephalography and Clinical Neurophysiology*, 1975, *38*:255–267.

Furst, C. EEG alpha asymmetry and visuospatial performance. *Nature*, 1976, *260*:254.

Gale, A. et al. Further evidence of sex differences in patterns of EEG asymmetry. *Biological Psychology*, 1978, *6*:203.

Galin, D., Johnstone, J., & Herron, J. Effects of task difficulty on EEG measures of cerebral engagement. *Neuropsychologia*, 1978, *16*:461.

Galin, D., & Ornstein, R. Lateral specialization of cognitive mode: An EEG study. *Psychophysiology*, 1972, *9*(4):412.

Gevins, A.S. Application of pattern recognition to brain electrical potentials *IEEE Transactions on Pattern Analysis and Machine Intelligence*, PAMI, 1980, *2*(5):383–404.

Gevins, A.S. The use of brain electrical potentials (BEP) to study localization of human brain function. *International Journal of Neuroscience*, 1981, *13*:27–41.

Gevins, A.S. et al. Automated analysis of the electrical activity of the human brain: A progress report. *IEEE Proceedings*, 1975, *63*(10):1382.

Gevins, A.S. et al. On-line computer rejection of EEG artifact. *EEG Clinical Neurophysiology*, 1977, *47*:704–710.

Gevins, A.S., Doyle, J.C., Cutillo, B.A. et al. Electrical potentials in human brain during cognition: New method reveals dynamic patterns of correlation. *Science*, 1981, *213*:18–922.

Gevins, A.S., Schaffer, R.E., Doyle, J.C., et al. Shifting lateralization of human brain electrical patterns during a brief visuomotor task. *Science*, submitted, 1982.

Gevins, A.S., Doyle, J.S., Schaffer, R.E. et al. Lateralized cognitive processes and the EEG. *Science*, 1980, *207*:1005–1008.

Gevins, A., Zeitlin, G., Yingling, C. et al. EEG patterns during "cognitive" tasks: 1: Methodology and analysis of complex behaviors. *Electroencephalography and Clinical Neurophysiology*, 1979a, *47*:693–703.

Gevins, A., Zeitlin, G., Doyle, J. et al. EEG patterns during "cognitive" tasks: 2: Analysis of controlled tasks. *Electroencephalography and Clinical Neurophysiology*, 1979b, *47*:704–710.

Gevins, A., Zeitlin, G., Doyle, J. et al. Electroencephalogram correlates of higher cortical functions. *Science*, 1979c, *203*:665–668.

Gevins, A.S., & Schaffer, R.E. A critical review of electroencephalograhic (EEG) correlates of higher cortical functions. *CRC Critical Reviews in Bioengineering*, October 1980, 113–164.

Glaser, E., & Ruchkin, D. *Principles of neurobiological signal analysis*. New York: Academic Press, 1976.

Glass, A., & Butler, S. Alpha EEG asymmetry and speed of left hemisphere thinking. *Neuroscience Letters*, 1977, *4*:231.

Grabow, J. et al. Summated potentials evoked by speech sounds for determining cerebral dominance for language. *Electroencephalography and Clinical Neurophysiology*, 1980a, *49*:38–47.

Grabow, J., Aronson, A., Offord, K. et al. Hemispheric potential evoked by speech sounds during discrimination tasks. *Electroencephalography and Clinical Neurophysiology*, 1980b, *49*:48–58.

Halgren, E. et al. Endogeneous potentials generated in the human hippocampal formation and amygdala by unexpected events. *Science*, 1980, *210*:803–805.

Hillyard, S. et al. Electrical signs of selective attention in the human brain. *Science*, 1973, *182*:177–180.

Ingvar, D.H. Localization of cortical functions by multiregional measurements of the cerebral blood flow. In M.A.B. Brazier & H. Petsche (Eds.), *Architectonics of the cerebral cortex*. New York: Raven Press, 1978, pp. 235–243.

Ingvar, D., & Lassen, N. *Brain work: The coupling of function, metabolism and blood flow in the brain*. New York: Academic Press, 1975.

Ingvar, D., Sjoland, B., & Ardo, A. Correlation between dominant EEG frequency, cerebral oxygen uptake and blood flow. *Electroencephalography and Clinical Neurophysiology*, 1976, *41*:268–276.

John, E. Functional neuroscience. In E. John & R. Thatcher (Eds.), *Neurometrics*, (Vol 2). Hillsdale N.J.: Erlbaum, 1977.

John E., Ruchkin, D., & Vidal, J. Measurement of event-related potentials. In E. Callaway, P. Tueting, & S. Koslow (Eds.), *Event-related brain potentials in man*. New York: Academic Press, 1978, pp. 93–138.

Just, M., & Carpenter, P. Eye fixations and cognitive processes. *Cognitive Psychology*, 1976, *8*:441–480.

Kahneman, D. *Attention and effort*. Englewood Cliffs, N.J.: Prentice-Hall, 1973.

Kooi, K., Tucker, R., & Marshall, R. *Fundamentals of electroencephalography* (2nd ed). New York: Harper & Row, 1978.

Lassen, N., Ingvar, D., & Skinhoj, E. Brain function and blood flow. *Scientific American*, 1978, *239*(4):62–71.

Leissner, P., Lindholm, L., & Petersen, I. Alpha amplitude dependence on skull thickness as measured by ultrasound technique. *Electroencephalography and Clinical Neurophysiology*, 1970, *29*:392–399.

Loomis, A. et al. Distribution of disturbance patterns in the human electroencephalogram with special reference to sleep. *Journal of Neurophysiology*, 1938, *1*:413.

Luria, A. *The working brain: An introduction to neuropsychology*. New York: Penguin, 1973.

Luria, A. *Higher cortical functions in man*. New York: Basic Books, 1977.

McKee, G., Humphrey, B., & McAdam, D. Scaled lateralization of alpha activity during linguistic and musical tasks. *Psychophysiology*, 1973, *10*:441.

Marsh, J., & Brown, W. Evoked potential correlates of meaning in the perception of language. *Progress in Clinical Neurophysiology*, 1977, *3*:60–72.

Matejcek, M., & Schenk, G. (Eds.). *Quantitative analysis of the EEG: Methods and applications*. Konstanz: AEG-Telefunken, 1975.

Mazziotta, J.C. et al. The metabolic map of the unstimulated normal human brain in transverse and coronal section. 3rd Annual Meeting of the American Academy of Neurology, New Orleans, La., 1980.

Mazziotta, J.C. et al. Tomographic mapping of human cerebral metabolism: Sensory deprivation. *Annals of Neurology*, 1981a, in press.

Mazziotta, J.C. et al. Tomographic mapping of human cerebral metabolism; auditory stimulation. *Neurology*, 1981b, in press.

Mazziotta, J.C., & Phelps, M.E. Human cerebral metabolism at rest, during physiological stimulation and with pathological lesions of the visual pathway. *Neurology*, 1981, in press.

Metter, E.J. FDG positron emission computed tomography in a study of aphasia. *Journal of American Neurological Association*, 1981, 173–183.

Molfese, D. Cortical involvement in the semantic processing of coarticulated speech cues. *Brain and Language*, 1979, *7*:86–100.

Molfese, D., Papanicolaou, A., Hess, T. and Molfese, V. Neuroelectrical correlates of semantic processes. In H. Begleiter (Ed.), *Evoked brain potentials and behavior*, New York: Plenum Press, 1979b.

Morgan, A. et al. Differences in bilateral alpha activity as a function of experimental task, with a note on lateral eye movements and hypnotizability. *Neuropsychologica*, 1971, *9*, 459.

Morrell, L., & Salamy, J. Hemispheric asymmetry of electrocortical response to speech stimuli. *Science*, 1971, *174*:164–166.

Moruzzi, G., & Magoun, H. Brain stem reticular formation and activation of the EEG. *Electroencephalography and Clinical Neurophysiology*, 1949, *1*:455.

Naatanen, R., Gaillard, A.W.K., & Mantysalo, S. Early selective-attention effect on evoked potential reinterpreted. *Actuae Psychologica*, 1978, *42*:313–329.

Naatanen, R., & Michie, P. Different variants of endogeneous negative brain potentials in performance situations: A review and classification. In D. Lehmann & E. Callaway (Eds.), *Human evoked potentials: Applications and problems*. New York: Plenum Press, 1979, pp. 251–267.

Neville, H.J. Event related potentials in neuropsychological studies of language. Unpublished manuscript, 1981.

Ornstein, R. et al. Differential right hemisphere engagement in visuospatial tasks. *Neuropsychologia*, 1980, *18*:49–64.

Parasuraman, R., & Beatty, J. Processing demands affect slow negative shift latencies and N100 amplitude in focussed and divided attention. Society for Psychophysiological Research, 20th Annual Meeting, October, 1980. (Abstract)

Phelps, M. Positron computed tomography studies of cerebral glucose metabolism in man: Theory and application in nuclear medicine. *Seminars in Nuclear Medicine*, 1981, *XI*(1)32–49.

Phelps, M.E. et al. Tomographic mapping of the metabolic response of the human visual cortex to stimulation and deprivation. *Proceedings of the 32nd Annual Meeting of the American Academy of Neurology*, Los Angeles, Calif., 1981.

Picton, T.W. et al. Methodology and meaning of human evoked potential scalp distribution studies. *Proceedings of the 4th International Congress on Event Related Potentials of the Brain*, Hendersonville, N.C., 1978, EPA-600/9-77-043, pp. 515–522.

Purpura, D. et al. Synaptic mechanisms in thalamic regulation of cerebrocortical projection activity. In D. Purpura & M. Yahr (Eds.), *The thalamus*. New York: Columbia University Press, 1966, pp. 153–172.

Rebert, C.S. Electrogenesis of slow potential changes in the central nervous system: A summary of issues. *Proceedings of the 4th International Congress on Event Related Slow Potentials of the Brain*, Hendersonville, N.C., 1978a, EPA-600/9-77-043, pp. 3–11.

Rebert, C.S., & Low, D. Differential hemispheric activation during complex visuomotor performance. *Electroencephalography and Clinical Neurophysiology*, 1978, *44*:724.

Rechtschaffen, A., & Kales, A. A manual of standardized terminology, techniques and scoring system for sleep stages of human subjects. *Brain information services*, Brain Research Institute, UCLA, Los Angeles, 1973.

Remond, A. (Ed.). *EEG informatics: A didactic review of methods and applications of EEG data processing*. New York: Elsevier, 1977.

Rohrbaugh, J.W., Lindsley et al. Synthesis of the contingent negative variation brain potential from arm contingent stimulus and motor elements. *Science*, 1980, *208*:1165–1168.

Roth, W.T. How many late positive waves are there? *Proceedings of the 4th International Congress on Event Related Potentials of the Brain*, Hendersonville, N.C., 1978, EPA-600/9-77-043, pp. 170–172.

Simon, O., Schultz, H., & Rassman, W., The definition of waking stages on the basis of continuous polygraphic recordings in normal subjects. *Electroencephalography and Clinical Neurophysiology*, 1977, *42*:48.

Simpson, R., Vaughn, H., & Ritter, W. The scalp topography of potentials in auditory and visual go/no go tasks. *Electroencephalography and Clinical Neurophysiology*, 1977, *43*:864–875.

Skinner, J.E., & Yingling, C.D. Central gating mechanisms that regulate event related potentials and behavior. In J.E. Desmedt (Ed.), *Attention, voluntary contraction and event related cerebral potentials,* (Vol. 1). Basel: Karger, 1977, pp. 30–69.

Sutton, S., John et al. Evoked potential correlates of stimulus uncertainty. *Science*, 1965, *150*:1187–1188.

Sutton, S., Tueting, P., & Hammer, M. Evoked potentials and feedback. *Proceedings of the 4th International Congress on Event Related Potentials of the Brain*, Hendersonville, N.C., 1978, EPA-600/9-77-043, pp. 184–188.

Teuting, P. Event related potentials, cognitive events and information processing. *Proceedings of the 4th International Congress on Event Related Potentials of the Brain*, Hendersonville, N.C., 1978, EPA-600/9-77-043.

Thatcher, R.W. EP correlates of delayed letter matching. *Behavioral Biology*, 1977, *19*:1–23.

Thatcher, R., & John, E. *Functional neuroscience: foundations of cognitive processes* (Vol. 1). Hillsdale, N.J.: Erlbaum, 1977.

Thatcher, R.W., & Maisel, E.B. Functional landscapes of the brain: An electrotopographic perspective. In H. Begleiter (Ed.), *Evoked brain potentials and behavior*. New York: Plenum Press, 1979, pp. 143–169.

Verzeano, M., Calma, I. Unit activity in spindle bursts. *Journal of Neurophysiology*, 1954, *17*:417–428.

Verzeano, M. et al. The activity of neuronal networks in the thalamus of the monkey. In K. Pribram & D. Broadbent (Eds.), *Biology of memory*. New York: Academic Press, 1970, pp. 239–272.

Walter, W. et al. Contingent negative variation: An electric sign of sensorimotor association and expectancy in the human brain. *Nature*, 1964, *203*:380–384.

Wood, C.C. Auditory and phonetic levels of processing in speech perception: Neurophysiological and information-processing analyses. *Journal of Experimental Psychology* [*Human Perception*], 1975, *104*(1):3–20.

Wood, C.C. et al. Auditory evoked potentials during speech perception. *Science*, 1971, *171*:1248–1251.

10

Laterality of Cerebral Function: Its Investigation by Measurement of Localized Brain Activity

Frank Wood

INTRODUCTION

Fundamental scientific advance sometimes occurs when a new measurement technique is applied to an old question. The contribution of the telescope to the development of astronomy and physics is the most familiar, classical example. It may be that the recent development of techniques for noninvasive observation of normal brain activity, with adequate spatial and temporal resolution, will enable fundamental, foundational progress in the neurosciences. The purpose of this chapter is to consider that possibility in the special context of the issue of lateralization of function in the human brain. That necessarily requires clarification of a range of philosophical, methodological, and practical questions that naturally arise when a branch of science is confronted with a promising new technology.

These pivotal intersections between a line of theoretical development and a line of technological progress have some inherent features that are instructive. First, new measurement techniques usually permit observations that are, in some sense, "closer" to the phenomenon in question. This "closeness," however, has some distinctive qualities. Higher spatial or temporal resolution is often involved but only if the important features of the phenomenon in question are well described at that higher level of resolution. The terms, "important" and "well described," are value judgments that must be made by reference, both to the current level of theoretical understanding and to the scientist's own ability to tolerate a large number of data points. For example, the microscope is not helpful in the study of the sizes and shapes of beaks in birds. Indeed, the understanding of this phenomenon is improved when it is reanalyzed, as Darwin did, at a much coarser level of resolution—not fine measurements on individual birds in present time but rough, overall descriptions of sizes and shapes of beaks in whole species of birds in evolution across relatively long time periods. The "closest" observation is thus the one for which spatial and temporal resolution, however fine or coarse, permits an effective combination of accurate prediction and simplified description of the phenomenon under study.

An improved measurement technique, permitting "closer" observation in the sense described above, usually also requires an accompanying mathematical development before the full possibilities of the new technology can be realized. Such mathematical developments, in turn, are usually not simple practical necessities of the new technology (as the geometry of light defraction was necessary for the telescope). Rather, the mathematical innovation is necessitated by the newly described scientific phenomena themselves (as the calculus, for example, was inherent and, therefore, necessary in Newton's attempts to describe the physics of falling objects, whether apples or planets). One could hardly consider the prospects of a new technology in the neurosciences, therefore, without considering the mathematical approaches that would likely be required.

Naturally, an evaluation of the prospects of a new technology also presupposes clarification of the particular scientific questions for which pursuit would be thus enabled or facilitated. As noted above, this involves clarification of the optimal level of temporal or spatial resolution. In a larger sense, it requires at least some intuition of where the fundamental scientific inquiry is going. Scientific history is replete with serendipitous discoveries, but the larger truth lies in the selection of those discoveries that are worth pursuing. The neurosciences, in their current fragmentation and lack of shared vocabulary, may be especially vulnerable to the squandering of a new technology on questions that are interesting but ultimately trivial. One cannot escape the requirement, therefore, of making some initial guesses, using the best information and insight available, about which questions are most worth pursuing with the new technology.

The converse of the above principle is that one must expect new discoveries not anticipated by the current, consensual scientific understanding. In one sense, that is trivially obvious; one would hardly call it a new technology if it did not ultimately permit new discoveries. Yet it is unsettling to notice how often new technologies, including those that are the subject of this chapter, are addressed not just to the old questions, which may still permit new answers, but to old versions of old questions, the answers to which have long ago been discovered. If one were at the absolutely first stages of the use of a new technology, one could hardly speculate about the new discoveries that are waiting. In the present case, however, there are already enough data to indicate what some of the new discoveries are and will be. One must consider, within the data already available, not only where new progress is likely to come but also where it has already taken place.

SPATIAL-TEMPORAL RESOLUTION AND THE PROBLEM OF COMPLEXITY

It is frequently remarked that the brain is a complex organ and that this complexity stands in the way of satisfactory scientific understanding. Reference is often made, for example, to the large number of functionally discrete sites in the brain (ten to the fourteenth synapses). This is actually an unenlightening tautology, however, since the simplified description of otherwise complex phenomena is virtually the definition of science itself. The perpetuation of this tautology, in scientific as well as popular discussion, therefore, merely indicates that the appropriate simplifying descriptions have not yet been devised. It does not indicate that such simplifying descriptions are impossible in principle or even infeasible in practice. As noted in the introduction, the problem may be an inappropriately fine degree of temporal and spatial resolution. If so, the techniques under discussion in this chapter will attract interest precisely because they describe brain function and activity in much coarser resolution than would be provided, for example, by electrophysiological measurements of the activity of single cells in the brain.

The coarser resolution is achieved by local, spatial summation of the activity of individual neurons. Except in quite unusual and special circumstances, this does sacrifice the ability to observe the coordinated activity of small networks of neurons, scattered across several different brain regions. The existence and functional significance of such networks is not disputed (Hebb, 1949), and these techniques for coarse, regional functional mapping of brain activity are inherently ill suited to the study of such networks. However, 150 years of research in the neurosciences has also established the functional significance of local small regions of cortex and of subcortical structures, as well. These are regions intermediate in size between single cortical columns of cells and whole lobes or hemispheres of cortex. This cortical mosaic model has often been debated, but it is finally an empirical question whether or not techniques designed to observe a functional cortical mosaic will prove to have appropriate power to describe reliable and valid phenomena of brain activity.

The existing techniques vary in the combinations of temporal and spatial resolution that they offer. Positron emission tomography provides three-dimensional spatial resolution on the order of a few millimeters, although this does vary with the sharpness of the structural or functional boundaries being observed. When used to assess local glucose utilization as an index of local metabolic activity, however, positron emission tomography has quite coarse temporal resolution, on the order of approximately 30 minutes. Regional cerebral blood flow by the inhalation method, however, is spatially quite irresolute, with circles of resolution on the cortical surface approximatley 1 to 1.5 inches in diameter. The temporal resolution is, however, more favorable; it is possible to estimate cortical gray matter flow in 11 minutes, and the behavorial activation task itself may only need to be carried on for approximately 3 to 4 minutes. Electrophysiological techniques go even further in this direction, with temporal resolution on the order of seconds or fractions of a second and spatial resolution no better than a few inches. Thus, while the spatial-temporal resolutions of these techniques are of a roughly similar order of magnitude, the techniques may lend themselves to somewhat different specialized uses in functional mapping of the brain, depending upon whether the spatial or temporal features are the most important.

The above analysis suggests that positron emission tomography and similar three dimensional techniques will be the methods of choice where a literal picture of the whole brain functional landscape is required. The behavioral state or task serving as the stimulus for this landscape of functional activity will necessarily be a simple one; sensitive manipulations of the nature of the task will ordinarily be swamped by the temporal irresolution of this technique. The requirement to sustain the task or the behavioral state for such a long time inherently confounds all but the simplest variations in such behavioral states or tasks. Questions such as, "What happens (in terms of overall glucose utilization) in the left thalamus during 30 minutes of sustained, repetitive motions of the right hand?" are uniquely suited to positron emission tomography. This is also true for questions about chronic behavioral or emotional states, such as anxiety, especially when questions are asked about subcortical structures and their overall level of activity during such states.

At the other extreme, the various electrophysiological techniques, including the study of event-related potentials and the use of power spectrum analysis of the ongoing EEG, allow for highly refined manipulation of stimulus properties as well as detailed temporal delineation of the unfolding brain response to those stimuli. To the extent that one gets even coarse geographical information from such studies, they also contribute to the general functional mapping enterprise. Their unique contribution lies in the precision of the experimental control; questions about the differential effects of various stimulus attributes on roughly localizable brain activation are best answered with these techniques (see Gevins, this volume).

Regional cerebral blood flow by the inhalation method, as noted above, occupies an intermediate position in the trade-off of spatial and temporal resolution. It has been previously argued (Wood, 1980) that this particular method has an optimal combination of spatial and temporal resolution in order to facilitate neuropsychological research that addresses the historic issues of localization of function. Because it is temporally much more resolute than emission tomography, inhalation regional cerebral blood flow can more easily assess the impact of major behavioral processes on localized brain functioning. While not suited for the delineation of detailed stimulus characteristics, the method is well suited to manipulation of basic cognitive activities such as speech comprehension, spontaneous speech expression, and certain types of verbal memory, to name only some obvious and familiar examples. Appropriate experimental design can be used to deconfound a variety of subprocesses and control processes, allowing the relative isolation of some of the basic processes under study.

Considerations of spatial and temporal resolution do not exhaust the overall issue of resolution. Complexity, or the number of dependent measures, is essentially a third dimension of resolution. As noted above, the study of brain activity has been bedeviled by the seemingly hopeless complexity of the phenomena in question. All of the above techniques involve major simplifications and, therefore, involve implicit strategies of complexity reduction. Such reduction is the essence of science, but, if carried too far, it does become trivial and unhelpful to further progress. To return to the earlier example of the telescope, it is fair to say that the taking of occasional photographs through the telescope would hardly advance the understanding of the solar system, after the initial curiosity about the new pictures was satiated. Analogously, the emission tomography technology is vulnerable to this casual approach, since the pictures themselves are so interesting. The very thing that makes them interesting to see is the most basic problem that they present; the pictures contain so much information that one is somewhat at a loss about how best to proceed to reduce, categorize, cross-refer, and thus understand them. To put it another way, the complexity dimension is transformed almost entirely into the spatial and, therefore, visual domain. Consensual techniques for analyzing and reducing such information are not available.

Inhalation regional cerebral blood flow studies, surprisingly, also exceed the normal visual channel capacity of scientific investigators, but the problem is perhaps enough smaller in that technique that one can begin to see some of the possible techniques that can be used to confront this rich complexity. Successful use of such techniques in regional cerebral blood studies may help to inform the development and use of similar techniques in emission tomography, since both are addressed to the same spatial complexity domain. The electrophysiological techniques have the most well worked out procedures for handling the complexity encountered in those types of investigations, but these are of less direct utility to regional cerebral blood flow and the emission tomography investigations. That is because electrophysiological techniques deploy almost all of their power in the temporal domain, and the issues that arise in spatial mapping do not usually reach serious proportions in electrophysiological investigations.

As a general principle, it would be fair to say that the issues surrounding spatial, temporal, and complexity resolution are fundamental issues for the use of any of these techniques in the study of lateralization of function. The more important principle, however, is the converse one. It states that the study of lateralization of function is favored by a set of techniques with just this general level of spatial, temporal, and complexity resolution. In some ways, this principle is obvious by definition. Laterality of function is probably a meaningless concept unless there is some geographically localized concentration of activity in one of the two hemispheres. Presumably, this concentration could range in scope from an entire hemisphere down to a few cortical columns, but it is usually thought of at a level intermediate between these two extremes. Thus, in most cases, lateralization of function also implies some intrahemispheric localization. This certainly leaves open the question of whether or not an entire hemisphere sometimes acts as a unit asymmetrical to the other hemisphere, and it leaves open the question of the nature and extent of diffuse neuronal networks that may play a role in either the lateralization or localization of function. Still, any researchable question about lateralization of function almost necessarily focuses on some subregions of a hemisphere, which serve as the pivot for these larger hemispheric and smaller cell assembly units of analysis. If the foregoing interpretation is correct, the conclusion is inescapable that the problem of lateralization of function is uniquely well suited for study by the techniques of localized measurement of brain activity being considered in this chapter. These techniques provide the appropriate level of spatial, temporal, and complexity resolution in order to permit major advances in the understanding of lateralization of function.

MATHEMATICAL PROBLEMS

Mathematical and statistical issues subdivide into two categories, which may be termed external and internal. External issues are concerned with the linkage between measurements of local brain activity and the corresponding physiological and environmental correlates. Internal issues have to do with relationships within the localized brain activity measurements themselves.

External Data Analysis

External issues of data interpretations naturally revolve around the experimental technique for isolating the environmental or physiological variables in question. These issues of experimental design are the province of classical experimental and physiological psychology, which have well worked out procedures for the isolation of independent variables. It is, furthermore, accurate to say that the study of localized brain activity, even in its infancy, has suffered greatly from lack of attention to basic techniques of experimental design. Formal group studies comparing an experimental and a control condition, either behaviorally or physiologically induced, are rare.

The other side of the question, however, is whether there is anything that can be learned from less systematic observations. Suppose, for example, that there is a single subject who is repetitively listening to sentences and signaling whether those sentences are true or false. An emission tomography scan, representing local glucose utilization in the brain, as summed across the duration of the execution of this task, might show an area of high metabolic activity in the left temporal lobe, at a level that seems to represent the temporal planum. This observation, standing alone, would have little scientific value by the usual standards of experimental psychology. One would have no idea whether the left temporal lobe activation was the result of some feature of the task itself, an enduring personality trait of the subject, or some feature of the immediate stimulus environment, such as a persistent noise; still, the scan is not utterly useless. It is at least the first exemplar of a category of pictures, a category whose boundaries will be successively refined as new observations are made.

The initial response to the picture, noticing the left temporal lobe hypermetabolism, is distinctive and characteristic; one notices the feature that stands out visually against a background of relatively undifferentiated levels of metabolism in most other areas of the scan. Thus, visual pattern recognition processes are at work, utilizing such component processes as figure-ground differentiation, contour or contrast enhancement, and local spatial summation. Were the results of the scan to have been presented in numerical or tabular, that is, nonspatial form, one might scarcely have notice or recognized the distinctive left temporal lobe activation. Even in a single case, therefore, the mere fact that the results are presented in pictorial form does constrain the initial interpretation by causing one to notice only the most visually salient features of the scan. This could certainly be deceptive; it could turn out that the visually salient feature was not the feature that was relevant to the intended task manipulation, namely, sentence comprehension. However, this visual reduction does something quite useful in providing a few salient features for which to look in the next scan.

To continue the hypothetical example, suppose that the same subject is then rescanned, this time under conditions of pictorial stimulation; the subject repeatedly sees pictures and signals, whether they are true in the sense of plausible or false in the sense of absurd. Suppose, then, that the scan shows a right parietal focus of activation. The category of scans now has two exemplars, and one is alerted to a host of task, subject state, and environmental variables that might correspond to the salient differences between the two scans. One is equally impressed, although less consciously so, by communalities between the two scans: regions whose level and landscape are the same in the two scans. It is now very much as though one is a subject in a simultaneous discrimination training and generalization training experiment. One is, in effect, being invited, on a trial-by-trial basis, to establish certain features of the functional landscape that are constant across a variety of task manipulations, hence, generalization training. At the same time, one has the opportunity to discover reasonably predictable features of the task manipulation that correspond to salient differences in the functional landscapes, hence, stimulus discrimination training. In the early stages of this process, one's confidence certainly does not approach the 0.05 or, still less, the 0.01 level. That is not to say, however, that one has no confidence at all. Indeed, studies of natural or artificial concept formation always show that the reliability of the concept, either generalized or discriminated, rises most rapidly in the first few trials, thereafter to rise more slowly. Even in a few trials, therefore, one does gain much informal information and certainty. The information is not yet fully reliable, and it is sometimes even difficult to verbalize, but it is the very information that tends to direct scientific intuition and leads to the formulation of specific hypotheses that can be subjected to formal experimental tests.

Naturally, lateralized asymmetries in the functional landscape are especially vivid and apparent to initial visual inspection. This suggests that hypotheses about lateral differences are especially likely to occur, even in the early stages of the examination of individual scans. Accordingly, by the analysis presented above, one should expect some new ideas about laterality to develop during the current phase of investigations in measurement of localized brain activity. Some of these will be considered later in this chapter. In summary, the most obvious external feature of data analysis is the visual-spatial reductionism that is involved. This biases the intuitive interpretation of the scans toward features that are visually salient, but it permits and encourages the early formulation of hypotheses that could later be tested by formal, controlled experiments.

A second set of external linkages, between the local measurements of brain activity and extrinsic factors, has to do with correlations between the task activity and local functional activity. The most familiar two aspects of task activity are speed and accuracy and the trade-off relationship between them. Correlations with task accuracy have already proved instructive in this literature, although correlations with speed have not yet been systematically attempted. The point is that quantitative features of the task and its performance may be systematically related to observable features of the functional landscapes induced by the tasks. Task difficulty, the range and probability relationships among stimuli, associated physiological responses such as heart rate, and strategy differences in task execution are simply some of the most obvious examples of variables that might have their own relationship to the functional landscape. The same is true for relationships to the host of personality or trait variables that characterize the subjects themselves; everything from level of anxiety to psychometrically measured intelligence is "fair game" for this line of research. Clearly, the logic of these inferences is correlational, but there is certainly much to be learned from systematic explorations of such variables and their impact on the functional landscapes.

Internal Data Analysis

Data obtained from localized measurements of brain activity are marked by several distinctive characteristics and problems of analysis. These arise whenever there is more than one subject or more than one functional landscape. Characterizations of groups of scans, with regard to internal features of the data, do provide some particularly useful information. Among the more interesting and important of these characteristics are the following.

The Correlation between Means and Variances

As is not at all uncommon in physiological measurements, local measurements of brain activity tend to show greater variance with higher mean values. Consider a group of subjects, all of whose scans were obtained under conditions of a quiet, resting baseline. Under these conditions, there is a tendency for activity to be somewhat higher in the frontal regions than in the posterior regions of the cortex. This higher mean, however, is also accompanied by higher variance in frontal activity; only some, not all, subjects show this hyperfrontality. When, across a group of subjects, a given region shows a higher variance as well as a higher mean, it actually indicates that region is less affected by the state or task in question; it is more free to show individual differences among subjects. It can be presumed that these individual differences reflect differences in the subjects' approach to tasks in question, in this case differences in "approach" to the resting baseline situation. Another way to conceptualize this is to regard the regions of high variance as regions that are disinhibited or set loose by the particular state in question, in this case, the resting baseline. Such disinhibition would naturally have a distinctive neurobehavioral interpretation, different from the interpretation that would be adopted if subjects in a given state tended uniformly to show higher metabolism in some areas than in others.

Correlations between means and variances are ubiquitous in the blood flow literature, although they are seldom mentioned. (The emission tomography literature does not yet contain enough formal groups, in which all subjects are in the same state, to permit such analyses.) There are several noteworthy details that attend these correlations between means and variances. First of all, there are sometimes striking hemispheric differences, so that within a hemisphere there might be a high correlation between means and variances, whereas in the other hemisphere there would be a low correlation between means and variances. Such differences can be used as grounds for inferring the extent to which the hemisphere reflects disinhibitory processes (high correlation between means and variances with some areas of high variance) versus constrained processes (low correlation between means and variances with some areas showing high means and low variances) during the state or activation task in question. The determination that a given hemisphere shows low correlation between means and variances can then be followed up with an inspection to determine which areas show not only high means but also low variances, with the inference that such regions are the particular ones most constrained and activated by the task itself.

Next, one can plot the regression line that describes the correlation between means and variances, extrapolating to the Y intercept and thus obtaining an indication of the level of metabolic activity that would be associated with zero variance. In most cases, these intercepts converge at a common point, across activation conditions and across laboratories, a point that apparently represents something near the physiological minimum of activation. An interesting issue then arises about the interpretation of a hemisphere in which the Y intercept (extrapolated level of mean functional activation under conditions of zero variance) is significantly higher than the Y intercept for the other hemisphere. Such a finding can be taken as an indication that there is a general hemispheric activation, extending essentially across all areas and not part of the localized disinhibition that gives rise to the high correlation between means and variances. Examination of these twin indexes—strength of correlation between means and variances and Y intercept of the regression line for describing that correlation—provides a useful way for characterizing and summarizing certain features of the hemispheric (and laterally asymmetrical) response to a given state or task.

The correlation between means and variances is sometimes so striking as to raise the possibility that a Poisson distribution underlies the data. Specifically, Poisson distributions are characterized by equal means and variances and reflect the likelihood of occurrence of a certain number of events per unit of time or space. Translated into the measurement of local brain activity, a Poisson process would imply several specific and interesting things. First, the particular metabolic index would be interpreted as an indirect reflection or summation of the number of discrete events (on or off) of activation within the site in question. A random process would then be assumed to distribute those events of activation across subjects, at the site in question, at an average number of events per site per unit of time. The randomness could be partly due to subject variables and also partly due to variations in the definition of the anatomical site in question. At that point, the shape of the distributions would become especially important. If the distributions all tended to be approximately normal, it would imply that the number of activation events within a probe site was relatively large (since the Poisson distribution assumes a normal shape after means of 12 or 15). However, if the sites showing low activation are strongly and positively skewed and if a Poisson process is responsible, it could only reflect the operation of a relatively small number of activation events within a single site (since the Poisson distribution assumes a highly positively skewed shape as the mean approaches zero).

Existing data have not yet been sufficiently described by reference to the shapes of the distributions in question, but if there was a systematic tendency for the sites of lower means to have positively skewed distributions, whereas sites with higher means had progressively more normal distributions, it would certainly imply a Poisson process as one possible explanation. An additional way to approach this problem would be to look at sites that vary in size. If smaller sites tend to show positively skewed distributions (since they have a smaller number of activation events in the site), whereas larger sites show more normal distributions, it is just possible that inferences could be drawn about the approximate number of functionally relevant activation events within a given site. This might then permit inferences about the "granularity" of the activation process. If "strong" versions of the cortical mosaic model are correct, these functionally discrete units or "grains" may be much larger than the cortical columns; they may number no more than dozens or hundreds across the cortical surface.

The Shape of the Distributions

Flow or metabolism values across subjects at a given site do not generally distribute normally. There are several reasons for this nonnormality. Floor and ceiling effects, familiar in certain other physiological measurement situations, are clearly present. Naturally, these effects operate to produce positively or negatively skewed distributions as the means approach the floor or ceiling, respectively. Large enough sets of data have not really been studied, at least in normal subjects, to establish clearly that such an effect is present. It remains an open, empirical question whether or not the typical nonnormality of these distributions can be explained by floor and ceiling effects. This would require systematic investigation of the shape of the distributions as a function of their means and would be considerably complicated by the possibility that the upper ceiling, at least, could vary across conditions of activation or even across sites in a given condition of activation. Under conditions of the resting baseline, for example, it may well be that the physiological limit of frontal lobe flow or metabolism is higher than the physiological limit of parietal lobe flow or metabolism. These differential ceilings could themselves be an effect of the resting baseline. Perhaps the better way to consider the question would be to say that a systematic trend for the higher means, in a given condition, in order to be negatively skewed while the lower means are positively skewed, would provide evidence of the existence and the approximate level of floor and ceiling effects. In turn, such floor and ceiling effects would have important physiological interpretations, particularly if the ceiling were differential as a function of different states of activation. If a certain activation establishes differential ceilings in different brain sites, that would suggest some further very interesting hypotheses about the mechanisms of local brain activation and the modulation of such activation. For example, it might well give rise to hypotheses about inhibitory as well as excitatory processes. It is an issue that cannot be settled until a sufficiently large number of normals is studied, with adequate controls for age, sex, and similar variables, but it is clearly an issue that would deserve just such careful attention.

Another interesting possibility regarding the shape of the distributions is that of multimodality. If distributions are bimodal, for example, in a given site but not in other sites, one is naturally led to a consideration of possible typologies of subjects whose activation of a given site, under the stated activation condition, is determined by some uniform, categorical attributes of the subjects. A discontinuity of this type would have special implications for classical questions relating to cerebral laterality. One thinks immediately of handedness, for example. Are left- and right-handers simply two or more groups along a continuum, however skewed? Or are they, instead, representative of fundamentally different types of cerebral organizations? If the latter, one should expect multimodal distributions in some areas, areas that presumably reflect the functional processes involved in handedness.

Of even greater interest than handedness, in this regard, is the question of speech representation. Formal group studies in regional cerebral blood flow and informal cases in emission tomography have certainly suggested that language activation does ordinarily result in some focal left hemisphere increases in flow or metabolism. If there are individual differences in "strength" of this left lateral asymmetry of language processing, one would expect those differences to be mapped along a dimension of flow or metabolism differences in the relevant cortical sites, for example, Wernicke's or Broca's areas. If the proposed dimension of lateralization is also discontinuous, bimodal distributions should be expected. Before reaching strong conclusions about underlying "strength" of laterality, however, one would obviously have to rule out differential strategy selection by the subjects; even though they have the "strength" to mobilize a certain area they may choose not to do so under given conditions. Here again, a typology of characteristic strategy choices by subjects could emerge from multimodal distributions in the areas in question.

It is clear, then, that a systematic examination of the distributions of flow or metabolism variances, across given sites, could be enormously instructive. An early goal of emission tomography research, therefore, should be to accumulate a large enough sample of carefully defined normal subjects to permit these distributions to settle out and to allow enough statistical power to analyze significant divergences from normality. Sample sizes in the middle 30s to 40s would seem to be only minimally adequate for this purpose; a standard reference group approaching 100 in size would be well worth the considerable expense, if only for the information that it would provide about the shape of distributions across subjects at various brain sites.

Intercorrelation among Brain Sites

Flow or metabolism values, distributed across subjects at a given site, may correlate more or less highly with the values obtained at another site. The complete intercorrelation matrix contains much information of great relevance for fundamental understanding of brain functioning and brain behavior relations. Obviously, the first possibility to consider is that of high intercorrelations among separate regions. This would be inherently uninteresting if the regions were adjacent; that would simply define the spatial extent of a single, functionally discrete site. When high correlations exist between noncontiguous sites, however, one is entitled to consider the possibility of a functional system that organizes the separate sites. The delineation of such factors, representing systems that are functionally coherent under those particular state or activation circumstances, would provide important information about the system-wide, organizational response of the brain to such states or conditions of activation.

The second feature of interest, in this regard, is clearly the definition of sites that have low correlations between them. When two such sites are adjacent to each other, they mark a boundary between one functionally discrete unit and the next, thus demarcating two regions that have considerable functional independence under the particular state or activation conditions employed. In this way, the demonstration of particularly low intercorrelations between some sites is required to give additional meaning to the factors of high intercorrelation. At least low intercorrelations help assure that a given highly coherent factor or cluster of sites is not simply a more sensitive indication of whole brain, system-wide activation.

Reliable description of an entire intercorrelation matrix for even the relatively few number of sites used in the inhalation regional cerebral blood flow technique—usually between 16 and 32 sites—would again require a sample size of between 70 and 100 subjects. If each pixel on an emission tomography scan is considered as a separate site, however, the number of subjects required to gain strong descriptive power from the massive intercorrelation matrix of all those sites would be astronomical. It is common and necessary, therefore, when using the emission tomography data, to consider combining adjacent pixels into larger functional or anatomical units. Sometimes this is done by examining the scans and attempting to identify anatomical landmarks and to plot the assumed boundaries of various neuroanatomical structures. Having done that, one then considers an entire structure (for example, the caudate nucleus) as a single unit, anatomically defined. It is agreed that this is a rough procedure and that anatomical boundaries can, at best, be only crudely estimated, not only because of inherent uncertainty about the location of structures in a given scan but also because of partial volume effects (these are the result of a given pixel straddling an anatomical boundary, summing the values on both sides of the boundary and thus blurring the boundary itself).

Another way to approach the same question is to begin with functional boundaries and to ask if those make any neuroanatomical sense. The question then is how to define those functional boundaries, and the most obvious technique is to consider correlations only betwen adjacent pixels. This implies that a suitable sample size is available, that is, between 50 and 100 subjects. To consider only the intercorrelation between adjacent pixels, looking for lines of low intercorrelation that could define functional boundaries separating independent regions, would be technically feasible in most computer installations. However, such a procedure would have two important drawbacks. First, one would have only minimal confidence that the same pixel represents anything similar to the same region of brain across many subjects. This is due to the inherent variability and to the size and shape of brains. That problem could be approached by "stretching" each scan to fit a common template, but this would then make the pixels of somewhat differing sizes, across subjects. The second drawback is the more serious: adjacent sites will have a tendency to be highly interrelated, simply because the individual pixels are close to the lower limits of resolution of the technique. This means that adjacent pixels will always, to some extent, be reflecting each other's activity, or the activity of a common region that overlaps both, thus ensuring high correlations. The approach to this problem, in turn, is to consider correlations between pairs of sites that have one or two pixels between them. This overcomes the problem of overlapping but, in so doing, naturally sacrifices some spatial resolution. The technique of using alternate sites, that is, skipping "in between" pixels in each case, would also help with the first drawback mentioned above. A pixel at a certain site, defined by some major landmarks and a coordinate system in relation to them, would still depict somewhat different parts of the brain for different subjects. However, if the "in between" gap is large enough, this variability will at least be unlikely to intrude on the next adjacent pixel in the correlation matrix. It would be necessary to extend the mapping into three dimensions, but in principle this would be feasible and would permit the delineation of rough functional boundaries between areas that have functional independence from each other.

Once these functional boundaries were established, it would be appropriate to consider the territory within the boundary—perhaps leaving a margin of one or two pixels around the territory just inside the boundary—as a single, functionally discrete area. Metabolic or flow values could then be summed within that area, and the set of such defined areas could become the basic elements of the data matrix.

The most exciting possibility is that the functional systems, thus defined, would reorganize and restructure themselves under different conditions of state or activation. One might expect, furthermore, to discover patterns of functional organization that characterize certain populations and that permit inferences about basic mechanisms at work in those populations. The implications for laterality research are enormous; if there are individual differences in some aspect of lateralization, these should be reflected in different types of functional organization. One would expect, furthermore, that these differences would be amplified and enhanced under conditions of task activation, challenging those particular processes such as language, which are assumed to relate to the underlying dimension of laterality.

Relation to External Factors

The above three features characterize interesting internal relationships, within the set of localized measurements of brain activity, across a group of subjects. The true power of these measurements is finally realized only when these internal analyses are properly related to external factors, as described above. More than anything else, it is the impact of a properly defined behavioral challenge task that offers the greatest gains in the mapping of brain behavior relations, including laterality phenomena. When that impact can be fully described, in terms of its effect on the variety of internal relationships within the data, one can expect large-scale advances in the understanding of brain function.

Not surprisingly, the full-scale, large-group studies advocated above have not been done. Enough has been done, however, partially utilizing many of the specific techniques described, that one can already begin to appreciate the sort of advances that lie in the future. Accordingly, some of these more important initial findings form the basis for the next section of this chapter.

REVIEW OF EXISTING DATA

In surveying the existing literature in such a new field of inquiry, one is tempted to want to inspect almost every single observation that has been made. In the emission tomography literature, this might still be feasible, but the regional cerebral flow literature is now old and stable enough to yield more integrated information from larger, formal groups. It is then more efficient to restrict attention to a handful of studies that meet certain criteria. These are: the use of normal subjects, rather than patients; the use of large enough sample sizes to permit stable, statistical analysis (or to provide replication of earlier studies); and the use of suitable experimental designs, especially those involving well-controlled behavioral activation.

Studies meeting the above criteria do not occur in the emission tomography literature; large enough sample sizes of normals, under carefully controlled conditions of behavioral activation, are not yet available. It is necessary to look to the noninvasive regional cerebral blood flow literature, therefore, with its capability for simultaneous bilateral measurements, for illustrative and informative studies. It is convenient to consider them, first of all, from the point of view of the particular methodologies that they illustrate and thereafter to summarize the contributions that they make to the study of cerebral laterality.

Studies Emphasizing External Data Analysis Factors

The historic first study of laterality of brain activation as a function of modality of tasks was done by Risberg, Halsey, Wills, and Wilson (1975), using 12 right-handed, normal volunteers. Subjects were solving either verbal analogy problems or visual perceptual closure problems under conditions of a substantial monetary reward for accurate performance. Under these conditions, the verbal task resulted in left postcentral flow increases from the resting baseline, whereas the perceptual tasks resulted in right parietal and frontal increases from the resting baseline. An earlier group of 12 subjects, who did not receive the reward, showed only small task-related increases, also tending in the same directions but not attaining statistical significance.

This study is the first to demonstrate lateralized activation according to the verbal versus the visual-spatial nature of the task. The tasks themselves are not particularly well controlled, thus in either task one cannot be sure exactly which aspect of the task (sensory or cognitive, for example) is responsible for the relevant flow increases. This difficulty is somewhat overcome, however, by the reward manipulation. One is able to conclude that the heightened task saliency or extra effort induced by the reward is isolable as the independent variable for the asymmetrical activations observed.

Subsequent laterality studies, attempting experimental control of the activating tasks, can be divided into two types: those controlling the laterality of the stimulus or response and those attempting to control the specifically cognitive component of the task. A recent study by Prohovnik, Risberg, Maximilian, and Hagstadius (1981, pp. 111–138) combined both techniques to yield some important findings. In this study, normal subjects were presented with tactile stimulation in either the left or right hand. The particular stimuli consisted of pressure from one or more elements in a 3 × 3 grid of small pistons resting on the surface of the hand. The experimental task was to monitor the repeatedly occurring stimuli, reporting with a verbal signal whenever the target stimulus occurred. The target was any stimulus that consisted of only one, instead of more than one, piston being pressed at a given time. The control condition consisted of passively receiving the stimuli but with no requirement to monitor and report them.

The design thus permitted blocked trials of left-hand versus right-hand attended stimulation. In this way, direct and well-controlled comparisons could be made between left- versus right-hand stimuli and between passive sensation and active attending.

The results were striking in showing that there was a much greater blood flow increase from resting baseline, under conditions of active attending, as compared with conditions of passive sensation. More striking still, from the point of view of laterality research, were two additional findings: even under conditions of right-hand stimulation and active attending, the right hemisphere showed greater blood flow response and activation than did the left; and the response to actively attended left-hand stimulation, while also marginally greater in the right than the left hemisphere, was strikingly large in both hemispheres—much greater than with actively attended right-hand stimulation.

This double asymmetry (greater right than left hemisphere response to either hand and greater bihemispheric response to the left hand) suggests not only a right hemisphere dominance for tactile pattern perception but also a disproportionately greater role of the right hemisphere in some aspects of lateralized attention. Later, the theoretical significance of this finding will be considered further; in the present context, it is of interest primarily because of its careful use of control conditions to isolate certain features of the task (side of stimulation and requirement for active, attentive pattern discrimination).

Let us now consider an experiment from the present author's work (Wood, Taylor, Penny, & Stump, 1980) illustrating not only a controlled behavioral task but also the use of correlations of flow with task accuracy. Subjects were first auditorally presented with a list of words, each one of which they repeated aloud twice. Later, during the measurement of blood flow, they heard another list of words, half of whose items were from the preceding list. The words were delivered at a rate of 1 every 2.5 seconds. Half the subjects were instructed to signal with their left hands if the word was from the preceding list. This was considered the recognition memory instruction. The other half of the subjects were asked to signal with their left hands if the word was a member or exemplar of a semantic category (in this case concrete nouns depicting objects small enough to fit inside an average living room). The latter instruction was considered to represent a semantic classification task. Both the stimulus and responsive components were identical in the two tasks; only the instruction—recognition memory versus semantic classification—was different. A direct comparison of the conditions, with regard to the blood flow patterns engendered by each, was then possible. The logic does not permit a "pure" isolation of the pattern engendered by a single task, but it does indicate with precision the contrast between the two tasks.

The finding was that the semantic classification task, in contrast with the recognition memory task, generated a left hemisphere flow increase over resting baseline. (This can just as plausibly be interpreted as a flow decrease generated by the recognition memory task. The latter possibility, that a recognition memory task, since it activated subcortical structures, would actually suppress cortical flow, was part of the theory of the experiment.)

Of special interest in this experiment were findings relating to the correlation between task accuracy and flow. The correlations between regional flow and accuracy on the semantic classification task were all positive, although none were significant. The correlations between flow and accuracy on the recognition memory tasks, however, were all negative, and several were highly statistically significant. The areas of especially high, inverse correlations between flow and recognition memory accuracy were the occipital poles bilaterally and the left temporo-occipital area. Thus, the subjects who performed the best on the recognition memory tasks were those whose flows during the tasks were the lowest in these particular posterior areas. Inverse correlations like this have been reported in other studies (Leli, Hannay, Falgout et al., 1982; Scott, Katholi, & Halsey, 1981). These inverse correlations alert us to the possibility that flow increases are not always interpretable as indicative of the activation of structures involved in the successful performance of the task in question. They may, instead, indicate that competing activity has been evoked and unsuccessfully inhibited.

An additional finding in the above experiment, relative to laterality, was that the left angular gyrus region was always higher than its right hemisphere counterpart, in all subjects under the recognition memory condition. This was a highly statistically significant asymmetry. Yet it suggests that, although there was no general hemispheric flow increase under the recognition memory task, there was nevertheless a left-right asymmetry in the angular gyrus region.

Studies Emphasizing Internal Data Analysis Factors

Gur and Reivich (1980) studied blood flow patterns in 36 male college students who were right-handed, with no first degree left-handed relatives. This is easily the largest and most homogeneous sample to be studied and reported in the literature on regional brain activation. It is large enough and homogeneous enough to permit stable, legitimate inferences about internal data analysis factors.

The subjects underwent blood flow measurements in three different conditions, for which ordering was counterbalanced. These conditions were: resting baseline, solving verbal analogies from the Miller Analogies Tests, and solving spatial closure problems on the Gestalt Completion Tests. This design is, therefore, very similar to the original design of Risberg et al. (1975), although it does not employ an explicit monetary reward condition.

The major interest lies in the correlation of means and variances and the impact of the behavioral activations on those correlations. These have been calculated from the results presented in the original Gur and Reivich paper and are summarized in Table 10-1. One wishes that there were more measurement sites, so that the correlations could each represent large Ns. However, despite this limitation the table is quite instructive.

Looking first at the resting baseline, one notes a modest correlation between means and variances when all 16 sites are considered in the correlation. When each hemisphere is considered separately, despite the fact that the correlations then represent only $N = 8$ each, it becomes clear that the two hemispheres are different. The left hemisphere shows a significant correlation, whereas the right does not. By the logic previously discussed, one can then infer that the differences in mean flow among right hemisphere sites are the result of a constraining type of activation process. By contrast, one can infer that the differences among mean flows in the left hemisphere are more the result of a process of disinhibition. This leads to the conclusion that the resting baseline selectively activates certain right hemisphere sites, while leaving the left hemisphere in a more disinhibited status.

This suggestion is supported by an examination of the spatial activation condition and very much resembles the resting baseline, inasmuch as the left hemisphere shows high correlation between means and variances, whereas the right hemisphere does not. The pattern obtained in the resting baseline closely resembles that obtained during a task already known to elicit focal right hemisphere activation. One can only speculate about the particulars of the way in which the resting baseline elicited a constrained mode of focal right hemisphere activation.

The verbal activation, however, tended to elicit relatively high correlations between means and variances in both hemispheres, although the correlation was marginally higher in the right. The expected low correlation in the left hemisphere is not seen, in order to reflect the presence of constrained focal processing there.

It is especially interesting that the conclusions flowing from the analysis of correlation between means and variances are virtually the opposite of those suggested in the analyses of mean hemispheric flow, as originally presented by Gur and Reivich. There had been a statistically significant change, from resting baseline to verbal activation, in a laterality index of hemispheric flow (right mean hemispheric flow – left mean hemispheric flow)/(right mean hemispheric flow + left mean hemispheric flow). No change in this laterality index, from resting baseline to spatial activation, was found. However, the use of such a difference measure (change in the laterality index from resting baseline to activation condition) is legitimate only for inferring differences between the two states; one cannot know from this which state is the "nonactivated" state. It could be that the baseline and spatial condition were both similarly activated. A simple inspection of the hemispheric means in the three conditions shows that, in the resting baseline and in the spatial activation condition, the right hemispheric mean was higher than the left hemispheric mean, whereas the opposite was true during the verbal activation. None of these differences, however, is statistically significant.

TABLE 10-1.
Parameters of the Intercorrelation and Regression of Means to Variances in the Gur and Reivich Study

Condition	Sites	Pearson r	y-Intercept	Slope	Standard error
Resting baseline	Left hemisphere; N = 8	.62	53.43	.054	1.83
	Right hemisphere; N = 8	.19	62.60	.014	1.93
	Both hemispheres; N = 16	.36	56.59	.030	2.04
Verbal activation	Left hemisphere; N = 8	.63	55.26	.111	2.45
	Right hemisphere; N = 8	.71	52.87	.118	2.07
	Both hemispheres; N = 16	.60	55.64	.098	2.27
Spatial activation	Left hemisphere; N = 8	.71	52.98	.117	1.77
	Right hemisphere; N = 8	.23	61.34	.031	2.24
	Both hemispheres; N = 16	.50	57.13	.072	1.98

403

The possibility that the verbal activation condition was the "nonactivated" condition is strongly confirmed by another analysis that Gur and Reivich presented, namely, the correlation of task accuracy with hemispheric flow. Again using the change from resting baseline, they showed a significant correlation between accuracy on the spatial task and change in laterality index from resting baseline to spatial activation. A nonsignificant, almost a zero, correlation was found between accuracy on the verbal task and the increase in laterality from resting baseline to verbal activation.

Another feature to be noted in Table 10-1 is the Y intercept, reflecting the extrapolated mean for a probe site that would be expected when the variance is zero. As can be seen in the table, both the resting baseline and the spatial activation condition show substantially higher Y intercepts in the right hemisphere than in the left. The left hemisphere Y intercepts in both cases, as well as both Y intercepts in the verbal activation condition, are all closely similar and are at a level that may represent something like a physiological minimum, under these conditions, for these subjects. Despite the fact that these Y intercepts appear to conform to the other converging evidence for selective right hemisphere activation of a constrained type, in the resting baseline and the spatial task, at present, it is necessary to be somewhat cautious of this index. First, it is not clear whether or not it can be interpreted as a stable value in a situation where the correlation itself is nonsignificant. Second, even if the Y intercepts are interpreted with the usual confidence bands for inferring significant differences, more experience with the practical or theoretical significance of this index would be needed before strong interpretations of these findings could be made. Nonetheless, it may prove useful to continue to calculate and consider these values in the normal course of data analysis, in both the emission tomography and regional cerebral blood flow techniques.

Studies reporting the entire matrix of intercorrelations among all sites have not been done. Some studies have selectively reported some particular sets of intersite correlations, however, especially those dealing with homologous left and right hemisphere regions. Prohovnik, Hakansson, and Risberg (1980) reported homologous site correlations for 99 measurements made on 22 subjects during a quiet resting baseline. They found the classical, tertiary association areas to be the ones that had the lowest, sometimes nonsignificant, correlations between homologous left and right hemisphere sites. However, sites appearing to represent the classical visual, auditory, tactile, and motor primary projection areas seemed to be those with the highest cross-hemispheric correlations. The authors interpreted this finding to suggest that, even in rest, lateral asymmetries in hemispheric activity would occur only in those areas specialized for higher, cognitive types of analyses.

This study has the considerable difficulty that individual subjects were measured between four and eight different times, with each measurement being entered as a separate case in the correlational analysis. This greatly complicates the interpretation of the findings; intersubject variance is confounded with intrasubject variance, and some individual subjects contribute more to the variance, by virtue of their greater number of measurements than do other subjects. The intrasubject variance is itself a major focus of the study, for example, in the demonstration that flows decrease generally but especially in the frontal areas from the first to the second baseline measurement. Given that the interpretation is exceedingly complex, the finding of lower interhemispheric correlations in the tertiary association areas cannot be generalized to a single measurement situation. Nonetheless, from the point of view of the investigation of cerebral laterality, the study has important heuristic value in suggesting that the factors that produce intrasubject as well as intersubject variance in resting baseline flows have unilateral impact primarily in the tertiary, not the primary processing areas.

There are no studies as yet analyzing the distributions of flow values at given sites in large samples. Maximilian, Prohovnik, Risberg, and Hakansson (1980) did report individual subject values for mean left hemispheric flow in their experiment on word learning and recall. If these values are plotted, it becomes apparent by inspection that, on both occasions when the subjects were actively recalling prior material, there was a distinct bimodality of hemispheric flows; subjects clustered either in a range of flow gray values in the 60s and low 70s or else in the 90s or 100s. One is tempted to suspect that the subjects with the higher flow may have been those who performed less well (Wood et al., 1980), but the more interesting question is whether or not this might reflect a typology of subjects or of strategies selected by subjects.

As is evident from the above two studies, which represent the best examples of analyses of correlations and distributions, much more can be done in future studies using these types of analyses. The existing studies only give hints of the contributions that could be made to the study of cerebral laterality.

Summary of Major Findings in Cerebral Laterality

The above studies are certainly not the only ones to have made important contributions to the understanding of cerebral laterality. While they are among the best examples of certain features of design and data analysis, there is more that can be inferred about the general state of brain activation studies of cerebral lateral asymmetries. Having already considered in detail some of the methodological issues, this section will summarize more concisely some of the major emerging trends in the literature.

Hyperfrontality

The original observations of this phenomenon are due to Ingvar (1976), who later reviewed the question (Ingvar, 1979) and concluded that the phenomenon represented "inner anticipatory programming." The ordinary resting hyperfrontality of flow is also seen in most states of activation, although in an important study by Risberg, Maximilian, and Prohovnik (1977), it was shown that the frontal component of task activation (solving Raven's matrixes) habituated upon a repeat execution of the tasks, using parallel forms on a second day. See the general review by Risberg (1980) for a discussion of other aspects of hyperfrontality, including pharmacological influences.

The implications of hyperfrontality for the study of laterality are considered by Prohovnik, Hakansson, and Risberg (1980), leading to the suggestion that the commonly seen hyperfrontality within a given hemisphere represents a control process that is specific to the specialized functions (verbal or visual-spatial) of that particular hemisphere. It can be expected that future studies, using careful design and analysis, may well be able to isolate a specifically frontal component of hemispheric functioning, a component that apparently has similarities to our notions of attention, set, anticipation, or similar control processes.

Negative Correlations with Task Accuracy

The first study to demonstrate this phenomenon was that of Wood et al., (1980), described above. More recently, Leli et al. (1982) have shown a similar phenomenon. In their study, subjects were shown slides of lateral body parts and asked to identify them as right or left. The task generated a bilateral parietal occipital increase in flow, relative to control conditions, but in the left hemisphere, this increase was strongly inversely correlated with task accuracy. The authors proposed that this might reflect the beneficial effects on visual-spatial performance of suppression of left hemisphere activity (Ray, Newcombe, Semon, & Cole, 1981).

While a variety of other explanations for the observed inverse correlations between task accuracy and flow must be considered, the general issue promises to add a new dimension to the studies of cerebral laterality. When excitation in one region can be contrasted with suppression in another, it is possible to have considerably more confidence in the understanding of the functional interrelationship among various brain structures involved in active cognitive processing.

Relative Difficulty of Showing Focal Left Hemisphere Activation in Verbal Tasks

Such activation tends to elicit small increases (Wood et al., 1980); to be difficult to distinguish from nonverbal tonal activation (Knopman, Rubens, Klassen et al., 1980); to show higher variances as well as means in the apparently focally activated sites, thus suggesting disinhibition (see especially Knopman et al., 1980, and Gur & Reivich, 1980); or to require high monetary reward to bring out a distinct effect (Risberg et al., 1975). There seems to be no doubt that verbal activation can generate left hemisphere flow increases, particularly in the temporal and frontotemporal areas. It is far from clear, however, what the specific ingredients of that verbal task activation are and how those ingredients may differ across subjects. It certainly appears that, when the verbal task is "easy" or somehow automatized, activation is difficult to observe, and there may be differences among subjects in the degree to which they confront such tasks in an automatized way. Therefore, the resolution of the considerable uncertainties surrounding verbal activation cannot be accomplished by single case studies or by small groups of subjects. Careful and reasonably extensive studies, permitting isolation of several different independent variables (especially task difficulty as distinguished from speed), correlation with subject variables, and various types of internal data analysis, are required.

Lateral Asymmetries in the Effects of Unilateral Stimuli or Responses

Halsey, Blauenstein, Wilson, and Wills (1979, 1980) have shown, in normal right-handed males, that left hand repetitive movement elicits substantially greater contralateral hemispheric activation than does right-handed movement. A further analysis of right- and left-handers, with inverted and noninverted posture, led to the conclusion that the greatest contralateral activation by a motor task occurs when the nonpreferred hand is used, contralateral to the nonspeech-dominant hemisphere. Hence, an interaction can be hypothesized between handedness and speech dominance in determining the apparent "difficulty" and consequent highest flow activation engendered by unilateral motor activity.

Similar or related phenomena seemed to have occurred on the sensory side, both tactile (Prohovnik et al., 1981) and auditory (Maximilian, 1980, pp. 103–121). The tactile study has been discussed in detail above, showing the greater flow increases, both bilateral and especially right hemispheric, under actively attended left- rather than right-hand tactile stimulation. The auditory study required active attention to linguistic features of words, presented monaurally either to the left or right ear. Both conditions resulted in unilateral, focal left temporoparietal flow increases. However, the activated left temporoparietal region was larger under left ear stimulation than it was under right ear stimulation. Moreover, there was a significant frontotemporal flow increase in the contralateral hemisphere, with only conditions of left but not right ear stimulation.

Sensory and motor studies of this type suggest that cerebral lateral asymmetries occur, in some form at least, with respect to lateralized, relatively simple sensory and motor processes. Here, as in the inverse correlation studies described above, greater activation is apparently a signal of greater difficulty in executing the task.

Lateralized Attentional Phenomena

The Prohovnik et al. (1981) study on lateralized tactile stimulation purports to show a greater role of the right hemisphere in certain attentional mechanisms. The study permits this conclusion only with respect to attention to spatial features and does not support the broader proposals that have been made for a right hemisphere role in generalized attention (Heilman & Van Den Abell, 1980). Clarification of this fact has recently been provided by an important study by Harter (1982), showing great evoked potentials over the right hemisphere under conditions of attention to the location of a stimulus but greater evoked potentials over the left hemisphere under conditions of attention to intralocation features of the stimulus (such as color).

What the current literature does suggest, then, is that different components of attention may be isolable and differentially referable to the two hemispheres. Naturally, that requires careful experimental design to isolate only the attentional ingredient. Brain activation studies in this particular area could well emulate the extremely careful design of the Harter study (1982).

This brief review ends where it began in considering the issue of hyperfrontality, namely, on the subject of possible lateralized components of attention. It is fair to say that the most impressive prospects for immediate progress in understanding of cerebral lateral asymmetries, at least by the brain activation methods considered in this chapter, lie in this area of specification of component processes of attention.

SUMMARY AND CONCLUSIONS

The advent of new technologies for studying localized brain activation, in response to specific behavioral processes, requires careful reconsideration and specification of a variety of methodological criteria that should attend such research. Some, but certainly not all, of these methodological issues have been reviewed in this chapter and illustrated by studies extant in the literature.

Some emerging contributions to the understanding of cerebral laterality have been identified, and the most immediately promising of these may well be in the area of attentional processes. While only regional cerebral blood flow studies have been reviewed, because of their greater number of subjects and suitable experimental designs, it can be stated that many of the conclusions drawn from that review are also indicated in the extant single case and small group studies of normals that have been reported, using the emission tomography technique. Thus, it should be the case that fundamental new progress in the understanding of cerebral lateral asymmetries in the normal human brain should be aided by the new techniques that are now available.

REFERENCES

Gur R.C., & Reivich, M. Cognitive task effects on hemispheric blood flow in humans: Evidence for individual differences in hemispheric activation. *Brain and Language*, 1980, *9*, 78–92.

Halsey J.H., Blauenstein U.W., Wilson E.M., & Wills, E.L. Regional cerebral blood flow comparison of right and left hand movement. *Neurology*, 1979, *29*, 21–28.

Halsey J.H., Blauenstein U.W., Wilson E.M., & Wills, E.L. Brain activation in the presence of brain damage. *Brain and Language*, 1980, *9*, 47–60.

Harter R. Lateralized asymmetries in event-related potentials as a function of attention to inter-location versus intra-location cues. *Neuropsychologia*, 1982.

Hebb, D. *The Organization of behavior*, New York: Harper, Row, & World, 1949.

Heilman K., & Van Den Abel T. Right hemispheric dominance for attention: The mechanisms underlying hemispheric asymmetries of inattention (neglect). *Neurology*, 1980, *30*, 327–330.

Knopman D.S., Rubens A.B., Klassen A.C. et al. Regional cerebral blood flow patterns during verbal and nonverbal auditory activation. *Brain and Language*, 1980, *9*, 93–112.

Leli D.A., Hannay M.J., Falgout J.C. et al. Focal changes in cerebral blood flow produced by a test of right-left discrimination. *Brain and Cognition*, 1982.

Maximilan V., Cortical blood flow asymmetries during monaural verbal stimulation. In Maximilian, V. (Ed.), *Functional changes in the cortex during mental activation: Application of regional cerebral blood flow measurements in neuropsychological research*. Lund, Sweden: University of Lund and CWK Gleerup, 1980.

Maximilian V.A., Prohovnik I., Risberg J., & Hakansson K. Regional blood flow changes in the left cerebral hemisphere during word pair learning and recall. *Brain and Language*, 1980, *6*, 22–31.

Prohovnik I., Hakansson K., & Risberg J. Observations on the functional significance of regional cerebral blood flow in "resting" normal subjects. *Neuropsychology*, 1980, *18*, 203–217.

Prohovnik I., Risberg J., Maximilian V., & Hagstadius S. Regional cortical activity during perception: Lateralized tactile sensation and attention. In Prohovnik I. (Ed.), *Mapping brainwork: Theoretical and methodological considerations in applying the regional cerebral blood flow method to neuropsychology*. Lund, Sweden: University of Lund and CWK Gleerup, 1981.

Risberg J. Regional cerebral blood flow measurements by Xe-inhalation: Methodology and applications in neuropsychology and applications in neuropsychology and psychiatry. *Brain and Language*, 1980, *9*, 9–34.

Risberg J., Halsey J.H., Wills E.L., & Wilson B.M. Hemispheric specialization in normal man studied by bilateral measurements of the regional cerebral blood flow. *Brain*, 1975, *98*, 511–524.

Wood F. Theoretical, methodological, and statistical implications of the inhalation rCBF technique for the study of brain-behavior relationships. *Brain and Language*, 1980, *9*, 1–8.

Wood F., Taylor B., Penny R., & Stump D. Regional cerebral blood flow response to recognition memory versus semantic classification tasks. *Brain and Language*, 1980, *9*, 112–113.

11

Hemisphere × Task Interaction and the Study of Laterality

Joseph B. Hellige

The present volume is a testimonial to the fact that a wide variety of research techniques is used to make inferences about cerebral hemisphere asymmetry. Each of these techniques is capable of providing useful information about hemispheric asymmetry. However, for each of the techniques or experimental paradigms, many factors can influence the magnitude and even the direction of observed, behavioral laterality. It is, therefore, difficult to sort out the contributing factors so that effects caused by cerebral hemisphere asymmetry can be distinguished from behavioral laterality effects caused by other factors. Furthermore, the precise way in which cerebral laterality determines behavioral laterality is a matter of some debate. As a consequence, the present chapter argues that investigation of the interaction of right versus left hemisphere with various task variables is often necessary for studying cerebral laterality. The first section of this chapter illustrates some of the ways in which the investigation of such Hemisphere × Task interactions is important by reviewing examples from several experimental paradigms.

When examining the interaction of two or more variables, it is necessary to consider issues related to the interpretability of interaction effects, especially issues surrounding the choice of an appropriate measure of behavior (i.e., dependent variable). Therefore, the second section of the chapter considers the kinds of interactions that are and are not interpretable, depending upon the assumptions one is willing to make about the precise relationship of the theoretical construct to be measured and the dependent variable that is actually observed. From this discussion emerge several suggestions about the interpretation of laterality experiments, including experiments that examine individual differences in the degree of hemispheric asymmetry.

The choice of an appropriate dependent variable in laterality research has been discussed by others who consider the merits of various "laterality indexes." The third section of this chapter discusses the relationship between the notions presented here and the concept of computing an appropriate laterality index. It will be seen that many of the same considerations that motivate the present discussion about interpretability of interactions have motivated computation of laterality indexes. Therefore, certain suggestions made here will be compared with various laterality indexes. This section will also consider the relative merits of computing an index of hemispheric difference versus preserving measures of both left and right hemisphere performance under a range of experimental conditions.

The final section of the chapter discusses the fact that it is possible to have agreement about the existence of a Hemisphere × Task interaction (in a statistical or measurement sense) but to have considerable disagreement about the best interpretation of the interaction. Accordingly, several factors related to the theoretical interpretation of laterality effects will be discussed. It is proposed that more emphasis should be given to incorporating cerebral laterality into more general theories of cognition and information processing than to formulating theories of cerebral laterality per se.

IMPORTANCE OF HEMISPHERE × TASK INTERACTION

An interaction of two variables is said to occur when the effect of one variable is not the same at all levels of the second variable. For example, in laterality research, a Hemisphere × Task interaction occurs whenever the difference between right and left hemisphere performance is not the same for all of the task conditions employed. Viewed another way, a Hemisphere × Task interaction occurs whenever the differences between task conditions are not the same for both hemispheres. For methodological and statistical purposes, it is desirable to obtain measures of performance for both hemispheres in each of the task conditions within a single factorial experiment, so that the reliability of the Hemisphere × Task interaction can be assessed more readily. However, on a conceptual level, it does not matter whether all of the task conditions are contained in a single factorial experiment or whether the hemisphere difference is compared across different experiments, with each experiment using a different task. For purposes of the present discussion, therefore, the term *Hemisphere × Task interaction pattern* refers to both single and multiple experiment research in which the goal is to consider the extent to which hemisphere differences change with variations in the task.

The whole notion of two cerebral hemispheres that are somehow asymmetrical in function requires the study of Hemisphere × Task interaction. As the following review of research indicates, the study of such interactions serves certain control functions as well as providing tests of theories about hemispheric asymmetry. It is probably impossible to separate these two functions. Perhaps the example most familiar to neuroscientists is the importance of "double dissociation" for making inferences about localization of function from studies of brain-damaged individuals (e.g., Teuber, 1955; 1964).

Suppose the goal of a study with brain-damaged patients is to test the hypothesis that performance of a specific task, A_1, depends upon the left cerebral hemisphere (but not on the right). In order to demonstrate this, some investigators would argue that it is necessary to demonstrate a double dissociation between hemisphere and task. Such double dissociation represents a particular type of Hemisphere × Task interaction and simultaneously serves both control functions and theoretical functions. Figure 11-1 plots an idealized representation of a double dissociation that would support the above hypothesis. For simplicity, only two levels of performance are considered, that is, performance on a task is simply classified as normal or impaired. For Task A_1, performance is impaired after left hemisphere damage but not after right hemisphere damage. Such a result is consistent with the above hypothesis, but it is also consistent with other hypotheses. For example, perhaps left hemisphere damage disrupts behavioral performance in general rather than specifically disrupting Task A_1. This possibility can be eliminated by showing that performance on some other task, A_2, is impaired by damage to the right cerebral hemisphere (but not the left). It is this particular form of Hemisphere × Task interaction in brain-damage studies that constitutes the prototypical double dissociation.

Hemisphere × Task interaction patterns can be extremely informative in separating effects of cerebral hemisphere asymmetry from behavioral laterality effects produced by other factors. This has been especially important in research with neurologically normal individuals, in whom both perceptual laterality and lateralized response effects are determined by a variety of cortical and peripheral factors. For example, it has been recognized for some time that many factors can influence the magnitude and direction of visual half-field differences in a visual laterality experiment. Therefore, if visual half-field asymmetry is to be useful as a tool for studying cerebral hemisphere asymmetry, it is necessary to sort out the contributions of the various factors. Although the visual half-field difference within any particular experimental

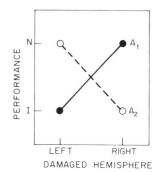

Figure 11-1. *Idealized representation of double disso-ciation. N and I refer to normal and impaired per-formance, respectively. See text for explanation.*

condition may represent the contribution of many factors, the various factors often make conflicting predictions about Visual Field (Hemisphere) × Task interactions. As a consequence, the study of such interactions is necessary to separate the effects of the various factors. It is instructive to briefly consider how cerebral laterality effects might be separated from two other factors known to influence visual half-field effects: peripheral visual pathway asymmetries and postexposure scanning biases.

There is anatomical and physiological evidence that the crossed visual pathways dominate the uncrossed visual pathways (see White, 1969, for a review). At least under conditions of monocular viewing, this peripheral pathway asymmetry may contribute to visual half-field differences. Even under binocular viewing conditions, peripheral pathway asymmetry, combined with dominance of one eye, may influence visual half-field differences (e.g., Hayashi & Bryden, 1967; Wyke & Ettlinger, 1961). However, there is little reason to think that effects caused by peripheral pathway asymmetry should change with the nature of the experimental task. This is especially true if the same physical stimuli (e.g., letters) are used for each of two or more tasks with different processing requirements. As a result, Visual Field × Task interac-tions are very difficult to account for by peripheral factors and are, therefore, more informative about hemispheric asymmetry than are the simple visual field effects within each task considered in isolation.

Another variable known to influence visual half-field differences is the postexposure scanning bias of the observers (see White, 1969). For English-speaking observers, early visual laterality experiments reported a right visual field word recognition advantage with unilateral presentation of a single word and a left visual field word recognition advantage when two words were presented simultaneously, one to each visual field (bilateral presentation). The opposite pattern of results was reported for Hebrew words (which are scanned from right to left) presented to Hebrew speakers. As White (1969) points out, the Visual Field × Unilateral versus Bilateral interaction for each language group is consistent with the hypothesis that observers are biased to scan the postexposure visual trace in the same direction in which they typically read. In contrast, left hemisphere specialization for verbal processing would predict a right visual field (left hemisphere) advantage, presumably of the same magnitude, for all of these conditions.

Rather than abandoning visual half-field studies of hemispheric asymmetry, investigators attempted to discover if certain parameters of visual presentation could reduce the contribution of scanning biases. Since White's (1969) review, many experiments have found a right visual field advantage in all of the conditions listed above when the stimulus duration is sufficiently short to prevent shifts in eye fixation, when there is adequate control for eye fixation (see McKeever, 1974; White, 1972), and even when the letters within a word are arranged vertically rather than horizontally (e.g., Turner & Miller, 1975). Note that the discovery of the optimal parameters of visual presentation required examination of several Visual Field (Hemisphere) × Task interaction patterns.

A variety of factors can also influence observed laterality effects in other experimental paradigms, as evidenced by most of the contributions to this volume. As in the preceding examples, separating the contributions of the factors relies heavily upon the study of interaction patterns. In some cases, it is even concluded that only certain Hemisphere × Task interactions provide evidence about cerebral hemisphere asymmetry. For example, several authors have discussed the importance of various control procedures in studies of asymmetry of the electrophysiological activity measured from the left and right sides of the scalp (e.g., Donchin, Kutas, & McCarthy, 1977; Gevins, this volume). Slight asymmetries in such things as electrode placement and skull thickness can influence the measured response asymmetry and can lead to inappropriate conclusions about hemispheric asymmetry. Accordingly, Donchin et al. (1977) argue that it is necessary to use at least two experimental tasks for each subject, with exactly the same electrode placement, and to demonstrate that the response asymmetry is not the same for both tasks; that is, only Side of Scalp (Hemisphere) × Task interactions are informative.

Thus far, the examples have emphasized the importance of focusing on Hemisphere × Task interactions to control for various determinants of measured laterality that have nothing to do with hemispheric asymmetry. The examination of these interactions is equally necessary for testing theoretical predictions related to cerebral laterality. As an example, consider various tests of Kimura's (1966) direct-access model of perceptual asymmetry versus Kinsbourne's (1970, 1973, 1975) attention gradient model.

According to the direct-access model, performance on a task will be better when the stimuli are presented directly to the cerebral hemisphere that is most efficient for the task than when the stimuli are presented to the less efficient hemisphere. Consequently, right ear and right visual field advantages for verbal tasks are thought to occur because right-side stimuli project directly to the left hemisphere, which has been thought to be specialized for verbal processing. Likewise, left ear and left visual field advantages are thought to occur for certain nonverbal tasks because left-side stimuli project directly to the right hemisphere, which has been thought to be specialized for certain nonverbal, perceptual functions.

According to the attention gradient model, perceptual laterality depends upon the balance of activation between the two hemispheres at the time when a stimulus is presented and not on the directness of the pathway to a specialized hemisphere. The fundamental notion is that asymmetric activation of the two hemispheres produces a gradient of attention across the body field, with attention being most easily directed toward locations in space contralateral to the more activated hemisphere. Right-side advantages are predicted for tasks that demand greater left than right hemisphere involvement (e.g., verbal tasks) because the ongoing processing activates the left more than the right hemisphere, thereby biasing attention to the right side of space. An analogous argument is advanced to explain left-side advantages when the task activates the right more than the left hemisphere.

Note that the direct access and attention gradient models, even in their original formulations, make many identical predictions. In order to differentiate between them, it is necessary to create conditions for which the two models make different predictions. One approach originally taken by Kinsbourne was to specify certain Hemisphere × Task interactions that were predicted by the attention gradient model but not by the direct access model. A complete review of the many experiments directed at distinguishing these models and the current status of the controversy is beyond the scope of this chapter (but see Hardyck's chapter in this volume; Bolles, 1979; Friedman & Polson, 1981; Hellige & Cox, 1976; Hellige, Cox, & Litvac, 1979; Moscovitch & Klein, 1980). However, the following examples should suffice to illustrate the importance of examining appropriate interaction patterns when trying to distinguish the models.

Many tests of the attention gradient model have been similar in logic to an experiment by Bruce and Kinsbourne (1974). They had observers attempt to recognize complex polygons presented to the right or left visual field and found a small, nonsignificant left visual field (right hemisphere) advantage when the task was performed alone. However, when observers were given a list of words to hold in memory during each polygon recognition trial, a significant right visual field (left hemisphere) advantage was obtained.

According to Kinsbourne, holding words in short-term memory activates the left more than the right hemisphere, biasing attention toward the right side of space. Because neither the underlying hemispheric asymmetry nor the structural connections between retina and hemisphere changed with imposition of a verbal memory load, the direct access model was seen to have difficulty with such Hemisphere × Concurrent Load interactions.

The attention gradient model also predicts that, when verbal and nonverbal stimuli are randomly intermixed, the same visual field advantage should be found for both stimulus types. This is because it is not possible in the randomly mixed condition to be selectively set for one type of stimulus or the other, that is, to selectively activate one hemisphere. Some experiments have demonstrated this effect (e.g., Cohen, 1975), others have not (e.g., Geffen, Bradshaw, & Nettleton, 1972), and still others find that randomly mixing verbal and nonverbal stimuli causes the laterality patterns for the two types of stimuli to become more similar but not identical (e.g., Dee & Fontenot, 1973; Hellige, 1978).

Unfortunately, neither the concurrent load studies nor the random mixing studies have produced unequivocal results (see the papers cited earlier for discussion of this fact). For example, the effect of a concurrent verbal memory load depends upon such things as the difficulty of the memory task, the level of processing required by the perceptual laterality task, and the amount of practice the observers are given on the task (e.g., Hellige et al., 1979). Furthermore, both the direct access and attention gradient models have been modified to accommodate many of the Hemisphere × Task interactions that once served to distinguish between them (e.g., Moscovitch & Klein, 1980). Consequently, it has become very difficult to provide empirical tests of these models.

Many other theoretical conclusions have also been based on Hemisphere × Task interaction patterns. Consider the following examples from visual laterality studies. Several studies have attempted to determine whether there is a relationship between hemispheric asymmetry and serial versus parallel processing by examining the manner in which reaction time to different numbers of stimuli interact with the visual field to which the stimuli are presented (e.g., Cohen, 1973; Polich, 1980). Sergent (1982a) concludes that features in faces are scanned by the left hemisphere serially from top to bottom while features are processed in their order of perceptual salience by the right hemisphere. This conclusion is based upon an appropriate Visual Field (Hemisphere) × Location of Critical Feature interaction, with reaction time as the dependent variable. On a different topic, Hellige (1980, in press) argues that reductions of perceptual quality shift visual field differences toward a left visual field–right hemisphere advantage, based upon Visual Field (Hemisphere) × Perceptual Quality interactions from a variety of experiments, using both response accuracy and response latency as measures of performance.

A slightly different way in which interactions have become very important is in the study of individual differences in the direction and magnitude of hemispheric asymmetry. When one asks whether an individual (or population of individuals) is differently lateralized for a task than is another individual (or population), one is asking whether or not there is a reliable Hemisphere ✕ Individual (Population) interaction for the task of interest. Although some of this research has involved computation of various transformations of left-right difference scores (i.e., laterality indexes), it is instructive to recognize that, on a logical level, it is a Hemisphere ✕ Population interaction that is in question. In one sense, then, there is nothing particularly special about the study of population differences; the same reliance on various interactions is found as when various tasks (rather than populations) are examined, and the same concerns about the interpretability of interactions apply.

INTERPRETABILITY OF INTERACTION PATTERNS

The previous section of this chapter has pointed out several ways in which contemporary laterality research depends upon the examination of Hemisphere ✕ Task interactions. Consequently, it is important to consider several issues related to the interpretability of interaction patterns. This topic has been discussed in a variety of contexts within psychology, including statistics and design textbooks (e.g., Winer, 1971) and the literature on such varied topics as measurement (e.g., Krantz, Luce, Suppes, & Tversky, 1971), human memory (e.g., Loftus, 1978; Postman, 1976; Underwood, 1964), and child development (e.g., Lawrence, Kee, & Hellige, 1980). The purpose of the present section is to consider the types of interaction patterns that are and are not interpretable, depending upon the assumptions that are made about the relationship of the theoretical construct to be measured and the dependent variable that is actually observed. This is done with a view toward developing guidelines for the design and interpretation of laterality research. First, an illustration of some of the problems involved in trying to interpret interactions.

Potential Problems of Interpretation

The primary purpose of experimentation dealing with cerebral hemisphere asymmetry is to test various hypotheses, models, theories, and so forth, that is, various conceptualizations about cerebral hemisphere asymmetry and its role in human information processing. Often, the conceptualizations do not dictate exactly what the measure of behavior (i.e., the dependent variable) must be. Rather, predictions are generated on a conceptual level and a dependent variable, such as percentage of correct responses or reaction time, is chosen for convenience or from habit. To illustrate this, consider the following hypothetical experiment.

Suppose an investigator hypothesizes, based upon some sort of conceptualization, that the left hemisphere is more specialized for the recognition of one set of stimuli (call it set A_1) than for the recognition of another set of stimuli (call it set A_2). What the investigator would most like to do would be to observe directly the subject's perception of both stimulus types, A_1 and A_2, after they have been presented to each of the two hemispheres, perhaps in a visual laterality experiment. Figure 11-2 shows a result that would be consistent with the experimenter's hypothesis and plots the subjects' perception (arbitrarily referred to as Perceptual Strength) for each of the two hemispheres of presentation. The parameter is the set of stimuli, condition A_1 versus condition A_2. For both conditions, the Perceptual Strength is higher for left hemisphere presentation than for right hemisphere presentation. However, as hypothesized, the left hemisphere advantage is larger for condition A_1 than for condition A_2.

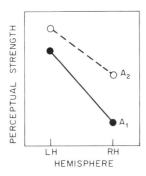

Figure 11-2. *Perceptual Strength in each of the two hemispheres for stimulus sets A_1 and A_2. LH and RH refer to left hemisphere and right hemisphere presentation, respectively.*

The experimenter encounters something of a problem insofar as the subjects's perception (what we have called Perceptual Strength) is not empirically observable. Therefore, in conducting the experiment, an observable dependent variable must be chosen that is related to Perceptual Strength. For the sake of example, suppose the experimenter chooses the probability of a correct response for each stimulus type presented to each hemisphere. Such a dependent variable seems reasonable because there is likely to be at least a monotonic relationship between Perceptual Strength and Probability Correct.

That is, as Perceptual Strength increases, it should lead only to increases in Probability Correct. However, it is important to keep in mind that the conceptual hypothesis involves a prediction about Perceptual Strength and that Probability Correct is simply a convenient empirical measure.

The left-most panels of Figure 11-3 plot a hypothetical outcome of an experiment to test the prediction. Probability Correct is plotted as a function of hemisphere of presentation for both conditions, A_1 and A_2. In terms of Probability Correct, the left hemisphere advantage is larger for condition A_1 than for condition A_2. The form of the interaction is identical to that in Figure 11-2. Assume that the interaction shown in Figure 11-3 is reliable, that is, either there is no error variability or the interaction is statistically significant by some appropriate test (e.g., analysis of variance or planned comparison). Does this result necessarily support the researcher's hypothesis? As one might imagine, if the answer were "yes," this chapter would be considerably shorter than it is.

One might well ask whether there are ceiling or floor effects in these results that becloud interpretation of the interaction. For example, left hemisphere performance appears very near perfect for condition A_2; perhaps if there were more room for improvement, the left hemisphere advantage would be as large for condition A_2 as for condition A_1. It is not too difficult to imagine two conditions in which the strength of the subject's perception (i.e., what we are calling Perceptual Strength) is not equal but for which even the lower Perceptual Strength value is sufficient to permit the Probability Correct to be equal to 1.0. It is this possibility that makes a ceiling effect difficult to interpret. In a similar manner, right hemisphere performance in condition A_1 is close to a Probability Correct of zero, and may reflect a floor effect. Attempts to interpret interactions in the presence of a ceiling or floor effect have created problems in past laterality research and were largely responsible for discussion of laterality indexes, a topic that will be discussed later.

Even if it is assumed that the interaction shown in the left-most panels of Figure 11-3 is not the result of ceiling or floor effects, there are still problems of interpretation. Recall that the conceptual hypothesis deals with what has been called Perceptual Strength (e.g., see Figure 11-2). Whether the interaction shown in the left-most panel of Figure 11-3, using Probability Correct as the dependent variable, is preserved at the level of Perceptual Strength depends upon the precise relationship between Probability Correct and Perceptual Strength. For example, if Probability Correct is a linear function of Perceptual Strength, the observed interaction will be preserved for Perceptual Strength. However, there are many plausible monotonic relationships between Probability Correct and Perceptual Strength that do not preserve the interaction. Two examples of this are illustrated in Figure 11-3.

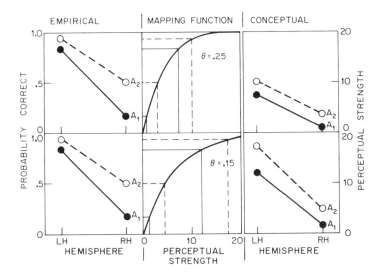

Figure 11-3. *The left-most panels plot Probability Correct as a function of left (LH) versus right (RH) hemisphere of presentation for two stimulus sets, A₁ and A₂. These are hypothetical results from an experiment described in the text. The middle panels plot Probability Correct as a function of the conceptual mechanism of interest, Perceptual Strength. The right-most panels plot Perceptual Strength as a function of left (LH) versus right (RH) hemisphere of presentation for the two stimulus sets, A₁ and A₂. The results in these right-most panels use the mapping functions shown in the middle panels to transform the Probability Correct results shown in the left-most panels into the appropriate results, in terms of Perceptual Strength.*

The middle panels of Figure 11-3 show two hypothetical functions for mapping between the unobservable Perceptual Strength and Probability Correct. In both cases, Probability Correct is a negatively accelerated function of Perceptual Strength, that is,

$$\text{Probability Correct} = 1.0 - e^{-\theta(\text{Perceptual Strength})}$$

The values on the Perceptual Strength scale were chosen arbitrarily, and θ is the rate parameter that determines how quickly the function rises toward a Probability Correct of 1.0. The general form of these negatively accelerated functions is such that equal increments in Perceptual Strength produce successively smaller changes in Probability Correct as Perceptual Strength becomes larger. The two middle panels of Figure 11-3 differ only with respect to the value of θ. It is possible to use the two hypothetical mapping functions shown in Figure 11-3 to indicate what the observed interaction using Probability Correct (shown in the left-most panel) indicates about the interaction in terms of Perceptual Strength (shown in the right-most panel).

Consider first the upper panels of Figure 11-3. The observed results indicate a greater left hemisphere advantage for condition A_1 than for condition A_2. If the mapping function is actually that shown in the middle panel, there is virtually no Hemisphere $\times$ Condition interaction in terms of Perceptual Strength. The situation can be even more serious, as shown in the three lower panels. With a slightly different mapping function, the observed interaction in the left panel produces a very different interaction in terms of Perceptual Strength, that is, in terms of Perceptual Strength, the left hemisphere advantage is larger for condition A_2 than for condition A_1, exactly the opposite of the experimenter's hypothesis.

The examples shown in Figure 11-3 illustrate that the interpretation of interactions can depend upon the precise relationship between the theoretical construct to be measured (e.g., Perceptual Strength) and the dependent variable observed (e.g., Probability Correct). Put another way, some interactions can be made to disappear or even reverse by monotonic rescaling of the dependent variable (e.g., Krantz et al., 1971; Loftus, 1978). If there are theoretical reasons why the dependent variable should not be rescaled, the problems of interpretation are not so great. However, it is often the case in laterality research that the dependent variable is chosen more for convenience than for theoretical reasons, and specific scale properties are unknown.

Although the example discussed was originally formulated in terms of two stimulus sets, it is worth noting that conditions A_1 and A_2 could just as easily refer to other variables, including population variables of the sort examined in studies of individual differences. That is, suppose that the investigator predicted that population A_1 was more lateralized for a task than population A_2. Exactly the same concerns about mapping functions, scaling, and so forth apply. This is particularly important because many of the Hemisphere $\times$ Population interactions reported in the literature are similar in form to that shown in the left-most panels of Figure 11-3 (e.g., see Chapters by Pirozzolo, Rayner, & Hynd and by Levy, this volume).

Dealing with the Problems

There are two general ways of dealing with problems of interpreting interaction patterns. The optimal strategy is to use dependent variables that are linear transformations of the unobservable, theoretical processes of interest. In such cases, all interaction patterns are interpretable, in a measurement sense. The other strategy is to take advantage of the fact that certain interaction patterns cannot be made to disappear by any monotonic rescaling of the dependent variable. That is, some interaction patterns will retain their form for any monotonic mapping function that relates the dependent variable to the theoretical construct to be measured. By separating interpretable from uninterpretable interaction patterns, it is possible to offer guidelines for interpretation, given only minimal assumptions about the dependent variable. Each of these two strategies will be considered in turn.

Theory-based Dependent Variables

There are cases in which a theory or theoretical framework dictates the use of a particular dependent variable. One example in the psychological literature is the Theory of Signal Detectability (see Massaro, 1975; Swets, Tanner, & Birdsall, 1961). A detailed review of the theory is beyond the scope of this chapter, but it is instructive to note that the theory proposes that each response given by an observer in a stimulus detection experiment is determined partially by the output of the observer's sensory system and partially by decision processes (e.g., response biases). Accordingly, the theory predicts that certain measures (e.g., d' and certain nonparametric analogs) will reflect the output of the sensory system, whereas other measures (e.g., Beta and certain nonparametric analogs) reflect the operations of the decision system. Other predictions involve such things as the exact shape of what is referred to as the receiver operating characteristic.

There are occasional examples of laterality research using measures derived from signal detection theory (e.g., Bryden, 1976; Gardner & Branski, 1976; Zaidel, this volume). The use of specific dependent variables in these studies has been justified by pointing to the need for separating response bias from other psychological processes and to the Theory of Signal Detectability as providing an appropriate way in which to make this distinction. Because certain dependent variables are required by the theory that is being used as a frame of reference, it would be inappropriate to do transformations. However, if the theory is grossly in error or is not applicable to the task being used, then measures such as d' and Beta are as arbitrary as other potential dependent variables.

Another example of a particular dependent variable dictated by a theoretical framework is the use of reaction time (RT) in studies of short-term memory scanning. Sternberg (1969, 1975) provides a theoretical framework in which RT, as a dependent variable, is assumed to be a linear function of processing time as a theoretical component. He argues that transformations of RT in tests of his theory (or in experiments to be interpreted within the framework of his theory) are not appropriate. Instead, interpretations of interactions and additivity are to be based directly upon RT as the dependent variable. Visual laterality experiments have recently had some success separating stimulus encoding processes from memory scanning processes by using memory scanning paradigms with RT as the dependent variable (e.g., Hellige, 1980; Madden & Nebes, 1980; O'Boyle & Hellige, 1982).

Many other laterality experiments have used RT as the dependent variable and typically have not used any transformations of the data. Although it is generally not discussed, RT in these studies is sometimes assumed to be a direct (linear) reflection of processing time, just as in the memory scanning experiments. Real time processing has become an important theoretical construct in the information-processing approach to psychology (e.g., Haber, 1969; Massaro, 1975; Posner, 1978). It seems only natural for studies of laterality effects to be similarly concerned with processing time, especially if one goal is to incorporate hemisphereic asymmetry into more general models of human cognition. However, as others have pointed out, RT is not always used to measure processing time as a specific theoretical construct. For example, in a particular experiment, RT may be used as an index of perceptual strength, memory strength, or some other construct (see Loftus, 1978, for a similar discussion). In such cases there is usually no basis for assuming a linear relationship between RT and the theoretical construct of interest, and interpretation of interaction patterns has the same problems that occur with any dependent variable that is chosen arbitrarily.

Arbitrary Dependent Variables and Interpretability

While there are instances of laterality research in which the dependent variable is chosen for some theoretical reason, in the majority of experiments the dependent variable is to some extent arbitrary. In such cases, some interaction patterns are more interpretable than others. This can be demonstrated most easily by examining possible interaction patterns for a 2 × 2 factorial experiment in which one variable is the hemisphere of stimulus presentation or the hemisphere responding. As will be discussed later, the principles derived from this simplest case can also be extended to more complex designs.

When the dependent variable is chosen arbitrarily, the only thing typically assumed about the function mapping between the dependent variable and the theoretical construct to be measured is that the function is monotonic. Figure 11-4 gives examples of interaction patterns that are interpretable with only this assumption of monotonicity. That is, none of the patterns shown can be changed qualitatively by any monotonic transformation of the dependent variable (assumed to be Probability Correct). The interaction patterns are assumed to be reliable (i.e., are accurate reflections of the population interaction pattern for the dependent variable shown) and free of ceiling and floor effects.

Figure 11-4 plots four hypothetical interaction patterns labeled a, b, c, and d. For each of the four patterns, the upper panel plots Probability Correct as a function of hemisphere with the parameter being conditions (A_1 versus A_2). Exactly the same results are shown in the lower panels plotted with conditions (A_1 versus A_2) on the abscissa and hemisphere as the parameter. Both types of graphical representation are about equally common in laterality research.

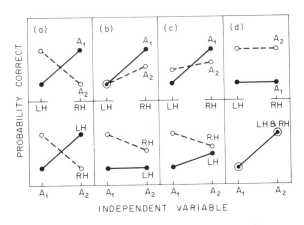

Figure 11-4. *Examples of interpretable interaction patterns, assuming only that the relationship between the theoretical construct to be measured and Probability Correct is monotonic. See text for additional details.*

Interaction patterns a, b, and c in Figure 11-4 are all examples of what have been referred to as crossover interactions, demonstrating what is also referred to as *ordinal nonindependence*. This situation exists whenever the ordering of observed data points corresponding to the levels of one variable (e.g., A_1 versus A_2) is not the same at all levels of the other variable (e.g., left versus right hemisphere). Monotonic transformation of the dependent variable cannot change the ordering of data points; thus, reliable interactions that demonstrate ordinal nonindependence cannot be scaled away by monotonic transformation (see Krantz et al., 1971; Winer, 1971).

Interaction pattern d does not show an interaction at all. Rather, there is only a main effect of the Task variable. This pattern is similar to the others in the sense that any monotonic transformation of the dependent variable must preserve the main effect of Task and cannot introduce any additional effects. However, as discussed earlier, in some cases the absence of a Hemisphere ×

Task interaction may be uninterpretable for other reasons, especially if the only main effect is a hemisphere difference. For example, recall the earlier discussion of electrophysiological studies of laterality.[1]

Figure 11-5 gives examples of the types of interaction patterns that are not interpretable in the sense that there are monotonic transformations of the dependent variable that can remove the interaction or introduce a very different one. Figure 11-5 plots three such interaction patterns in the same manner as the patterns in Figure 11-4. None of the patterns shown in Figure 11-5 demonstrates ordinal nonindependence (i.e., even when there is an interaction, the curves do not touch or cross). Patterns a and b of Figure 11-5 are similar to each other in that there is a hemisphere difference in the same direction for both tasks (A_1 and A_2), but of different magnitudes. In both cases, the two tasks are also of different levels of difficulty. It is this combination that produces the difficulty. Patterns a and b differ in that, in pattern a, the hemisphere difference is larger for the less difficult task, but in pattern b the hemisphere difference is larger for the more difficult task. Interaction pattern c of Figure 11-5 shows two main effects but no interaction. Most common monotonic transformations of the dependent variable will introduce an interaction into a pattern of this sort. This happens because equal intervals in terms of the theoretical component typically produce either systematically larger or systematically smaller changes in the dependent variable as performance becomes better (e.g., see Figure 11-3).

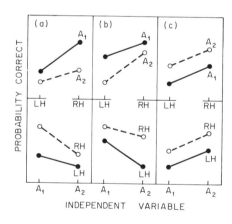

Figure 11-5. *Examples of uninterpretable interaction patterns, assuming only that the relationship between the theoretical construct to be measured and Probability Correct is monotonic. See text for additional details.*

As more is assumed (in addition to monotonicity) about the relationship between the dependent variable and the theoretical construct to be measured, interaction pattern a or b of Figure 11-5 can become interpretable, even though the assumed relationship is nonlinear. For example, assume that changes in a theoretical component of interest (e.g., Perceptual Strength) produce successively smaller changes in Probability Correct as the value of the theoretical component increases. Negatively accelerated functions such as those shown in Figure 11-3 fall into this category. Under this assumption, interactions such as that shown in Figure 11-5, a cannot be removed when Probability Correct is transformed into the appropriate theoretical construct; in fact, such interactions are enhanced. This would be true of any interaction for which the hemisphere difference is larger for that condition (Task or Population) leading to overall better performance. Similarly, if it is assumed that changes in the theoretical component produce successively larger changes in Probability Correct as the theoretical component becomes larger (e.g., inverse functions), interactions such as that shown in Figure 11-5, b become interpretable. Unfortunately, there is often no basis for assumptions beyond monotonicity; thus, extreme caution is best exercised when dealing with any of the interaction patterns shown in Figure 11-5.

The examples given thus far to illustrate the interpretation of interactions have all been based upon a hypothetical 2 × 2 factorial experiment. While such designs are sufficient for illustrating the potential problems, it is important to consider briefly how the points raised here generalize to more complex designs. One way in which a design could become more complex is to increase the number of levels of the independent variables. In laterality research, the Hemisphere variable will always have two levels, but there is no limit on the number of levels of the Task or Population variable. In general, we might consider the interpretability of interactions in a 2 (Hemisphere) × m (Task) design. It should be obvious that, even though this design is somewhat more complex than a 2 × 2, reliable interactions that demonstrate ordinal nonindependence cannot be removed by a monotonic transformation of the dependent variable while reliable interactions that do not demonstrate ordinal nonindependence might be removed. The issue is again whether or not the ordering of data points for the levels of one independent variable (e.g., Hemispheres) is exactly the same for all levels of the second independent variable (e.g., Task).

The design of a laterality experiment becomes even more complex by adding additional independent variables, for example, a 2 (Hemisphere) × m (Task Variable 1) × n (Task Variable 2) design. In such a design, the interpretation of two-factor interactions has already been discussed,[2] but there is a three-factor interaction that merits some consideration. A reliable three-factor interaction indicates that one of the two-factor interactions (e.g., the Hemisphere × Task Variable 1 interaction) is not the same at all levels of the remaining variable (e.g., Task Variable 2). Consequently, to understand a three-factor interaction, it is often useful to examine one of the two-factor interaction patterns at each level of the third variable to see how the two-factor interaction pattern changes. A reasonable rule of thumb to follow would be to exercise the same caution in interpreting each of these two-factor components as discussed earlier for any two-factor interaction.

Guidelines for Design and Interpretation of Laterality Experiments

In view of the preceding discussion about interpretability of interactions, the following guidelines can be offered for the design and interpretation of laterality experiments. Whenever possible, the dependent variable should be chosen for theoretical reasons, and any assumptions about the relationship of the dependent variable to a specific theoretical construct should be made explicit. Even in these cases, it is critical to avoid ceiling and floor effects, for their presence always beclouds interpretation of any interaction pattern. If a particular dependent variable is not dictated by a theoretical framework, at least it may be possible to take steps to use tasks for which performance is the same when averaged across hemispheres. In such cases, if an interaction is observed, it will be of the crossover type. That is, as Figures 11-4 and 11-5 illustrate, problems of interpretability arise when a Hemisphere × Task interaction is accompanied by large main effects of both variables.

Unfortunately, it is often not possible to equate the overall level of difficulty for all tasks. In fact, some task manipulations are intended to change the level of task difficulty. For example, it was noted earlier that attention has recently been given to the effect of perceptual quality on visual half-field effects. Specifically, it has been predicted and reported that, when some types of visual stimuli are perceptually degraded, visual laterality patterns shift toward a left visual field (right hemisphere) advantage (e.g., Hellige, 1980, in press; Sergent & Bindra, 1981; Sergent, 1982a, 1982b). By its very nature, degrading a visual stimulus worsens the overall level of performance on a task. If it did not do so in a particular experiment, one could reasonably question whether perceptual quality was actually manipulated. Other examples include such things as the introduction of a concurrent task designed to interfere with performance (e.g., Friedman & Polson, 1981) or embedding auditory stimuli in noise (e.g., Berlin, 1977).

In these cases, where a main effect of task is expected, it is particularly important to use theory-based dependent variables and to find at least some interactions of the type shown in Figure 11-4, b and c, in which the interaction still demonstrates ordinal nonindependence despite a main effect of task. It is also useful to test the conceptual prediction across several paradigms and with more than one dependent variable. To the extent that these various experiments all produce similar conceptual results, confidence in the theory is greatly increased.

Another case in which it is difficult to equate overall performance is in studies of individual differences. There is never any guarantee that different subject populations will find a particular task equally difficult. There is no entirely satisfactory way to deal with this problem. Consider a study designed to determine whether laterality for a task changes with age. If exactly the same task is used for all ages, younger children will probably not perform as well as older children. Unless there is an actual crossover interaction (which is generally neither predicted nor found in developmental studies of laterality), the interaction pattern falls into the uninterpretable category. Often there is some aspect of the basic task that can be manipulated to equate overall performance for all ages (e.g., stimulus duration, intensity, size, familiarity, etc.). In a sense, the equating of difficulty across age makes the interaction pattern more interpretable. However, this assumes that the manipulation to equate performance levels does not also change the task in any important way related to cerebral hemisphere asymmetry. Unfortunately, this is often difficult to know. One possible solution to this dilemma is to examine the Hemisphere × Population interaction for several levels of task difficulty. If the interaction pattern is the same over the several levels of difficulty, the pattern can be accepted with some confidence. If not, the specific nature of the results is likely to be helpful in formulating a reasonable conclusion.

INTERACTION AND THE CONCEPT OF A LATERALITY INDEX

To the extent that issues similar to those raised in the preceding section have been discussed in the laterality literature, it has been primarily under the topic of computing an appropriate "laterality index." A laterality index is intended to provide a single value that directly reflects the magnitude as well as the direction of hemispheric asymmetry for a particular task performed by a particular individual or group of individuals. If an index can be computed that actually satisfies all of these criteria, almost any Hemisphere × Task interaction pattern would become interpretable. To a large extent, the same considerations that were raised about the interpretability of interaction patterns have led to considerations of various laterality indexes. However, the suggested solutions have typically been rather different, emphasizing certain data transformations rather than design changes. To illustrate this, we will begin with a brief review of the factors motivating the computation of a laterality index and some of the suggested indexes.

Computing a Laterality Index

In early studies of dichotic listening, the dependent variable reported was typically the number of correct identifications of right ear stimuli (Rc) and the number of correct identifications of left ear stimuli (Lc). In order to provide some estimate of the magnitude of hemispheric asymmetry for a task, the difference between Rc and Lc was often computed (e.g., Rc – Lc). That is, Rc – Lc was used as a laterality index, as defined earlier. In order to determine whether two tasks or two subject populations were differentially "lateralized," Rc – Lc difference scores were compared across tasks or subject populations. This procedure worked reasonably well when the various tasks or subject populations were lateralized in opposite directions. However, problems arose as soon as the questions of interest dealt with comparing magnitudes of cerebral laterality, when lateral differences were present and in the same direction for all tasks or subject populations. Included were questions about whether the right ear (left hemisphere) advantage is greater for consonants than for vowels or whether the left hemisphere advantage for certain verbal tasks is larger for males than for females or for adults compared with young children.

To a large extent, investigators became concerned about Rc – Lc as a laterality index because its possible values are not independent of overall accuracy. Consider a hypothetical dichotic listening experiment in which 100 stimuli are presented to each ear. If overall performance is at 90% (180 correct identifications of 200 stimuli), the maximum possible value of Rc – Lc is 20. However, if overall performance is at 50% (100 correct identifications of 200 stimuli), the maximum possible value of Rc – Lc is 100. To put the problem another way, there is no guarantee that a one-unit change in Rc – Lc represents the same amount of change in cerebral laterality across all levels of overall performance. This was identified as problematic because overall performance was found to differ, sometimes rather widely, across tasks or subject populations.

Several authors have attempted to deal with this problem by computing alternative laterality indexes. For example, in addition to Rc – Lc, Harshman and Krashen (1972) consider the following two alternatives that take overall performance into account when measuring laterality:

$$\text{Percent of Correct (POC)} = \frac{Rc}{Rc + Lc} \text{ , and}$$

$$\text{Percent of Error (POE)} = \frac{Le}{Le + Re} \text{ , where}$$

Le = number of errors for left-ear stimuli and Re = number of errors for right-ear stimuli. The POE value is computed with Le in the numerator so that, for both POC and POE, scores range from 0.0 to 1.0; 0.0 indicates a perfect left-ear advantage, 0.5 indicates no laterality effect, and 1.0 indicates a perfect right-ear advantage. Of these indexes, Harshman and Krashen preferred POE, largely because POE was the index least correlated with overall accuracy in their survey of dichotic listening studies.[3]

Marshall, Caplan, and Holmes (1975) pointed out that, while the possible values of POC are not constrained at levels of overall performance below 50%, the value becomes severely limited as overall performance increases from 50% to 100%. The opposite is true of POE (see also Repp, 1977). Therefore, Marshall et al. prefer the following laterality index, which they refer to as f:

$$\text{if overall accuracy} < 50\%, \text{ then } f = \frac{Rc - Lc}{Rc + Lc}, \text{ and}$$

$$\text{if overall accuracy} > 50\%, \text{ then } f = \frac{Rc - Lc}{Le + Re}$$

Note that, for all levels of accuracy, f is equal to Rc − Lc divided by the maximum possible valve of Rc − Lc for that level of accuracy, that is, f is the observed proportion of the maximum possible laterality effect. Note also that, when accuracy is less than 50%, f is a linear transformation of POC ($f = 2(\text{POC}) - 1$), and when accuracy is greater than 50%, f is a linear transformation of POE ($f\,2(\text{POE}) - 1$). Additional properties of f and similar indexes can be seen in discussions by Repp (1977), Colbourne (1978), Kuhn (1973), Eling (1981), Stone (1980) and in chapters by Porter and Hughes, Sprott and Bryden, and Levy in this volume.

At this point it is instructive to note that comparing Rc − Lc difference scores for different tasks or subject populations is equivalent to examining Hemisphere × Task or Hemisphere × Population interaction patterns with number of correct responses (or any linear transformation such as percentage or probability correct) as the dependent variable. It can be seen that, when such a dependent variable has been arbitrarily chosen, certain interaction patterns are not interpretable, in the sense that they can be changed qualitatively by monotonic transformation of the dependent variable (see Figures 11-3 and 11-5). It is exactly the situations that produce these uninterpretable interaction patterns that also create problems for Rc – Lc as a laterality index. For example, ceiling or floor effects place artificial limits on the maximum possible value of Rc – Lc. Even in the absense of ceiling and floor effects, it cannot be assumed that equal changes in the value of an arbitrarily chosen dependent variable reflect the same magnitude of change in some theoretical component across all levels of overall performance (see Figure 11-3). If this is true of number of correct responses as a dependent variable, it has the same implications for computing Rc – Lc as a measure of laterality.

In the preceding section of this chapter, it was argued that the only way to make the problematic interaction patterns interpretable is to use a dependent variable for which the particular scale properties can be explicitly assumed. Short of this, such interaction patterns must be treated with extreme caution. In terms of comparing laterality index values across conditions, the problematic cases only become interpretable if the index is actually a direct (i.e., linear) reflection of the theoretical component it is intended to measure, in this case, the magnitude of cerebral hemisphere asymmetry for some specific set of psychological processes. Any transformation of Lc and Rc involves implicit assumptions about the function mapping between number or percentage correct and the specific psychological processes of interest and often involves further assumptions about such things as the relationship between hemispheric asymmetry and overall accuracy. These assumptions are often more arbitrary than based on theory (see Colbourne, 1978; Eling, 1981; Richardson, 1976). Consequently, it is not possible to treat any of these transformations of Rc – Lc as a "true" laterality index of the sort defined at the beginning of this section.

For example, choosing one laterality index over others because empirical studies find it to be less correlated with overall accuracy than other indexes carries an implicit assumption that the magnitude of hemispheric asymmetry is independent of task difficulty. This is a difficult assumption to justify in light of suggestions noted earlier that certain manipulations such as perceptual degradation of visual stimuli reduce overall accuracy and also change the laterality effect. It would seem, therefore, that the development of any laterality index must follow or accompany the emergence of theories relating cerebral hemisphere asymmetry to such things as overall accuracy, not vice versa.

In the laterality index literature, Richardson (1976) probably comes closest to some of the suggestions made in this chapter. He points out the arbitrary nature of the laterality indexes but still sees a need for developing what he calls a theory-independent measure of laterality. Richardson recommends attending only to ordinal properties of laterality data. In many ways, his recommendations are similar to treating only certain Hemisphere × Task interaction patterns as interpretable, although he does not discuss his proposal in such terms. For comparing two tasks or subject populations, he proposes that the set of scores (Lc, Rc) from condition A_1 represents a greater degree of right-side lateralization than the set (Lc', Rc') from condition A_2 if, and only if, Lc is less than Lc' and Rc is greater than Rc'. Note that, conceptually, this pattern of results is identical to the types of crossover interactions shown in Figure 11-4, panels a and c. It is unclear why Richardson does not include a result such as that shown in Figure 11-4, panel b, where, in his terms, Lc equals Lc' and Rc is greater than Rc'. Richardson does conclude, however, that, if one task has both a higher Lc and a higher Rc than the other task (see Figure 11-5 for examples), questions about the relative magnitude of laterality cannot be answered. Essentially, Richardson's position argues against computing a numerical index of the magnitude of laterality.

Limitations of Laterality Indexes

There are two other problems of focusing attention exclusively on laterality indexes that are especially important to consider. One is that almost all of the numerical transformations of Rc – Lc are based upon accuracy as the dependent variable (but see Levy, this volume). In many cases, other measures such as RT are used, and the same concerns about interpretability are relevant. This is obvious when right and left hemisphere scores are preserved and the form of the interaction pattern is considered when trying to interpret the data. This has not been so obvious or dealt with in the laterality index literature.

The second problem with laterality indexes that is particularly important is that an index completely obscures the left and right hemisphere scores from which the index is derived. Consequently, when the laterality index has a different value for different experimental conditions, it is often impossible to determine the form of the interaction pattern. For example, suppose a reasonable laterality index indicates a right hemisphere advantage for each of two conditions, A_1 and A_2, but the advantage is larger for condition A_1. Because the left and right hemisphere scores are obscured, it cannot be determined whether the data represent a crossover interaction (as illustrated in Figure 11-4, panel c) or not (as illustrated in Figure 11-5, panel a). It has been argued previously that the former type of interaction is more interpretable than the latter. Therefore, given the arbitrary nature of the laterality indexes, obscuring the form of the Hemisphere × Task interaction is not wise.

Preserving the actual left and right hemisphere data points is also important for theoretical reasons. That is, it is often important to know whether any changes in performance are restricted to one hemisphere or are present in different magnitudes for both hemispheres. Consider a recent experiment examining the effect of concurrent activity on dichotic listening (Wexler & Heninger, 1980), which is characteristic of the way in which laterality is reported in many experiments.

Wexler and Heninger (1980) had subjects attempt to report dichotically presented consonant-vowel syllables in each of three conditions: syllable task alone, with a concurrent verbal processing task, and with a concurrent spatial processing task. For each of these three conditions, a "laterality score" was reported, which is equal to $\frac{Rc - Lc}{Rc + Lc} \times 100$. The mean laterality score was significantly larger in the verbal and spatial concurrent activity conditions (11.8 and 11.5, respectively) than in the absence of concurrent activity (7.4), with larger values indicating a greater right ear advantage. One conclusion reached by the authors is that both the verbal and spatial concurrent tasks led to an increase in "perceptual asymmetry." If the laterality index used is assumed to be a linear transformation of "perceptual asymmetry," this conclusion is clearly appropriate. However, as discussed earlier, such an assumption may not be warranted. Furthermore, although Wexler and Heninger do report overall error rates for each of the three conditions, it is impossible to judge whether or not there were ceiling effects in the syllable-alone condition that produced this interaction or to know the form of the Hemisphere × Task interaction. For example, it is unclear whether imposing a concurrent verbal task reduced the performance of both hemispheres but by different magnitudes, or whether, instead, left hemisphere performance remained unchanged or even improved when the concurrent task was employed. Although such information is theoretically important, it cannot be obtained from the report of a laterality index and overall accuracy.

This brief review of the concept of a laterality index has, of necessity, been illustrative rather than exhaustive. The purpose has not been so much to argue for or against any particular index as to argue in favor of preserving the left and right hemisphere data points from which all of the indexes are computed. This is not to say that all of the proposed indexes are of equal merit (see Sprott & Bryden and also Levy, this volume). When used in conjunction with observations of the actual left and right hemisphere scores, certain indexes may serve a useful function. For example, it may be easier to test the statistical significance of a lateral difference within a single subject by converting the data to a laterality index (see Kuhn, 1973; Sprott & Bryden and also Levy, this volume). However, it should be kept in mind that, despite occasional claims to the contrary, there is no such thing as a "theory-independent" laterality index that should be applied indiscriminately to all studies. If the design and procedures of a study permit such things as ceiling and floor effects to occur, there is simply no way to eliminate problems of interpretation by rescaling Rc – Lc. Instead, to the extent that such problems can be solved, it must be at the time when the studies are designed.

THE CONCEPTUALIZATION OF INTERACTIONS

The primary purposes of this chapter have been to illustrate the importance of examining Hemisphere × Task interaction patterns and to point out that only those patterns that demonstrate ordinal nonindependence are interpretable when the dependent variable is arbitrarily chosen and that the computation of an arbitrary laterality index is not a solution to problems of interpretability. It is possible to have agreement about the existence of a Hemisphere × Task interaction in a statistical or measurement sense and, at the same time, have considerable disagreement about the theoretical mechanism responsible for the interaction. The present section considers some general issues related to the conceptualization of Hemisphere × Task interactions and considers the importance of designing studies to incorporate cerebral hemisphere asymmetry into established theories and models of human cognition.

As noted earlier, there are two general ways of conceptualizing any Hemisphere × Task interaction. One might emphasize the fact that the laterality effect (i.e., hemisphere difference) is not the same for all levels of the task variable. Conceptually, this is similar to comparing a laterality index across conditions. Alternatively, one might emphasize the fact that the task effect is not the same for both levels of the hemispheric variable. In one sense, these two ways of thinking about an interaction are equivalent to each other, and the emphasis is arbitrary. However, there seem to be subtle biases in the approach taken to interpret an interaction that are related to the choice of emphasis. To illustrate this, consider a recent experiment on face recognition reported by Sergent (1982a, Experiment 1).

Sergent (1982a, Experiment 1) required subjects to indicate whether or not a probe face presented to the left or right visual field was identical to a target face presented previously in the center of a viewing screen. The two schematic faces were either identical or differed in only one or two features; the four relevant features were hairstyle, eyes, mouth, and jaw. All faces had the same ears and nose. For purposes of illustration, only those trials on which the two faces were different by a single feature will be considered.

Sergent reports a reliable Visual Field × Location of Different Feature interaction with RT as the dependent variable. One way to describe the interaction is in terms of the visual field difference for each of the four feature locations. This way of describing such interactions has been the more common in previous laterality research and probably stems from a conceptualization of the experiment as a comparison of the relative efficiency of the two hemispheres. Note also that this way of thinking about the interaction is closely related to the concept of comparing a laterality index across experimental conditions, with the RT difference between visual fields treated as such an index.

In Sergent's experiment, RT was significantly faster on right visual field (left hemisphere) trials than on left visual field (right hemisphere) trials when the only difference between the two faces was in the hairstyle or eyes. In contrast, there were nonsignificant laterality effects in the opposite direction when the faces were different in mouth or jaw features. In terms of hemispheric efficiency for face recognition, these results might be viewed as inconclusive because there was no main effect of visual field (hemisphere). Beyond that, this particular way of thinking about the interaction might lead to the conclusion that the left hemisphere is more efficient for recognizing hairstyle and eyes while, if anything, the right hemisphere is more efficient for recognizing mouths and jaws.

In this case, considerable insight is gained by organizing the information contained in the interaction in a somewhat different way. Specifically, on right visual field (left hemisphere) trials, RT was significantly faster if the different feature occurred in the upper part of the face than if the different feature occurred in the lower part of the face. Based on this result, Sergent suggests that, on these trials, the faces are compared in a serial fashion from top to bottom; this conclusion is further justified by her subsequent experiments. In contrast, on left visual field (right hemisphere) trials the feature location effect was quite different, and subsequent experiments suggest that on these trials the features are compared in their order of perceptual salience. Based on these results, Sergent concludes that both hemispheres can process information about faces with equal overall efficiency but do so in qualitatively different ways.

In these experiments, the direction of hemisphere differences within any specific feature location condition is not very important in a theoretical sense. Yet much laterality research has been biased toward reporting only lateral differences for each condition or toward thinking of interactions with an emphasis on the lateral differences for each condition. Sergent's work clearly demonstrates the importance of examining carefully the task effects for each hemisphere of presentation to consider for each visual field (hemisphere) what sort of processing model could account for the pattern of task effects. In this sense, it is useful to think of the experiment just described as an experiment about mechanisms for perceiving and comparing faces; where one purpose is to incorporate hemispheric asymmetry into a general theory of face processing.

The importance of designing experiments to incorporate cerebral hemisphere asymmetry into general models of cognitive processing has been recently discussed in several other places (e.g., Friedman & Polson, 1981; Hellige, 1980, in press; Madden & Nebes, 1980). It is acceptance of this goal that led to the earlier suggestions about the choice of a dependent variable in studies of hemispheric asymmetry. For example, if one thinks of an experiment as an investigation of detection processes, signal detection theory provides a framework in which certain dependent variables are required (e.g., Gardner & Branski, 1976). If an experiment is designed to study encoding versus memory scanning processes, a framework is available in which RT is the measure of choice (e.g., Hellige, 1980; Madden & Nebes, 1980; Sternberg, 1969). Even when a particular dependent variable is not dictated by a theory, existing models of psychological processes have been developed, using particular dependent variables. For example, models of face recognition and comparison have been successfully tested using RT as the dependent variable (e.g., Smith & Neilsen, 1970). When designing experiments to investigate the role of cerebral hemisphere asymmetry in such processes, it would seem reasonable to use those dependent variables and experimental manipulations that have been useful in building existing theories about the processes of interest, even though these theories to date have ignored hemispheric asymmetry. At least the existing theories with their, albeit imperfect, dependent variables provide an initial framework for examining quantitative and qualitative differences between the cerebral hemispheres.

The point of view just expressed is somewhat different from a point of view that has characterized most of the laterality index literature. It has been written several times that, to be a theoretically based dependent variable for laterality research, a dependent variable must be based upon a detailed theory about cerebral laterality per se (see the many references cited in the preceding section). It is this belief and the acknowledged absence of such a theory that has led to the strong emphasis on searching for a "theory-independent" measure of "laterality." As seen earlier, there is no such index, but, even more important, the search for such an index obscures an important point.

Investigators are interested in studying and measuring specific psychological processes and should try to choose dependent variables that are related in known ways to the processes of interest. "Laterality" is not such a process. Rather, "laterality" refers to some reflection of the difference in a process, depending upon which cerebral hemisphere receives the stimulus material or initiates the response or both. Unless the actual dependent variable used accurately reflects the processes of interest, there is little hope that any transformation of the right minus left difference score will reflect those processes. Therefore, rather than searching for an atheoretical measure of laterality, investigators must choose the most theoretically justifiable dependent variable available to measure the processes of interest. This choice should be based upon theories about those processes, regardless of whether the theories currently have anything to do with cerebral laterality. In conjunction with appropriate caution in the interpretation of interaction patterns, this strategy for choosing dependent variables offers reasonable hope for continued progress.

CONCLUDING COMMENTS

Over the last two decades, interest in cerebral hemisphere asymmetry and its implications for human cognition have increased greatly. With the increasing interest has come a vast and growing research literature. As the present review illustrates, most of these studies involve the examination of Hemisphere × Task or Hemisphere × Population interaction patterns. Along with the other methodological issues discussed in this volume, it is important to consider issues surrounding the study of such interactions and the choice of dependent variables. Heretofore, these kinds of issues have been discussed only in terms of computing an appropriate laterality index rather than in terms of the interpretability of interactions. For several reasons, an overemphasis on "atheoretical" laterality indexes can be detrimental by providing a false sense of security and by encouraging investigators to present findings in a way that makes it impossible to recover the actual data points. Nevertheless, the problems that led to discussions of alternative laterality indexes are very real and must be considered in the interpretation of laterality experiments. This chapter illustrates that it is possible to consider the same problems in terms of Hemisphere × Task interaction patterns that preserve the left and right hemisphere data points. This way of thinking about the interpretation problems makes aspects of experimental design that serve to minimize them more apparent. Rather than emphasizing the desirability of atheoretical measures of performance, this chapter stresses the importance of using existing theories about specific psychological processes to provide appropriate dependent variables. Although doing so will not eliminate all problems of interpretability, it will increase our ability to understand cerebral hemisphere asymmetry within the framework of contemporary cognitive psychology.

NOTES

1. All of the interaction patterns illustrated in Figures 11-4 and 11-5 occur rather regularly in laterality research. Perusal of recent issues of a single journal, *Neuropsychologia*, produced several examples of the patterns shown. For example, Type 11-4, a occurs in the Hand × Type of Warning Stimulus interaction reported by Bowers and Heilman (1980); Type 11-4, b occurs in the Memory Set Size × Visual Field interaction for Yes responses shown in Figure 1 of Madden and Nebes (1980); Type 11-4, c is similar to the Concreteness × Visual Field interaction reported by Elman, Takahashi, and Tohsaku (1981); Type 11-4, d, with a main effect of visual field and no Visual Field × Cuing Condition interaction, is reported by Schwartz and Smith (1980); Type 11-5, a is represented by the Ear × Presentation Modality interaction shown in the proportion correct data of Table 1 in Tweedy, Rinn, and Springer (1980); Type 11-5, b occurs in the Visual Field × Category interaction for males reported by Graves, Landis, and Goodglass (1981); and Type 11-5, c occurs with two main effects and the absence of an Age × Ear interaction reported by Borod and Goodglass (1980).

2. If both m and n are greater than two, another characteristic in addition to ordinal nonindependence is sufficient to indicate that no monotonic transformation can completely remove the two-factor Task Variable 1 × Task Variable 2 interaction. This characteristic is the failure of double cancellation as discussed in the conjoint measurement literature (e.g., Krantz et al., 1971; see Loftus, 1978, for an illustration). The failure of double cancellation is a different criterion than the lack of ordinal independence. For example, an interaction pattern can produce a failure of double cancellation and still show ordinal independence but not vice versa.

3. The empirical analyses reported by Harshman and Krashen (1972) are difficult to interpret because the raw data on which their correlations were computed were the left and right ear means from each of 45 previously published studies. Recent analyses suggest that the pattern of correlations is quite different when the raw data for the correlations are the left and right side scores from individuals who have all been exposed to the same task (e.g., Birkett, 1977; Hellige, Zatkin, & Wong, 1981). Furthermore, it is the case that the expected values of the correlation between various indexes and overall accuracy is not zero even when "laterality" is, in reality, independent of "accuracy" (see simulations by Stone, 1980).

REFERENCES

Berlin, C.I. Hemisphere asymmetry in auditory tasks. In S. Harnad, R. Doty, L. Goldstein, J. Jaynes, & G. Krauthamer (Eds.), *Lateralization in the nervous system*. New York: Academic Press, 1977.

Birkett, P. Measures of laterality and theories of hemispheric processes. *Neuropsychologia*, 1977, *15*, 693–696.

Bolles, D.B. Laterally biased attention with concurrent verbal load: Multiple failures to replicate. *Neuropsychologia*, 1979, *17*, 353–361.

Borod, J.C., & Goodglass, H. Lateralization of linguistic and melodic processing with age. *Neuropsychologia*, 1980, *18*, 79–84.

Bowers, D., & Heilman, K.M. Material-specific hemispheric activation. *Neuropsychologia*, 1980, *18*, 309–320.

Bruce, R., & Kinsbourne, M. Orientational model of perceptual asymmetry. Paper presented at the Psychonomic Society Convention, Boston, November, 1974.

Bryden, M.P. Response bias and hemispheric differences in dot localization. *Perception and Psychophysics*, 1976, *19*, 23–28.

Cohen, G. Hemispheric differences in serial versus parallel processing. *Journal of Experimental Psychology*, 1973, *97*, 349–356.

Cohen, G. Hemisphere differences in the effects of cuing in visual recognition tasks. *Journal of Experimental Psychology: Human Perception and Performance*, 1975, *1*, 366–373.

Colbourne, C. Can laterality be measured? *Neuropsychologia*, 1978, *16*, 283–289.

Dee, H.L., & Fontenot, D.J. Cerebral dominance and lateral difference in perception and memory. *Neuropsychologia*, 1973, *11*, 167–173.

Donchin, E., Kutas, M., & McCarthy, G. Electrocortical indices of hemispheric utilization. In S. Harnad, R. Doty, L. Goldstein, J. Jaynes, & G. Krauthamer (Eds.), *Lateralization in the nervous system*. New York: Academic Press, 1977.

Eling, P. On the theory and measurement of laterality. *Neuropsychologia*, 1981, *19*, 321–324.

Elman, J.L., Takahashi, K., & Tohsaku, Y. Lateral asymmetries for the identification of concrete and abstract *Kanji*. *Neuropsychologia*, 1981, *19*, 407–412.

Friedman, A., & Polson, M.C. The hemispheres as independent resource systems: Limited capacity processing and cerebral specialization. *Journal of Experimental Psychology: Human Perception and Performance*, 1981, *7*, 1031–1058.

Gardner, E.B., & Branski, D.M. Unilateral cerebral activation and perception of gaps: A signal detection analysis. *Neuropsychologia*, 1976, *14*, 43–54.

Geffen, G., Bradshaw, J.L., & Nettleton, N.C. Hemispheric asymmetry: Verbal and spatial encoding of visual stimuli. *Journal of Experimental Psychology*, 1972, *95*, 25–31.

Gevins, A.S. Brain potential (BP) evidence for lateralization of higher cognitive functions, this volume.

Graves, R., Landis, T., & Goodglass, H. Laterality and sex differences for visual recognition of emotional and non-emotional words. *Neuropsychologia*, 1981, *19*, 95–102.

Haber, R.N. Introduction. In R. Haber (Ed.), *Information processing approaches to visual perception*. New York: Holt, Rinehart and Winston, 1969.

Hardyck, C. Seeing each other's point of view: Visual perceptual lateralization, this volume.

Harshman, R., & Krashen, S. An unbiased procedure for comparing degree of lateralization of dichotically presented stimuli. *UCLA Working Paper in Phonetics*, 1972, *24*, 63–70.

Hayashi, T., & Bryden, M.P. Ocular dominance and perceptual asymmetry. *Perceptual and Motor Skills*, 1967, *25*, 605–612.

Hellige, J.B. Visual laterality patterns for pure- versus mixed-list presentation. *Journal of Experimental Psychology: Human Perception and Performance*, 1978, *4*, 121–131.

Hellige, J.B. Effects of perceptual quality and visual field of probe stimulus presentation on memory search for letters. *Journal of Experimental Psychology: Human Perception and Performance*, 1980, *6*, 639–651.

Hellige, J.B. Visual laterality and cerebral hemisphere specialization: Methodological and theoretical considerations. In J.B. Sidowski (Ed.), *Conditioning, cognition, and methodology: Contemporary issues in experimental psychology*. Hillsdale, N.J.: Erlbaum, in press.

Hellige, J.B., & Cox, P.J. Effects of concurrent verbal memory on recognition of stimuli from the left and right visual fields. *Journal of Experimental Psychology: Human Perception and Performance*, 1976, *2*, 210–221.

Hellige, J.B., Cox, P.J., & Litvac, L. Information processing in the cerebral hemispheres: Selective hemispheric activation and capacity limitations. *Journal of Experimental Psychology: General*, 1979, *108*, 251–279.

Hellige, J.B., Zatkin, J.L., & Wong, T.M. Intercorrelation of laterality indices. *Cortex*, 1981, *17*, 129–134.

Kimura, D. Dual functional asymmetry of the brain in visual perception. *Neuropsychologia*, 1966, *4*, 275–285.

Kinsbourne, M. The cerebral basis of lateral asymmetries in attention. *Acta Psychologica*, 1970, *33*, 193–201.

Kinsbourne, M. The control of attention by interaction between the hemispheres. In S. Kornblum (Ed.), *Attention and performance IV*. New York: Academic Press, 1973.

Kinsbourne, M. The mechanism of hemispheric control of the lateral gradient of attention. In P.M.A. Rabbitt & S. Dornic (Eds.), *Attention and performance V*. New York: Academic Press, 1975.

Krantz, D.H., Luce, R.D., Suppes, P., & Tversky, A. *Foundations of measurement*. New York: Academic Press, 1971.

Kuhn, G.M. The phi coefficient as an index of ear differences in dichotic listening. *Cortex*, 1973, *9*, 450–457.

Lawrence, V.W., Kee, D.W., & Hellige, J.B. Developmental differences in visual backward masking. *Child Development*, 1980, *51*, 1081–1089.

Levy, J. Individual differences in cerebral hemisphere asymmetry: Theoretical issues and experimental considerations, this volume.

Loftus, G. On interpretation of interactions. *Memory and Cognition*, 1978, *6*, 312–319.

Madden, D.J., & Nebes, R.D. Hemispheric differences in memory search. *Neuropsychologia*, 1980, 665–674.

Marshall, J.C., Caplan, D., & Holmes, J.M. The measure of laterality. *Neuropsychologia*, 1975, *13*, 315–321.

Massaro, D.W. *Experimental psychology and information processing*. Chicago: Rand McNally, 1975.

McKeever, W.F. Does post-exposure directional scanning offer a sufficient explanation for lateral differences in tachistoscopic recognition? *Perceptual and Motor Skills*, 1974, *38*, 43–50.

Moscovitch, M., & Klein, D. Material specific perceptual interference for visual words and faces: Implications for models of capacity limitations, attention, and laterality. *Journal of Experimental Psychology: Human Perception and Performance*, 1980, *6*, 590–604.

O'Boyle, M.W., & Hellige, J.B. Hemispheric asymmetry, early visual processes, and serial memory comparison. *Brain and Cognition*, 1982, *1*, 224–243.

Pirozzolo, F.J., Rayner, K., & Hynd, G.W. The measurement of hemispheric asymmetries in children with developmental reading disabilities, this volume.

Polich, J.M. Left hemisphere superiority for visual search. *Cortex*, 1980, *16*, 39–50.

Porter, R.J., & Hughes, L.F. Dichotic listening to CVs: Method, interpretation, and application, this volume.

Posner, M.I. *Chronometric explorations of mind*. Hillsdale, N.J.: Erlbaum, 1978.

Postman, L. Methodology of human learning. In W.K. Estes (Ed.), *Handbook of learning and cognitive processes* (Vol. 3), *Approaches to human learning and motivation*. Hillsdale, N.J.: Erlbaum, 1976.

Repp, B.H. Measuring laterality effects in dichotic listening. *Journal of the Acoustical Society of America*, 1977, *62*, 720–737.

Richardson, J.T.E. How to measure laterality. *Neuropsychologia*, 1976, *14*, 135–136.

Schwartz, M., & Smith, M.L. Visual asymmetries with chimeric faces. *Neuropsychologia*, 1980, 103–106.

Sergent, J. About face: Left hemisphere involvement in processing physiognomies. *Journal of Experimental Psychology: Human Perception and Performance*, 1982a, *8*, 1–14.

Sergent, J. The cerebral balance of power: Confrontation or cooperation? *Journal of Experimental Psychology: Human Perception and Performance*, 1982b, *8*, 253–272.

Sergent, J. & Bindra, D. Differential hemispheric processing of faces: Methodological considerations and reinterpretation. *Psychological Bulletin*, 1981, *89*, 541–554.

Smith, E.E., & Neilsen. G.D. Representation and retrieval processes in short-term memory: Recognition and recall of faces. *Journal of Experimental Psychology*, 1970, *85*, 397–405.

Sprott, D.A., & Bryden, M.P. Measurement of laterality effects, this volume.

Sternberg, S. Memory scanning: Mental processes revealed by reaction time experiments. *American Scientist*, 1969, *57*, 421–457.

Sternberg, S. Memory scanning: New findings and current controversies. *Quarterly Journal of Experimental Psychology*, 1975, *27*, 1–32.

Stone, M.A. Measures of laterality and spurious correlation. *Neuropsychologia*, 1980, *18*, 339–446.

Swets, J.A., Tanner, W.P., & Birdsall, T.G. Decision processes in perception. *Psychological Review*, 1961, *68*, 301–340.

Teuber, H.L. Physiological psychology. *Annual Review of Psychology*, 1955, 267–296.

Teuber, H.L. The riddle of frontal lobe function in man. In J.M. Warren & K. Aker (Eds.), *The frontal granular cortex and behavior*. New York: McGraw-Hill, 1964.

Turner, S., & Miller, L.K. Some boundary conditions for laterality effects in children. *Developmental Psychology*, 1975, *11*, 342–352.

Tweedy, J.R., Rinn, W.E., & Springer, S.P. Performance asymmetries in dichotic listening: The role of structural and attentional mechanisms. *Neuropsychologia*, 1980, *18*, 331–338.

Underwood, B.J. Degree of learning and the measurement of forgetting. *Journal of Verbal Learning and Verbal Behavior*, 1964, *3*, 112–129.

Wexler, B.E., & Heninger, G.R. Effects of concurrent administration of verbal and spatial visual tasks on a language related dichotic listening measure of perceptual asymmetry. *Neuropsychologia*, 1980, *18*, 379–382.

White, M.J. Laterality differences in perception: A review. *Psychological Bulletin*, 1969, *72*, 387–405.

White, M.J. Hemispheric asymmetries in tachistoscopic information processing. *British Journal of Psychology*, 1972, *63*, 497–508.

Winer, B.J. *Statistical principles in experimental design* (2nd ed.). New York: McGraw-Hill, 1971.

Wyke, M., & Ettlinger, G. Efficiency of recognition in left and right visual fields. *Archives of Neurology*, 1961, *5*, 659–665.

12

Measurement of Laterality Effects

D.A. Sprott
M.P. Bryden

In the two decades since Kimura's (1961) report of a relation between dichotic listening performance and cerebral speech lateralization, behavioral techniques for assessing lateral cerebral specialization have proliferated widely. This proliferation has brought with it a number of statistical and analytical problems that cloud the interpretation of laterality experiments. For example, researchers have long been aware of the fact that absolute differences in laterality are correlated with overall level of performance on the task; subjects who find the task easy and approach perfect performance are likely to show small absolute differences between left and right visual fields or ears, while those who find the task more difficult are more likely to show large absolute differences. Thus, in Kimura's (1964) classic study of the development of the dichotic right ear effect, younger children show larger absolute laterality effects than do older children. Few would argue that cerebral specialization for language diminishes with age. A careful examination of Kimura's data indicates that the problem arises simply because the younger children find the task relatively difficult and, therefore, have ample room to manifest a large laterality effect, while the older children correctly identify most of the items from both left and right ears, leaving little room for a difference in accuracy between the two ears.

Over the years, a number of suggestions have been offered as to methods of coping with this correlation between overall accuracy and the magnitude of the observed laterality effect (e.g., Bryden & Sprott, 1981; Halwes, 1969;

Kuhn, 1973; Marshall, Caplan & Holmes, 1975; Repp, 1977). The objectives of this chapter are to review the various measures that have been used to assess the degree of laterality, to consider the statistical assumptions of the various experimental procedures that have been employed, and to offer some suggestions as to appropriate procedures.

MEASURES OF LATERALITY

The Difference Score

In the following, p_R is the probability of identifying the stimulus on the right, and p_L is the probability of identifying the stimulus on the left.

The simplest index of laterality is the difference between performance on the two sides:

$$d = p_R - p_L \tag{1}$$

It is this measure that is most commonly reported in the literature and that is commonly analyzed by standard analysis of variance techniques. However, as Halwes (1969) pointed out and is evident from an examination of Kimura's (1964) data, the value d, is severely limited by the overall performance level, p_o, where:

$$p_o = \frac{1}{2}(p_R + p_L) \tag{2}$$

For example, if p_o is close to 1.00 then d must be small. In general, if p_o exceeds 0.5, d must lie between $-(2 - 2p_o)$ and $+(2 - 2p_o)$, while if p_o is less than 0.5, d must fall between $-2p_o$ and $+2p_o$. An alternative way of looking at this constraint, following the convention adopted by Marshall et al. (1975) and Repp (1977), is to examine the isolaterality contours. Isolaterality contours are obtained by plotting the possible values of p_R and p_L for a given fixed value of the laterality index. Thus, the lines in Figure 12-1 connect points that have the same value of d. As shown, isolaterality contours for the d index are a set of lines parallel to the major diagonal. From this figure, it can be seen that large values of d can be obtained only when p_o is intermediate in value.

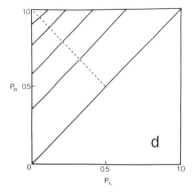

Figure 12-1. *Isolaterality contours for the (R – L) difference scores. Points connected by a line have the same value of d. The lines shown are all for situations in which $P_R > P_L$; when $P_L > P_R$ the line would fall below the main diagonal.*

POE and POC

One way of correcting for some of the limitations of d is to express the observed difference as a proportion of total accuracy. Krashen (1973) for example, has suggested using POC (percentage of correct responses) or POE (percentage of errors) as a measure of laterality, where:

$$POC = p_R / (p_L + p_R) \tag{3}$$

$$POE = (1 - p_L) / (2 - p_L - p_R) \tag{4}$$

A related measure is the ratio of the difference score to the total correct:

$$D = (p_R - p_L) / (p_R + p_L) \tag{5}$$

This, however, is the POC for the right side minus the POC for the left side, and since POC (L) = 1 – POC (R),

$$D = 2 \; POC \; (R) - 1$$

Therefore, D is equivalent to POC and presents the same problems.

The problem is that POC has a limit of 1 if p_o is less than 0.5 but a limit of $(1-p_o)/p_o$ when p_o exceeds 0.5. Similarly, POE has a limit of 1 when p_o exceeds 0.5, but a limit of $p_o/(1-p_o)$ when p_o is less than 0.5. The constraints are shown in the isolaterality contours of Figures 12-2 and 12-3.

Krashen (1973) attempted to choose between various measures of laterality on empirical grounds and recommended POE. However, the data that he used were obtained from a dichotic listening study in which p_o was almost always above 0.5; therefore, the limitation on POE was not evident.

Similarly, POE would correct the declining laterality effect in Kimura's (1964) data but only because p_o is always close to or above 0.5. Furthermore, Krashen's approach confuses mathematical limitations on a laterality index with empirical ones. The mathematical fact is that POE (and POC) do not have the same limits for all values of p_o. No empirical study of POE in any particular laterality experiment can alter this fact.

The *e* Index

Halwes attempted to solve the problem of the constraints on various laterality indexes by recommending that POC be used when p_o was less than 0.5 and that POE be used when p_o was greater than 0.5. Thus, he recommended a measure that Repp (1977) has termed *e*:

$$e = (p_R - p_L) / (p_R + p_L) \quad \text{if } p_o \leq 1/2 \tag{6a}$$

$$e = (p_R - p_L) / (2 - p_L - p_R) \quad \text{if } p_o \geq 1/2 \tag{6b}$$

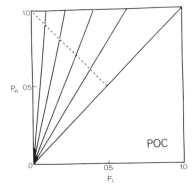

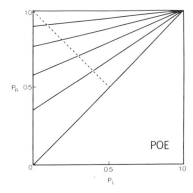

Figure 12-2. *Isolaterality contours for POC. Note that there are upper limits for any given value of POC.*

Figure 12-3. *Isolaterality contours for POE. Note that there are lower limits for any given value of POE.*

The resulting measure has a range of $(-1,1)$, irrespective of p_o. Isolaterality contours for this measure are shown in Figure 12-4. Marshall et al. (1975) and Repp (1977) have argued in favor of this measure, on the grounds that it at least approximates the familiar ROC curve of signal detection theory. However, the mathematical expression (6) is complicated and, as seen from Figure 12-4, there is a discontinuity in the slope at $p_o = 0.5$. For this reason, *e* is less convenient than other measures to be discussed.

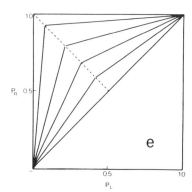

Figure 12-4. *Isolaterality contours for* e. *Note the inflection point on the minor diagonal.*

The Phi Coefficient

Kuhn (1973) has recommended the phi coefficient as a measure of laterality:

$$\text{phi} = (p_R - p_L) \, / \, \left\{ (p_R + p_L) \, (2 - p_R - p_L) \right\}^{1/2} \tag{7}$$

Like POE and POC, it can be shown that the range of the phi coefficient is dependent upon p_o.

The "Equivalent Normal Deviate" Measure

The general problem in constructing a laterality index is the transformation of the two parameters (p_R, p_L) into two functions, λ (p_R, p_L) and $p(p_R, p_L)$, whose ranges of possible values are mutually independent and where λ measures the "distance" between p_R and p_L, while p is a complementary measure of the sum of p_R and p_L, or the overall level of performance. Of the foregoing measures, only e accomplishes this, but it has the mathematical inconvenience of the abrupt change in shape at $p_o = 1/2$. Further, its range is finite ($-1 \leq e \leq 1$), and, as will be seen, it is statistically convenient to have a measure with an infinite range ($-\infty, \infty$). The convenience of an infinite range is exemplified by the correlation coefficient, where the r to z transformation facilitates statistical analyses.

A measure that is preferable to *e*, in light of the above discussion, is $\delta = \delta_R - \delta_L$, based on signal detection theory, where δ_i is the "equivalent normal deviate" given by:

$$p_i = \frac{1}{\sqrt{2\pi}} \int_{-\infty}^{\delta_i} \exp(-t^2/2)dt, \quad (i=R,L) \tag{8}$$

The use of (8) apparently dates back to Fechner (1860); it was rediscovered by biologists in the middle 1930s and has been widely used since under the name of "probit" (Bliss, 1935a, 1935b; Gaddum, 1933). Its use in biology arises in bioassay, that is, in assaying the strength of drugs. Such usage has been justified by assuming that the effects of a drug (e.g., death) occur if a certain quantity (e.g., the drug dose) exceeds some hypothetical tolerance assumed to be normally distributed in the population. Its use in signal detection theory is justified in a similar but even more sophisticated way (Green & Swets, 1966). Obviously, an infinity of such measures could be generated by replacing the normal distribution in equation (8) by any arbitrary distribution, $f(t)$.

It should be emphasized that a justification of such a measure in terms of the distribution of hypothetical tolerances described above or the more sophisticated argument of signal detection theory is by no means required. On whatever grounds such a measure has been put forward, its only justification is its empirical performance (see Finney, 1971, chap. 17). Is it measuring a real reproducible natural phenomenon?

MEASURES BASED ON LOG ODDS

A similar measure that has occasionally been used in signal detection theory, is increasingly used in bioassay, and has gained popularity from the development of "log linear models" is $\lambda = \lambda_R - \lambda_L$, where:

$$\lambda_i = \log\left\{p_i/(1 - p_i)\right\}, \quad i = (R,L) \tag{9}$$

This can be obtained from Equation (8) by replacing the normal distribution with the "logistic" distribution, $f(t) = \{[\exp(t)]/[1 + \exp(t)^2]\}$. It should be noted that, in this equation and throughout this chapter, natural logarithms are used. Because of computers, such a measure is now more convenient than (8). Tables are no longer as convenient as the use of pocket calculators, by which (9) can easily be calculated. Further, the numerical difference resulting from the use of (8) or (9) is small.

Perhaps the basic difference between λ and the preceding measures is that λ is based on odds, $p_R/(1-p_R)$, rather than on absolute probabilities, p_R. The laterality measures based on equations (8) and (9) are not constrained by p_0 and have an infinite range ($-\infty \leq \delta, \lambda, \leq \infty$).

The fact that a laterality measure is not constrained by p_0, that is, its range of possible values is independent of p_0, is merely a mathematical assertion. Nothing is thereby implied about the empirical independence of laterality and performance; the latter requires experimental demonstration. To study the possibility of the independence of laterality and overall performance requires that they be measured by parameters that are mathematically independent.

It is the purpose of the rest of this chapter to introduce statistical considerations and to derive and exemplify the use of laterality measures based on equation (9).

STATISTICAL ASPECTS

A notable characteristic of most of the previous treatment of laterality measures is the omission of any discussion of their statistical properties, such as their standard errors. One exception is provided in Kuhn (1973), where significance levels are derived for testing the phi coefficient, based upon the relationship of phi to the χ^2 test of independence in a 2 × 2 contingency table. His use of the procedure is incorrect, however, since different cells of the 2 × 2 table have observations in common, as described later. Further, as Levy (1977) has noted, phi is not independent of overall accuracy.

Other exceptions are found in papers by Studdert-Kennedy and Shankweiler (1970) and by Wexler, Halwes, and Heninger (1981). Their approaches will be discussed in a later section.

In order to develop a statistical analysis, a statistical model of the experiment must be assumed. This will entail assumptions as to the statistical characteristics of successive trials. Such assumptions lead not only to a statistical analysis but will also serve to focus attention on specific aspects of the observations that need examination and that have been ignored in the past.

Specifically, the simplest assumption is that the results of successive trials on an individual are statistically independent. That is, the successive trials behave like the tosses of a coin. If there are n_R trials on the right side, if it is assumed that there are constant probabilities p_R, $1-p_R$ of a correct, incorrect response, the same for all trials, and if it is assumed that the trials are independent, then the probability of observing exactly y_R correct responses is given by the binominal distribution:

$$\binom{n_R}{y_R} \; p_R^{\,y_R} \, (1 - p_R)^{\,n_R - y_R} \tag{10}$$

where $\binom{n_R}{y_R}$ is the number of ways of ordering the y_R correct and $n - y_R$

incorrect responses. Thus, under these assumptions, (10) is the statistical model. This is essentially the probability of observing y_R heads in n_R independent tosses of a coin whose probability of heads on a single toss is p_R. (For an unbiased coin, $p_R = 1/2$.)

It should be emphasized that the assumption of independence of trials in equation (10) does not mean that the responses need be independent. It implies that the correctness of the responses is independent. That is, being correct on the i'th trial is not affected by the correctness of the preceding trials. For example, in tossing a coin a subject might always respond "heads." The responses are then clearly not independent. However, provided the coin is tossed randomly, the successive outcomes of the tosses are independent and, hence, the correctness of the response, "heads," on successive trials is independent. Viewed in this light, it is seen that the validity of the independence assumptions rests in part on the design of the experiment. The successive trials should simulate the randomness of tosses of a coin.

From equation (9), it follows that not only is $\lambda_R = \log p_R/(1-p_R)$ estimated by:

$$\hat{\lambda}_R = \log(y_R/(n_R - y_R)) \tag{11a}$$

but also the estimated variance of $\hat{\lambda}_R$ is:

$$\hat{\sigma}^2_{\lambda_R} = (1/y_R) + 1/(n_R - y_R) \tag{11b}$$

It is the calculation of variances and standard errors of the estimates of laterality measures, $\hat{\lambda}_R$, on an individual that have been ignored in the literature and that depend upon the setting up of a statistical model such as (10).

It is also the variance (11b) that accounts for the convenience of laterality measures based upon equation (9). It is certainly true that the equivalent normal deviate (8) or Repp's (1977) e (6a, 6b) could also be similarly used. They would lead to formulas different from the above, but at least in the case of (8), the numerical results would be very similar. However, the resulting formulas are not as convenient and, in the case of (6a, 6b), probably quite complicated and inconvenient because of the awkward mathematical expression.

The quantities in (11) can be combined in the usual way to form the quantity:

$$u(\lambda_R) = (\hat{\lambda}_R - \lambda_R)/\hat{\sigma}_{\lambda_R} \tag{12}$$

If n_R is not too small, (12) will have an approximate standard normal distribution. This allows the testing of hypotheses $\lambda_R = \lambda_{R_o}$ merely by calculating the numerical value of the resulting $u(\hat{\lambda}_R, \lambda_{R_o})$ and referring the result to tables of the normal distribution. For instance, the test that λ_R deviates from zero is simply a test of $u(\hat{\lambda}_R, o) = \hat{\lambda}_R/\hat{\sigma}\lambda_R$. More importantly, approximate confidence intervals for λ_R can be obtained. For example, an approximate 95% confidence interval is $\lambda_R = \hat{\lambda}_R \pm 1.96\hat{\sigma}\lambda_R$.

It is the ease of calculation of $\hat{\lambda}_R$, $\hat{\sigma}_R$ of (11) and the approximate normality of (12) that suggest the use of laterality measures based upon odds ratios (9). As stated previously, equation (8) could equally be used but produces results very similar to (9) and is not as computationally convenient on pocket calculators. The normality of both (8) and (9) is enhanced by their range being infinite, $-\infty \leq \delta, X \leq \infty$, thus resembling ordinary physical measurements in this respect. Repp's quantity e (6), however, is forced to lie between $(-1,1)$. If e is close to either boundary, it is unlikely that a normal approximation will be very good. Because of the mathematical nature of e, it is unlikely that either its standard error is easily obtainable or that the corresponding quantity (12), $u(e)$, will have an approximate normal distribution. This makes e very difficult to use in a statistical analysis. The above statistical considerations thus present a strong case for basing laterality measures on equation (9), used in conjunction with (11) and (12).

The following sections discuss the laterality measures based on (9) and the statistical analysis based on (11) and (12), resulting from common types of laterality experiments.

EXAMPLES

Binomial Response Experiments

Perhaps the simplest type of experiment is one to which the binomial distribution model (10) and, hence, the resulting analysis in terms of (11) and (12) apply directly. This is an experiment in which a correct response is given on every trial, and one only wishes to know whether responses are given more frequently to items on the right side than to items on the left side. An example is Repp's (1978) dichotic fusion procedure, in which a pair of syllables presented dichotically fuse perceptually, so that only a single response is given to each stimulus pair. There are, thus, only two possible responses, right and left, with probabilities, p_R, $1-p_R$. The assumptions discussed previously then lead to (10) and, hence, to equations (11) and (12). Thus, an appropriate measure of laterality is equation (11a) with variance as in equation (11b).

Some other investigators have tested whether or not the dichotic laterality effect is significantly different from zero by comparing the frequency of correct responses on the right ear to the frequency of correct responses on the left ear in situations in which only a single response was given on each trial. Studdert-Kennedy and Shankweiler (1970) scored only those trials on which a single correct response had been made and compared left and right ear scores with the binomial test. Wexler et al. (1981) used Repp's (1978) fusional procedure and applied a χ^2 test of significance. These procedures are similar to ours, in the special case of testing only the existence of a laterality effect in a single response experiment. They do not, however, provide more general confidence limits on the magnitude of a laterality measure, such as (11a).

Comparison of Two Binomial Response Experiments

A more common experiment is one in which two sets of trials are intermingled and the subject is asked to respond to a right side item on some trials and to a left side item on the others. Dichotic monitoring tasks, in which the subject attends to one ear on some trials and to the other ear on other trials is one example of such an experiment. Here there are n trials on the right side, with probability p_R of a correct and $(1-p_R)$ of an incorrect response. The corresponding observed frequencies are y_R, $n-y_R$. There are n left side trials with corresponding probabilities p_L, $1-p_L$ and observed frequencies y_L, $n-y_L$. This gives rise to two binomial response models (10), one for each side.

Using (9), the accuracy on the right is λ_R and that on the left is λ_L, and their difference, the laterality, is:

$$\lambda = \lambda_R - \lambda_L = \log p_R (1 - p_L) / p_L (1 - p_R) \qquad (13a)$$

Using (11) in an obvious way, this is estimated by:

$$\lambda = \hat{\lambda}_R - \hat{\lambda}_L = \log y_R (n - y_L) / y_L (n - y_R) \qquad (13b)$$

with estimated variance:

$$\hat{\sigma}_\lambda^2 = \hat{\sigma}_{\lambda_R}^2 + \hat{\sigma}_{\lambda_L}^2 = 1/y_R + 1/(n - y_R) + 1/y_L + 1(n - y_L) \qquad (13c)$$

This is the situation used for discussion in the introduction, leading to the variety of measures mentioned there. Thus, the quantity (13a) is directly comparable to those measures. In particular, λ varies between $(-\infty, \infty)$, whatever the value of the performance level $p_o = (1/2) (p_R + p_L)$, and is zero only if $p_R = p_L$. As discussed earlier, it is preferable to Repp's (1977) e in leading to a mathematically simpler estimate (13b) with an easily calculable standard error (13c), for which the quantity $u(\lambda) = (\hat{\lambda} - \lambda)/\hat{\sigma}\hat{\lambda}$ corresponding to (12) is more nearly normally distributed (see Figure 12-5). As illustrated earlier, this leads directly to the assessment of the laterality λ of any specified subject via test of significance (e.g., H: $\lambda = 0$) and confidence intervals for λ (e.g., $\lambda = \hat{\lambda} \pm 1.96 \hat{\sigma}\lambda$).

Unilateral visual field studies (e.g., Bryden, 1965) are also amenable to this analysis. Such experiments provide separate estimates of the odds of identifying items presented in the left visual field and the odds of identifying items in the right visual field.

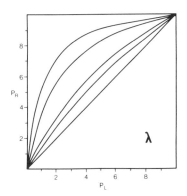

Figure 12-5. *Isolaterality contours for* λ.

Multinomial Response Experiments

The above analyses may arise in other guises. For example, there may be more than two possible responses. In the dichotic monitoring task, for instance, the incorrect responses (that occur with probabilities $1-p_R$, $1-p_L$) actually consist of two separate categories, namely, complete misses and incorrect lateralizations (see Bryden, Munhall, & Allard, 1980). The latter are reports of the item that was actually presented to the unattended ear while the former are reports of an item that was presented to neither ear. Let p_{IR} be the probability of an incorrectly localized response when the subject was asked to identify the right ear stimulus (that is, the stimulus actually identified occurred on the left). Let p_{IL} be the corresponding probability for the left side. There are now three possible responses with probability p_R, p_{IR}, $1-p_R-p_{IR}$ for the right side trials and p_L, p_{IL}, $1-p_L-p_{IL}$ for the left side trials and with corresponding observed frequencies $(y_R, y_{IR}, n-y_R-y_{IR})$, $(y_L, y_{IL}, n-y_L-y_{IL})$. However, if complete misses (which occur with probabilities $1-p_R-p_{IR}$, $1-p_L-p_{IL}$) are regarded as neutral with respect to lateralization, the resulting measure of laterality will be based upon p_R, p_L, p_{IR}, p_{IL} and will be essentially (13a) in a different guise:

$$\lambda = \lambda_R - \lambda_L = \log p_R p_{IL}/p_L p_{IR}$$

Then (13b) and (13c) are correspondingly modified:

$$\hat{\lambda} = \hat{\lambda}_R - \hat{\lambda}_L = \log y_R y_{IL}/y_L y_{IR}$$

$$\hat{\sigma}_\lambda^2 = 1/y_R + 1/y_{IR} + 1/y_L + 1/y_{IL}$$

Although there are three possible responses, the analysis is that of the comparison of binomial response models, arising from restricting attention to the two classes, p_R, p_{IR}, on the right side trials and p_L, p_{IL} on the left side trials.

Complete misses can be analyzed similarly by combining the classes, R, IR, and L, IL, giving another comparison of two binomial response models, $p_R + p_{IR}$, $1 - p_R - p_{IR}$ versus $p_L + p_{IL}$, $1 - p_L - p_{IL}$. This is suitable for comparing the frequencies of misses on both sides.

TWO-RESPONSE PROCEDURES

Another guise under which the single binomial response model occurs is the two-response procedure. One example of this is the dichotic task of Studdert-Kennedy and Shankweiler (1970). They presented a single pair of nonsense syllables dichotically, with the subject being required to identify both syllables. In this procedure there were four categories of response: both correct, left correct and right incorrect, right correct and left incorrect, and neither correct, with probabilities p_{RL}, p_L, p_R, and p_O, respectively, with $p_{RL} + p_L + p_R + p_O = 1$. The corresponding observed frequencies can be denoted as y_{RL}, y_L, y_R, y_O with $y_{RL} + y_R + y_L + y_0 = n$.

Although this experiment is quite different from the binomial response experiment illustrated earlier, since it gives rise to four categories, Studdert-Kennedy and Shankweiler (1970) correctly noted that the categories (RL) and (O) are neutral with respect to laterality. Thus, the appropriate measure of laterality should involve only the single-correct trials and be based upon p_R, p_L. This leads to $\lambda_R = \log p_R/p_L$ with $\hat{\lambda}_R = \log y_R/y_L$ and $\hat{\sigma}_R = 1/y_R + 1/y_L$, which are essentially (9), (11a), and (11b) of the binomial response model.

It is usually within the context of the dichotic two-response situation that the various measures of laterality have been discussed (e.g., Marshall et al., 1975; Repp, 1977). Unfortunately, this has usually been done by considering overall accuracy on the left and on the right, leading to the classification:

Stimulus	Response	
	Correct	Incorrect
Left	$y_{RL} + y_L$	$y_R + y_0$
Right	$y_{RL} + y_R$	$y_L + y_0$

Such a table cannot be analyzed by the above methods because cells 1 and 3 have observations y_{RL} in common and cells 2 and 4 have y_0 in common. In particular, as mentioned earlier, this violates the significance levels of the phi coefficient (7) proposed by Kuhn (1973). The whole purpose of the derivation of phi in Kuhn's paper appeared to be to use all four observations. This does not appear to be feasible, since it is difficult to see what information y_{RL} and y_0 contain concerning laterality. The above experiment exemplifies the important fact that the different response categories used to classify the possible observations must be mutually exclusive and exhaustive. The classification often used, as set out above, violates this and makes a statistical analysis quite difficult.

This analysis need not be confined to dichotic situations. For instance, bilateral visual field experiments of the sort pioneered by McKeever and Huling (1971) often yield data appropriate for this analysis. Likewise, Gibson & Bryden (1982) have employed this analysis in a tactual analogue of the dichotic task.

HETEROGENEITY OF LATERALITY MEASURES: COMBINATION OF LATERALITY MEASURES

The preceding discussion has been restricted to the analysis of a single experiment on a single subject. Suppose now that an experiment on a given subject is replicated r times, leading to laterality measures $\hat{\lambda}_i$, with corresponding estimated variances $\hat{\sigma}_i^2$, $i = 1,2, \ldots ,r$. As before, the $\hat{\lambda}_i$ are the estimates of the subject's true laterality measures, λ_i. The simplest hypothesis concerning the λ_is is that these are all equal: $\lambda_i = \lambda(i = 1,2, \ldots , r)$.

Using (12), the r $\hat{\lambda}_i$s and $\hat{\sigma}_i^2$s can be combined to form the corresponding r approximate standard normal quantities, $u(\lambda_i) = u_i$. Then assuming the r experiments are independent, the u_i^2 are independent χ^2 variates with one degree of freedom, so that Σu_i^2 is a χ^2 variate with r degrees of freedom. Under H: $\lambda_1 = \lambda_2 = \ldots = \lambda_r = \lambda$, the quantity Σu_i^2 is a function of the common λ. An estimate of the common λ is:

$$\hat{\lambda} = \sum_i \hat{\lambda}_i/\hat{\sigma}_i^2 / \sum_i 1/\hat{\sigma}_i^2 \tag{14a}$$

Inserting this into each $u_i(\lambda)$ gives $u_i(\hat{\lambda}) = \hat{u}_i$, and the resulting $\Sigma \hat{u}_i^2$ is numerically calculable and has an approximate $\chi^2_{(r - 1)}$ distribution, one degree of freedom being lost in estimating λ. Thus to test for homogeneity, H: $\lambda_i = \lambda$, the quantity $\Sigma \hat{u}_i^2$ can be calculated and referred to the χ^2 distribution with (r - 1) degrees of freedom. If the resulting $\Sigma \hat{u}_i^2$ is not significantly large, the combined experiments yield the estimate $\hat{\lambda}$ for the subject, with variance:

$$\hat{\sigma}_\lambda^2 = 1/ \sum_i (1/\hat{\sigma}_i^2) \tag{14b}$$

COMPARING EXPERIMENTS ON DIFFERENT SUBJECTS: THE RANDOM EFFECTS MODEL

If the r experiments above involve r different subjects, the above combination based on equality $\lambda_i = \lambda$ may be artificial, since it is not to be expected that different subjects have identical λ_is (any more than they have identical heights or weights). Thus, a more complicated model is required to reflect this possibility.

If it is not realistic to assume $\lambda_1 = \lambda_2 = \ldots = \lambda_r$, the next simplest assumption is that the different λ_is are normally distributed about the common λ with unknown variance σ^2. This is similar to the usual "random effects" model for normally distributed observations. However, its use in the above context appears new, and its analysis requires further research. It appears that the normality of $u(\lambda_i)$, of (12), along with the normality of λ_i leads to the quantity,

$$u_i(\lambda,\sigma) = (\hat{\lambda}_i - \lambda) / (\hat{\sigma}_i^2 + \sigma^2)^{1/2} \tag{15}$$

having an approximate standard normal distribution. However the appropriate way of using this fact to estimate λ, σ, based on the results $u_1,...,u_r$ arising from the group of r subjects, requires further investigation.

The most usual way of comparing λ values for different groups of subjects or for the same subjects tested under different conditions is to employ the individual laterality measures, for example, $\hat{\lambda}_i$ in a conventional analysis of variance. Such an analysis, however, fails to make use of the estimated precision, σ_i, of the individual estimate and, in particular, fails to take into account the fact that they differ. In effect, such an analysis assumes infinite precision, $\sigma_i = 0$.

The use of λ as a measure of the degree of laterality provides a measure that is mathematically independent of overall accuracy and can provide significance tests on each individual. For these reasons, it is to be preferred to previous measures suggested in the literature.

Bryden and Sprott (1981) have also shown how λ can be applied to complex laterality tasks such as the free recall of dichotically presented lists of numbers. However, the analysis of such situations becomes exceedingly complex, and it is difficult to argue that the result would be worth the effort. For situations such as this, where the derivation of the appropriate multinomial response model would be difficult, the estimated standard errors, $\sigma \lambda^2$, and resulting analysis will not be easily available. However, laterality measures, $\hat{\lambda}$, can still be constructed in terms of odds ratios, for which estimates will be readily available. These would still seem preferable to the previous measures (1) to (6).

RESPONSE TIME EXPERIMENTS

In recent years, it has become increasingly popular to use response time rather than accuracy as the dependent measure in laterality studies (e.g., McKeever & Jackson, 1979; Moscovitch, 1979; Springer, 1973). Such studies differ from accuracy studies in that the measure or metric is already available, namely, the response time or some simple function of it, such as its reciprocal or logarithm. Thus, many of the problems discussed in the preceding sections do not arise.

However, it is customary in response time studies to collapse over the individual response times in a particular cell and to use the median or mean response time as the primary entry in the data matrix. Such a procedure is obviously discarding a great deal of information and making it impossible to provide a statistical test on the individual subject. It is clear that one should move toward analyses that make fuller use of the data. In quite a different context, Treisman, Squire, and Green (1974) have shown that an analysis of the distribution of individual response times can lead to important psychological information.

How can one incorporate individual response times into an analysis? Assuming the response times, y, or some transform of them, f(y), are normally distributed with constant variance, the analysis would be the usual analysis of variance. The difficulty is that subjects make errors in laterality experiments, and a distinction must be made between trials on which a correct response is made and those on which an incorrect response is made. This leads to situations in which there are unequal numbers of observations per cell. For example, in a two-way classification, the (i, j) cell contains n_{ij} correct responses with corresponding response times, y_{ijk} ($i = 1, 2, j = 1, 2, k = 1, 2, \ldots, n_{ij}$). Then, under the preceding normality assumption, the cell means, $\overline{y}_{ij} = \Sigma_k y_{ijk} / n_{ij}$, will be normally distributed about the population mean, μ_{ij}, with unequal variances, σ^2 / n_{ij}. The analysis of variance is complicated by this fact. A general application of maximum likelihood estimation or a weighted least squares analysis is required; in complicated experiments, great care must be taken. However, with modern computers such analyses are feasible and generally more informative than replacing the observations by their mean or median and performing a standard analysis on them.

AN ILLUSTRATIVE EXAMPLE

After besieging the reader with mathematical formulas, it is perhaps wise to show how our calculations might be applied to an actual laterality experiment. In Table 12-1, the data from an unpublished experiment on single letter recognition conducted by one of the authors (M.P.B.) are shown. In this study, single capital letters were exposed approximately 3° to the left or right of fixation for 10 msec. Subjects were simply asked to identify the letter shown. The study was similar to those previously reported by Bryden (1965) and Bryden and Allard (1976) and involves a task that generally shows a weak right visual field superiority.

Since only a single letter was exposed on any one trial, left and right visual field trials can be treated as giving independent estimates of recognition accuracy. In this case, formula (13b) provides an appropriate measure of laterality. Table 12-1, first presents the distribution of correct and incorrect responses for each visual field. From these data, the value of $\hat{\lambda}$ for each subject has been computed. In the case of Subject 2, for example,

$$\lambda = \log \left(\frac{13 \times 18}{27 \times 22} \right) = \log (.394) = -0.932$$

The data also permit the calculation of a standard deviation for each $\hat{\lambda}$.

Again, for Subject 2,

$$\hat{\sigma}_\lambda = \sqrt{\frac{1}{18} + \frac{1}{13} + \frac{1}{22} + \frac{1}{27}} = 0.464$$

Finally, the individual λ values may be tested for deviation from zero by testing them against their own standard deviation. In the case of Subject 2,

$$z = \frac{-0.932}{0.464} = -2.009$$

Calculations of $\hat{\lambda}$, $\hat{\sigma}_\lambda$, and z_λ for all 16 subjects are shown in Table 12-1. By conventional standards, only four subjects show significant visual field effects: subjects 3, 6, and 9 show a significant right visual field superiority, while subject 2 shows a significant left visual field effect. Even using a much less stringent criterion, such as $p < .25$, would add only subject 15 to the group showing a right visual field effect. Such a finding is not uncommon in laterality studies; most researchers achieve statistical significance by testing large numbers of subjects rather than by using a sufficient number of trials to ensure that individual subjects show significant laterality effects.

TABLE 12-1.
Sample Calculation of Lambda in a Visual Hemifield Experiment

Subject	Left visual field Correct (A)	Left visual field Incorrect (B)	Right visual field Correct (C)	Right visual field Incorrect (D)	$\hat{\lambda}_i$ $\ln\left(\dfrac{B \cdot C}{A \cdot D}\right)$	$\hat{\sigma}_\lambda$	z_i
1	21	19	19	21	-0.2001	0.4477	-0.4470
2	22	18	13	27	-0.9315	0.4636	-2.0091
3	11	29	25	15	1.4802	0.4817	3.0727
4	26	14	28	12	0.2282	0.4784	0.4770
5	6	34	10	30	0.6359	0.5739	1.1081
6	6	34	14	26	1.1155	0.5531	2.0167
7	19	21	21	19	0.2001	0.4477	0.4470
8	25	15	28	12	0.3364	0.4750	0.7082
9	7	33	16	24	1.1451	0.5266	2.1745
10	19	21	17	23	-0.2021	0.4500	-0.4492
11	21	19	24	16	0.3053	0.4521	0.6754
12	27	13	29	11	0.2385	0.4892	0.4875
13	5	25	9	31	0.3726	0.6191	0.6018
14	24	16	23	17	-0.1031	0.4543	-0.2270
15	20	20	27	13	0.7308	0.4625	1.5800
16	17	23	18	22	0.1016	0.4509	0.2253

If the overall significance of the right visual field effect is tested by the conventional use of the t-test, the result is $t(15) = 2.30$, $p = .036$. It is interesting to note that a similar test on the difference scores yields $t(15) = 2.15$, $p = .048$, which is essentially the same result. As mentioned previously, however, more work needs to be done on this problem, since none of the approaches in the literature cited earlier take into account the finite and differing precisions of individual laterality measures [as given, for example, by (11b) for the case of measure (11a)].

Finally, it is necessary to reiterate that the λ value is mathematically independent of overall accuracy. In general, as the right minus left difference score increases, so does the λ value, and there are not likely to be any striking differences between the two analyses. However, if one wishes to go on to relate lateral differences to overall accuracy, for example, λ does not have a spurious correlation with accuracy built into it. Further, λ does provide a metric of the degree of lateralization that makes it a convenient choice if one wishes to relate the degree of lateralization to performance on other behavioral tasks.

ACKNOWLEDGMENTS

Preparation of this chapter was aided by grants to the authors from the Natural Science and Engineering Research Council of Canada.

REFERENCES

Bliss, C.I. The calculation of the dosage-mortality curve. *Annals of Applied Biology*, 1935a, *22*, 134–167.

Bliss, C.I. The comparison of dosage-mortality data. *Annals of Applied Biology*, 1935b, *22*, 307–333.

Bryden, M.P. Tachistoscopic recognition, handedness, and cerebral dominance. *Neuropsychologia*, 1965, *3*, 1–8.

Bryden, M.P. & Allard, F. Visual hemifield differences depend upon typeface. *Brain and Language*, 1976, *3*, 191–200.

Bryden, M.P., & Sprott, D.A. Statistical determination of degree of laterality. *Neuropsychologia*, 1981, *19*, 571–581.

Bryden, M.P., Munhall, K., & Allard, F. Attentional biases and the right-ear effect in dichotic listening. Paper presented at the annual meeting of the Canadian Psychological Association, Calgary, June 1980.

Fechner, G.T. *Elemente der psychophysik*. Leipzig: Breitkopf und Hartel, 1860.

Finney, D.J. *Probit analysis* (3rd ed.). Cambridge: Cambridge University Press, 1971.

Gaddum, J.H. Reports on biological standards III. Methods of biological assay depending on quantal response. Special Report Series, Medical Research Council, London, No. 183, 1933.

Gibson, C., & Bryden, M.P. Cerebral lateralization in deaf children using a dichhaptic task. Paper presented at the annual meeting of the International Neuropsychology Society, Pittsburgh, February 1982.

Green, D.M., & Swets, J.A. *Signal detection theory and psychophysics*. New York: John Wiley & Sons, 1966.

Halwes, T.G. Effects of dichotic fusion on the perception of speech. *Supplement to status report on speech research*. New Haven, Conn.: Haskins Laboratories, 1969.

Kimura, D. Cerebral dominance and the perception of verbal stimuli. *Canadian Journal of Psychology*, 1961, *15*, 166–171.

Kimura, D. Left-right differences in the perception of melodies. *Quarterly Journal of Experimental Psychology*, 1964, *16*, 355–358.

Krashen, S.D. Lateralization, language learning and the critical period: Some new evidence. *Language Learning*, 1973, *23*, 63–74.

Kuhn, G. The phi coefficient as an index of ear differences in dichotic listening. *Cortex*, 1973, *9*, 450–457.

Levy, J. The correlation of the phi function of the difference score with performance and its relevance to laterality experiments. *Cortex*, 1977, *13*, 458–464.

Marshall, J.C., Caplan, D., & Holmes, J.M. The measure of laterality. *Neuropsychologia*, 1975, *13*, 315–322.

McKeever, W.F., & Huling, M.D. Lateral dominance in tachistoscopic word recognition performance obtained with simultaneous bilateral input. *Neuropsychologia*, 1971, *9*, 15–20.

McKeever, W.F., & Jackson, T.L. Cerebral dominance assessed by object- and color-naming latencies: Sex and familial sinistrality effects. *Brain and Language*, 1979, *7*, 175–190.

Moscovitch, M. Information processing and the cerebral hemispheres. In M.S. Gazzaniga (Ed.), *Handbook of behavioral neurobiology* (Vol. 2), *Neuropsychology*. New York: Plenum Press, 1979.

Repp, B.H. Measuring laterality effects in dichotic listening. *Journal of the Acoustical Society of America*, 1977, *62*, 720–737.

Repp, B.H. Stimulus dominance and ear dominance in the perception of dichotic voicing contrasts. *Brain and Language*, 1978, *5*, 310–330.

Springer, S.P. Hemispheric specialization for speech opposed by contralateral noise. *Perception and Psychophysics*, 1973, *13*, 391–393.

Studdert-Kennedy, M., & Shankweiler, D. Hemispheric specialization for speech perception. *Journal of the Acoustical Society of America*, 1970, *48*, 579–594.

Treisman, A.M., Squire, R., & Green, J. Semantic processing in dichotic listening? A replication. *Memory and Cognition*, 1974, *2*, 641–646.

Wexler, B.E., Halwes, T., & Heninger, G.R. Use of a statistical significance criterion in drawing inferences about hemispheric dominance for language function from dichotic listening data. *Brain and Language*, 1981, *13*, 13–18.

13

Individual Differences in Cerebral Hemisphere Asymmetry: Theoretical Issues and Experimental Considerations

Jerre Levy

When neuroanatomy students are first presented with brain specimens, they may perceive little relation between the complex patterns of gyri and sulci in the wet mass before them and the nice drawings in their textbooks. Inspections of other brains in the laboratory reveal enormous variations from specimen to specimen in total size, in geometry of sulcal patterns, in relations of one gyrus to another, or in size of particular regions. In their physical configurations, human brains differ at least as much as human faces, and this is true even of brains from right-handers of the same sex.

There are certain statistical regularities observed in the dextral brain, but a quite substantial minority differs from the group-typical pattern. McRae, Branch, and Milner (1968) found in 87 right-handers that the occipital horn of the lateral ventricle was longer on the left in 60%, equal in 30%, and longer on the right in 10%. Hochberg and LeMay (1975) found that somewhat over two-thirds of right-handers had a larger left than right parietal operculum, but in the remainder, there was either no asymmetry or a reversal of the majority pattern. LeMay (LeMay, 1976, 1977; LeMay & Kido, 1978) found in a large series of dextrals that the right frontal lobe and the left occipital lobe were wider than those on the opposite side in about two-thirds of the sample. About 15% showed a reversed asymmetry, and the remainder displayed no asymmetry.

These large anatomical diversities in the right-handed brain contrast with neurological studies showing that almost all (98% to 99%) dextrals have speech lateralized to the left hemisphere. The homogeneity of right-handers in having verbal processes specialized in the left hemisphere and certain nonverbal processes specialized in the right hemisphere is one of the most striking characteristics of the dextral population and contrasts greatly with the heterogeneity of left-handers with respect to lateral specialization of function. It is difficult to believe that the anatomical variations would not have functional consequences, and there is some data to show that they do.

Schenkman, Butler, Naeser, and Kleefield (1981) examined nine patients with left hemisphere lesions and global aphasia and assessed functional ability on nine activities (e.g., bed mobility, feeding, driving) one to three months after insult. The greatest improvement was found in three patients with reversals of the typical frontal/occipital width asymmetries, whereas little improvement was found in patients with the typical asymmetry or no asymmetry. Hier, LeMay, Rosenberger, and Perlo (1978) studied occipital width asymmetry in 24 people with developmental dyslexia and found a great increase in the proportion with reversed asymmetry (42%). Those with reversed asymmetries had lower verbal IQs, as compared with those with the typical asymmetry, but the two groups scored the same for performance IQ. Luchins, Weinberger, and Wyatt (1979) found that right-handed schizophrenics had increased frequencies of asymmetry reversals, both for occipital width and for frontal width. The reversed asymmetries were concentrated in those schizophrenics without cerebral atrophy. These relations were subsequently confirmed in a larger sample of schizophrenics (Luchins, Weinberger, & Wyatt, 1981).

Although the data that relate anatomical to functional diversities in right-handers are still meager, they rather strongly suggest that there are aspects of lateral hemispheric functioning that are considerably more diverse among right-handers than specialization itself (considered in the classical sense). Thus, although language functions may be left hemisphere specialized and certain nonverbal functions may be right hemisphere specialized in the vast majority of right-handers, there appear to be other characteristics of lateral hemispheric functioning, related to anatomical asymmetries, that are considerably more variable.

This possibility is of great interest because normative studies of lateralization, although typically revealing the expected perceptual asymmetry on dichotic or lateralized tachistoscopic tasks for the sample of subjects as a whole, almost always find that a significant minority of subjects fails to display a significant asymmetry and that, even among those manifesting the expected direction of asymmetry, there is a large variability in magnitude. At least in some cases, laterality measures have been shown to be highly stable, so the diversities among subjects cannot be attributed to random error of measurement. It is always possible that an experimenter is reliably measuring factors having nothing to do with hemispheric lateral functioning and that differ among subjects. There is also the possibility that the laterality index is inappropriate so that it reflects a generic correlation with performance levels rather than real differences in asymmetry among subjects. However, the possibility that right-handers actually vary in important aspects of hemispheric functioning that are more or less independent of classical conceptions of hemispheric specialization and that standard laterality indexes are sensitive to these characteristics, as well as to the classical specialization factor, cannot be ruled out.

The normative study suffers from different interpretative difficulties than the neurological study, but the problems are at least or more severe. Correct inferences depend upon the assumptions that the test is reliable, that it validly reflects hemispheric functioning, that it validly measures the process it was designed to measure, and that, given validity in the data base, a valid laterality index has been employed. It is difficult to know whether these assumptions are met, and it is difficult to generate paradigms that can effectively evaluate the validity of the assumptions. Particularly when the issue of individual differences is addressed, one is faced with determining whether, even if group averages can be accepted as real, variations among subjects are meaningful. Do diversities among subjects in ear or visual field asymmetries represent real underlying differences in brain organization, or, alternatively, are they due to insufficient reliability and/or validity? Although the problems confronted in attempting to answer such questions have no easy solutions, they are not insolvable, and in the section to follow, suggestions are offered for disentangling hemispheric effects from other sources of variance.

SOURCES OF ERROR AND SUGGESTIONS FOR CONTROL

Reliability of the Measure

The reliability of a measure (e.g., RVF scores) is the ratio of true score variance to true score plus error variance. Thus, if the reliability of a measure is 0.85, 15% of the observed variance arises from error. The reliability of a difference score is given by the true score variance for one component score (e.g., RVF scores) plus the true variance for the other component score (e.g., LVF scores), minus twice the covariance between components, all divided by these factors plus the error variances for each component score.

For simplicity, let it be assumed that the observed variances of the RVF and LVF scores are equal, that their reliabilities are both 0.85, and that the covariance between RVF and LVF scores is half the true variance for either component. If the observed variance is set to unity, the reliability of the difference score would be:

$$r_{d,d'} = \frac{0.85 + 0.85 - 2(0.425)}{0.85 + 0.15 + 0.15} = 0.74$$

As the correlation between LVF and RVF scores increases in a positive direction, the reliability of the difference score decreases. At the limit, if the correlation of true scores between fields is unity, given the assumptions stated, all the variance in difference scores arises from error, and the reliability of the difference score is zero.

One can see immediately, therefore, that, even when the reliabilities of component scores are high, the reliability of the difference score can be quite low. However, note that, if the correlation between component scores is zero, the reliability of the difference score equals the reliability of a component score (where reliabilities of component scores are equal). Further, if there is a negative covariance between component scores, the reliability of the difference score will be greater than the reliability of a component score. In the example given, if the covariance in the numerator of the equation were negative, the value of the numerator would be 2.55 and the value of the denominator would be 2.85, giving a reliability for the difference score of 0.895. Thus, factors that would tend to put the two sensory half-fields in competition (dichotic paradigms, bilateral visual-field presentations, titration of exposure duration or of other factors affecting clarity of the stimulus in accordance with overall accuracy or speed of response averaged across fields, etc.) would be expected to counteract positive between-field correlations and to increase the reliability of the difference score.

In addition, since error, by definition, is uncorrelated with true scores, the more trials that are given, the smaller is the proportion of variance due to error since errors in one direction or the other are random and will tend to cancel. With a sufficiently large number of trials, the error component of variance will approach zero. The effect of trial number can easily be seen by comparing reliabilities for ear asymmetries on CV syllables, using stop consonants when trial number varies. Shankweiler and Studdert-Kennedy (1975) administered 120 dichotic CV trials on each of 2 days to one group of 22 subjects varying in handedness and to another group of 30 subjects who were right-handed. For both groups, the test-retest reliability for ear asymmetry was a quite respectable 0.70 for both groups. In contrast, Teng (1981) administered only 58 trials of dichotic CV syllables to 51 right-handed subjects at each of 2 test sessions and found a test-retest reliability for ear asymmetry of only 0.36.

The difference in reliabilities for Shankweiler and Studdert-Kennedy (1975) versus Teng (1981) is, however, only partially due to trial number. When a test is doubled in length, the true score variance is quadrupled, but the error variance is only doubled (Magnusson, 1967). If we set the observed variance to 1 for a test of a given length and if the reliability of the measure is 0.36, doubling test length will give a true score variance of 1.44, an error variance of 1.28, a total variance of 2.72, and a reliability of 0.53. The observed reliability found by Shankweiler and Studdert-Kennedy is higher than predicted from Teng's (1981) result, suggesting that additional sources of error were present in the Teng study, as compared with the Shankweiler and Studdert-Kennedy study, beyond simple test length.

The effect of trial number on reliability entails the assumption that all factors affecting performance remain invariant except for trial number itself. This is rarely, if ever, true. Subjects may be unstable during early trials before they adopt a consistent strategy of response (suggesting the importance of practice trials). Second, even after an initial stability is achieved, new cognitive operations may subsequently come into play as stimuli become increasingly familiar. Third, as trials proceed, fatigue may set in, introducing another source of variance. Fourth, time of day when the test and retest are run can affect performance if subjects are at different points in their circadian rhythms, and control over these factors may differ for different experiments that use different trial numbers. Detailed experimental factors may also differ for different experiments, such as those of Shankweiler and Studdert-Kennedy (1975) and that of Teng (1981). The former authors, for example, reversed earphones at the midway point in trials to control for possible differences between channels. Teng (1981), however, states that she set the amplication of the two channels to be identical and left them unchanged. With no switching of channels between ears and no recalibration of the earphones between sessions, it would not be surprising to find that channel amplitudes could change between sessions, with effects on subjects' asymmetries. In any case, all other things being equal, the administration of a relatively large trial number in laterality experiments will do much to overcome the problem of low reliabilities.

The Laterality Index

When laterality experiments are performed, the experimenter has performance measures [either accuracy or reaction time (RT)] for each sensory half-field and, from these measures, wishes to derive an index of lateralization that will be linear with respect to cerebral asymmetry of function. Linearity means that if a subject is one-half standard deviation more asymmetric on the index than the mean of the sample, the subject is also one-half standard deviation more asymmetric in hemispheric differentiation than the mean of the sample. In order to convert performance measures into an index with this characteristic, as Birkett (1977) has noted, a theory of brain function that will specify the appropriate transformation equation is required.

Thus, suppose on a go-no-go RT experiment involving a tachistoscopic lexical decision task, subject A has a 15 msec advantage in favor of the right visual field (RVF) and subject B has a RVF advantage of 20 msec. If the simple difference in RTs between fields is taken as the laterality index, we would conclude that B is more asymmetric than A. However, if A has a mean RT of 500 msec., the RVF advantage is 3% relative to the mean RT for the LVF, and if B has a mean RT of 700 msec, the RVF advantage is also 3% relative to the mean RT for the LVF. From this measure, one could conclude that the two subjects have equal degrees of hemispheric differentiation. It could also be found that for A, only 20% of LVF trials are faster than the mean of RVF trials, whereas for B, 30% of LVF trials are faster than the mean of RVF trials; if this index were used, one could conclude that A is more asymmetric in hemispheric function than B. Inconsistent conclusions are reached from the three different indexes, and without a theory of brain function, the correct one cannot be specified.

When accuracy is the dependent variable, one is not only confronted with inconsistent inferences from different laterality indexes (Birkett, 1977; Colbourn, 1978; Harshman & Krashen, 1972; Krashen & Harshman, 1972; Kuhn, 1973; Marshall, Caplan, & Holmes, 1975; Richardson, 1976) but also with the fact that, for some subjects, the performance measures are not valid reflections of hemispheric asymmetry (i.e., the measures themselves are invalid), due to near-ceiling or near-floor performance. When this occurs, no possible transformation can yield a valid laterality index since no mathematical legerdemain exists that can create validity from invalidity. The best that any laterality measure can do is to preserve the valid information in the data. If, for any subject, the total number of trials correct or incorrect (summed across sensory half-fields) is less than about nine or ten, it is futile to try to generate a laterality index for that subject since the error on the measure would be extremely large (if a small trial number has been given). If a large trial number has been given, the subject is close to ceiling or floor performance, making asymmetry of performance highly insensitive to differences between hemispheres.

It should be kept in mind, therefore, that there is a strong distinction between validity of a transformation function versus validity of the data base from which it is derived. Even if the transformation function is valid, an index for a given subject may be completely invalid because the data base for that subject is invalid. In specifying an appropriate laterality index, it must be assumed that the data contain valid information. When that assumption is not met, no index is valid and no justified conclusions can be drawn.

In almost all cases, laterality indexes that have been suggested rest on an unacknowledged theory of functional asymmetry. This theory can be called "the anatomical model," since it assumes that functional differences between hemispheres, like anatomical differences between hemispheres, have some fixed and unvarying value that is specified by the mean of the distribution of performance measures for each sensory half-field. Variability in performance over trials within a sensory half-field is assumed to be random and independent of the characteristics of the system being measured. Thus, an anatomist who has a brain specimen and wants to specify the relative sizes of the left and right temporal planes might take ten measurements on each side, with the mean of each set of measurements being taken to represent the best estimate of the anatomical region. The anatomist assumes that measurement-to-measurement variation results from the limitations of the instruments and from the limitations in accuracy of measurement and assumes that the size of the anatomical region remains completely fixed over measurements; the variation of anatomical measurements has nothing to do with any variation of the thing being measured. The anatomist is, consequently, justified in taking the mean of the sets of measurements as being the only relevant factor in designating the asymmetry of the planum temporale.

I believe this anatomical model is completely unjustified in attempts to specify functional differentiation between hemispheres. A functional system is, by its very nature, dynamic, and its level of processing can vary from moment to moment (trial to trial) in consequence of such factors as general activation, attentional focusing, degree of distraction, and other neuropsychological variables. Further, there is no reason to suppose that the effects of such factors on the functioning of each side of the brain are invariant, and if not, asymmetry of function can be similarly variable. This is to suggest that some fixed processing level of a hemisphere cannot be specified, since processing competency, although having some mean level for the given conditions of the experiment, also has some distribution that is as characteristic of the hemisphere as its average. I would claim, in other words, that, even if two subjects both have a mean RT of 500 (averaged across sensory half-fields) and even if both have a 20 msec advantage in favor of the RVF, it would be illegitimate to conclude that they have the same level of hemispheric differentiation of function if 30% of LVF trials are faster than the mean of RVF trials for one subject but if only 10% of LVF trials are faster than the mean of RVF trials for the other subject.

Under the dynamic model, the degree (and direction) of functional hemispheric differentiation is specified by the correlation between performance on each trial and sensory half-field (dichotomized as zero and one). For RT data, this yields the point-biserial correlation, r_{pb}, and for accuracy data, this yields the fourfold point correlation, r_p, also known as the phi coefficient. These correlations designate the importance of sensory half-field in affecting performance and, by inference, the importance of the hemispheric factor. Their squares specify the proportion of total variation in performance that derives from sensory half-field. These correlations not only reflect the mean performance for each sensory half-field but also the variability in performance for each sensory half-field.

As an analogy, one may consider the problem of gender differentiation for a given cognitive function. Many have noted that, even when there is a relatively large difference between the average of the sexes in performance on some task, there is tremendous overlap. In understanding how distinct the sexes are and how differentiated they are with respect to some cognitive process, appreciation of the degree of overlap is central to any specification that might be given. Thus, if the means of the two sexes are separated by even as much as 1 standard deviation, relative to within-sex variation (and assuming equal within-sex variances), 80% of the total variation in performance is within-sex variance and only 20% derives from the between-sex difference. This is equivalent to a point-biserial correlation between gender and performance of $r_{pb} = 0.447$ (since $r^2_{pb} = 0.20$). In considering gender differentiation, it is recognized that there are large and real diversities within the sexes, that some members of the inferior sex will surpass the average of the superior sex, and that the importance of the gender factor in performance can only be specified by a statistic that shows the difference between sexes relative to the variation within sexes.

Under the dynamic model of hemispheric function, trial-to-trial variations in performance within sensory half-fields are just as real and meaningful as person-to-person variations in performance within sexes, and the importance of the sensory half-field factor is specified by a statistic that reflects the difference in sensory half-fields, relative to variation within sensory half-fields.

The two correlations can be simply derived from:

$$\phi = r_{\mathrm{p}} = \frac{P_{\mathrm{R}} - P_{\mathrm{L}}}{2\sqrt{PQ}} \, , \tag{1}$$

when accuracy is the dependent variable, where P_{R} and P_{L} are proportions correct for the right and left sensory half-fields, respectively, P is the total proportion correct (summed across fields), and $Q = 1 - P$ is the total proportion incorrect (summed across fields), and from

$$r_{\mathrm{pb}} = \frac{\overline{RT}_{\mathrm{L}} - \overline{RT}_{\mathrm{R}}}{2s} \, , \tag{2}$$

when RT is the dependent variable, where $\overline{RT}_{\mathrm{R}}$ and $\overline{RT}_{\mathrm{L}}$ are the mean RTs for the right and left sensory half-fields, respectively, and s is the standard deviation computed over all trials. It may be noted that the two equations are structurally identical since $\sqrt{PQ}$ is the standard deviation, computed over all trials, of the proportions, a structural identity that is expected, given that both correlations are product-moment relations. When correlations have been computed for each subject in the sample, parametric treatment of the data can be carried out, once the correlations have been z-transformed by Fisher's method:

$$z = 1/2 \ln_{\mathrm{e}}(1 + r) - 1/2 \ln_{\mathrm{e}}(1 - r) \, . \tag{3}$$

The z-transformed correlations are additive and have a Gaussian distribution; the z-transforms may be used to compare subjects under different conditions or to compare different groups of subjects or both.

Others may disagree regarding my proposed dynamic model of hemispheric differentiation and may believe that the various "anatomical models" yield measures closer to their intuitions. It might be noted that, when accuracy is the dependent variable, the simple difference in proportions correct for the two sensory half-fields is identical to $r_{\mathrm{p}}(\phi)$ when overall performance is at 50% accuracy and differs little from r_{p} unless performance approaches ceiling or floor. Although $r_{\mathrm{p}}(\phi)$ gives the exact laterality index under a dynamic model, the simple difference in proportions correct (for a valid data base) is so close to r_{p} that it may be used with little concern. However, the discrepancy in conclusions reached for RT data, depending upon whether one uses an "anatomical" or a dynamic model of hemispheric functioning, can be very large, and therefore, it becomes highly important for researchers to consider the issues in some detail and to reach clear decisions regarding their own conceptualizations of hemispheric function. I have presented my own perspective, but it may be wrong, and only the collaborative efforts of the research community will be able to lead to a consensus that all can accept with comfort.

Validity of the Measure

Assuming that one has identified a highly reliable asymmetry measure and has adopted an appropriate laterality index, there is still the question of whether one is actually measuring properties of differential hemispheric functioning, and if so, what properties are being assessed. One could, for example, be reliably measuring biases in subjects for a left-to-right scan of iconic images, complex sensory differences between the two ears, or the relative efficiency of ipsilateral versus contralateral auditory pathways (Teng, 1981). Researchers might believe that they are indexing lateralization for face recognition when, in fact, they are assessing ability and lateralization for salient-feature detection. Obviously, certain of these differences (e.g., acuity differences between ears) are easy to detect and control, but other sources of error may not be so easy to identify.

There are two quite separate and distinct aspects of differential hemispheric functioning that are likely to affect performance on laterality tasks. The normative literature on laterality makes it clear that the vast body of researchers who attempt to assess functional asymmetry with dichotic listening, tachistoscopic, or dichhaptic methods seek to measure hemispheric specialization of function. The central premise is that, if one hemisphere is more specialized than the other for a given task, performance should be superior for stimuli presented in the contralateral sensory half-field. Different researchers have offered different models regarding the mechanisms by which hemispheric specialization results in perceptual asymmetries. These include the "split-brain" model, which says that the hemisphere initially receiving sensory information processes it and that differences between fields directly reflect differences in processing ability for the two sides of the brain. The "transfer" model proposes that, regardless of the sensory half-field in which a stimulus occurs, it is processed by the specialized hemisphere and that differences in performance between fields result from a delay or information loss in the course of transcommissural transfer. Activation or arousal models suggest that the specialized hemisphere becomes differentially aroused by tasks within its particular domain of abilities, biasing attention toward the contralateral half of space and yielding perceptual asymmetries that reflect greater attention for information in one field than in the other. It is probable that all these mechanisms operate, to one degree or another, in most laterality tasks, but the central point is that all the models of perceptual asymmetry ultimately derive from differences in the specialized abilities of each side of the brain. They all assume, in other words, that the sole aspect of hemispheric functioning reflected on laterality tasks is hemispheric specialization. If true, this would mean that, were it possible to control for scanning factors, acuity factors, processes entailed in the task, and so forth, the pattern of perceptual asymmetry shown by a subject would be a reflection of the differences between hemispheres in specialization. In this case, one should observe asymmetries that are perfectly congruent with inferences drawn from the neurological literature, not only with respect to the average performances of subjects, but also with respect to variations or their lack across subjects.

I believe that hemispheric specialization is only one aspect of hemispheric functioning that affects perceptual asymmetries and that, even with the most conceptually perfect task, one can never observe patterns of performance having perfect congruence with neurological inferences. I do not believe that studies of unilaterally brain-damaged patients versus normative studies with dichotic or tachistoscopic techniques measure the same factors in individual patients or subjects. The consistency that appears is a consistency with respect to statistical averages; neurological investigations reveal that language is specialized to the left hemisphere in the vast majority of right-handers while normative studies show that, on appropriate verbal tasks, there is a right sensory field advantage for right-handers, as a group. The group inference from normative studies supports neurological findings, and in both cases, I believe hemispheric specialization is being reflected. However, not all right-handers show the expected perceptual asymmetry, and even among those who do, there is a large variation in the degree of asymmetry observed.

What is responsible for this diversity? Is this merely error variance, or are there real individual differences among right-handed subjects in some aspect of hemispheric functioning? If there are real individual differences, it seems highly unlikely that these are differences in hemispheric specialization itself. Such differences should appear in studies of neurological patients but, in fact, do not. I am convinced, for reasons to be discussed in detail in later sections, that people have characteristic, habitual, and stable patterns of asymmetric hemispheric arousal, ranging from differentially high right-hemispheric arousal, through approximate equality of hemispheric arousal, to differentially high left-hemisphere arousal. If true, consider the effects of the arousal pattern on standard measures of laterality. If a verbal test is presented to a right-hander with asymmetrically high right hemisphere arousal, the hemispheric-specialization effect would operate to produce a right sensory field advantage, but the arousal factor would operate to produce a left sensory field advantage, with the two effects canceling each other to varying degrees (depending upon the magnitude of asymmetric arousal). This subject would manifest either a small right field advantage, no asymmetry, or a small left field advantage. The same subject, given a face recognition task, would be expected to show a very large left field advantage because the hemispheric-specialization effect and the arousal effect would summate. The reverse situation would occur for a subject having differentially high left hemisphere arousal.

Thus, the average pattern of asymmetry for a group of right-handers would reveal the dextral pattern of hemispheric specialization, but diversities among right-handers in the direction and/or magnitude of perceptual asymmetries would reflect variations in patterns of asymmetric hemispheric arousal that were superimposed on a relatively invariant pattern of hemispheric specialization characteristic of dextrals. If such habitual arousal asymmetries, varying in direction and degree, occur among people, dichotic or tachistoscopic measures must necessarily reflect both this factor and hemispheric specialization itself. One cannot, in other words, develop a "pure" measure of the latter, even in principle. This means that the validity of laterality indexes, as a measure of hemispheric specialization, cannot be perfect. Similarly, the validity of laterality indexes, as a measure of characteristic patterns of asymmetric arousal, must also be imperfect.

Given the fact that the laterality index is a "mixed measure" of two different aspects of hemispheric functioning, one can nonetheless assess how well the index measures the specialization factor by comparing different groups of subjects. If the measure is sensitive to hemispheric specialization, differences in asymmetry between right- and left-handed groups should be observed. Further, within a group of right-handers, average asymmetry patterns should differ for tasks designed to assess left hemisphere function versus those designed to assess right hemisphere function. If the task reflects hemispheric factors rather than scanning effects, the same asymmetry pattern should be observed for subjects who read from left to right and for those who read from right to left (e.g., Israelis). These and other types of checks on what a given task is measuring are highly important in laterality investigations. If only a single task, having a single measure for each sensory half-field, is given to one homogeneous group of subjects, there is no way of knowing whether the asymmetry observed has anything to do with hemispheric function or not. At earlier times, it was assumed that any asymmetries observed on lateralized tachistoscopic tasks derived from left-to-right scanning. Currently, it is generally assumed that any such asymmetries necessarily derive from hemispheric specialization; it is important that the validity of this assumption be empirically evaluated.

The major consideration to be kept in mind is that the experimental procedure should be such as to provide relevant information for deciding

whether the average performance of the group and the variations in performance among subjects are likely to reflect hemispheric specialization, characteristic patterns of asymmetric hemispheric arousal, or factors having nothing to
do with asymmetric functioning of the cerebral hemispheres. It is of crucial
importance that an experimenter recognize the distinction between a perceptual asymmetry for a given task and asymmetric hemispheric functioning for
some postulated process and, of equal importance, distinguish subject-to-
subject variations that may safely be regarded as random error versus those
that arise from real individual differences.

VARIATIONS AMONG RIGHT-HANDERS IN PATTERNS OF FUNCTIONAL BRAIN ASYMMETRY

Emotion and Personality

Models of Hemispheric Function in Emotion

The role of the two hemispheres in emotional/personality function is
currently a matter of serious debate. The most prevalent view, and one with
which I concur, is that the right hemisphere plays a special role in the
experience, expression, and discrimination of all emotion, whether dysphoric
or euphoric. Thus, in normal right-handed subjects, the majority displays a
left ear advantage in discrimination of the emotional tone of voice (Safer &
Leventhal, 1977), an LVF advantage in recognizing facial expressions
(Buchtel, Campari, De Risio, & Rota, 1978; Heller & Levy, 1981; Safer,
1981); and an asymmetry in favor of the left side of the face in the production
of expressions (Campbell, 1978; Chaurasia & Goswami, 1975; Heller & Levy,
1981; Moscovitch & Olds, 1979; Sackeim & Gur, 1978).

In clinical investigations, right hemisphere damage impairs story recall
for stories with emotional content (Wechsler, 1973); produces a specific deficit
in judging the emotional mood of the speaker when listening to spoken
sentences (Heilman, Scholes, & Watson, 1975); is associated with disabilities
in comprehending emotional expression on faces, over and above any general
impairment in facial recognition (Cicone, Wapner, & Gardner, 1979, cited in
Tucker, 1981); and causes difficulties in expressing emotion through tonal

inflections in speech (Ross & Mesulam, 1979). Under this model of hemispheric differentiation of emotion, variations in emotional/personality characteristics of normal right-handers would arise from differences in the affective
tone and related characteristics of the right hemisphere. Thus, those with the
critical, depressive, inward-looking, and untrusting attitudes of introverts
would have a dysphoric right hemisphere, while those with the uncritical,
optimistic, outward-looking, and trusting attitudes of extraverts would have a
euphoric right hemisphere (see, e.g., Eysenck's, 1967, characterization of these
polar personality types).

Alternative views hold that the two hemispheres play equal roles in
emotion but that the emotional valence of each side differs. Sackeim,
Greenberg, Weiman et al. (1982) propose that the left hemisphere tends
toward euphoria and the right hemisphere toward dysphoria, whereas Tucker
(1981) proposes that it is the right hemisphere that tends toward euphoria and
the left hemisphere toward dysphoria. Sackeim et al. base their interpretation
on findings that catastrophic/depressive reactions are associated with left
hemisphere damage and that complacency/euphoric reactions are associated
with right hemisphere damage (Alford, 1933; Gainotti, 1969, 1972; Hall,
Hall, & Lavoie, 1968; Hécaen, 1962); on reports that brief unilateral
inactivation of the left hemisphere with barbiturates is related to dysphoric
reactions as patients are recovering from the anesthesia, with euphoric
reactions related to right hemisphere inactivation (Rossi & Rosadini, 1967);
and on their own analysis of case reports of patients displaying pathological
laughing or crying resulting from brain damage, where crying was found to
occur with left side damage and laughing with right side damage (Sackeim et
al., 1982). Their interpretation is that damage to one or the other side results
in disinhibition of the intact hemisphere, so that the pathological emotion
displayed characterizes the emotional valence of the undamaged side.

Tucker (1981) interprets these same data in a radically different way. He
suggests that cortical damage results in disinhibition of ipsilateral limbic
regions, with brain damage exaggerating the emotional tone of the damaged
hemisphere. He points out that the emotional effects of unilateral hemispheric
inactivation are not observed when anesthesia is complete, but rather only as
patients are recovering, that is, during that time when it is reasonable to
suppose that the subcortical regions have regained function but prior to
cortical recovery. If Tucker's description of the time course of events is correct,
the observations pose major difficulties for the Sackeim et al. (1982)
hypothesis.

Both lateralized-valence models conflict, however, with the proposal that
the right hemisphere predominates in all emotions. If either of the former is
correct, data that appear to support the right hemisphere–predominance model
demand some account, and if, alternatively, these latter data are an accurate

description of reality, observations suggesting different emotional valences for the two hemispheres require explanation. One possibility that could reconcile the various findings incorporates both the idea, in accordance with Sackeim et al. (1982), that arousal relations between hemispheres are reciprocally inhibitory, and the idea, in accordance with Tucker (1981), that cortical regions exercise a modulatory and inhibitory influence over ipsilateral subcortical areas, while also holding that the right hemisphere is crucial for the regulation of all emotion.

The central hypothesis of this model is that the arousal level of the right hemisphere determines the nature of its affective tone: when arousal is high, affect tends toward euphoria and when arousal is low, affect tends toward dysphoria. The tonic arousal system not only involves ascending input to higher regions from the midbrain activating system but also descending input from higher regions to the midbrain, which serve to maintain arousal in the absence of sensory stimulation. Such a loop, however, is reciprocally facilitatory, involving a positive feedback pathway, and if unmodulated, would result in runaway hyperarousal and mania. I would speculate that limbic areas are crucially involved in the tonic arousal pathway, receiving activating input from the midbrain and sending signals to the midbrain for the maintenance of arousal, with certain neocortical regions (prefrontal areas?) serving to inhibit and modulate limbic and midbrain activity. Thus, the corticolimbic and corticomidbrain pathways would serve to regulate the arousal level in order to prevent a runaway hyperactivation. Disorders in control pathways could result in pathologically low or high arousal levels, and differences among people in the relative predominance of various components of the tonic arousal system could result in differences in average arousal levels. Trevarthen (1974) has concluded, from studies of split-brain patients, that brainstem commissures mediate a reciprocal inhibition of arousal between the two sides of the nervous system. If so, this would mean that high right hemisphere arousal would tend to occur with lower levels of left hemisphere arousal and vice versa.

Trevarthen's (1974) conclusion was based upon findings that, in split-brain patients, there are pervasive hemi-inattention phenomena, seen both with auditory and visual input. Although these patients can verbally report monaural left ear input with perfect accuracy, there is a total left ear suppression with dichotic listening. With bilateral visual input, patients are aware of the stimulus in only one visual field, the RVF for tasks calling on specialties of the left hemisphere and the LVF for tasks calling on specialties of the right hemisphere. This radical attentional bias for one sensory half-field under conditions of bilateral input, with complete suppression of one half of space, contrasts greatly with normal people who can attend to information on both sides of space simultaneously, at least to a significant extent. The hemi-inattention phenomena can be explained under the supposition that brain stem commissures mediate a reciprocal inhibition of arousal, producing strong asymmetries of arousal between the two sides of the brain, asymmetries that are greatly reduced and controlled in the normal brain through cross-facilitation via the neocortical commissures.

Thus, in the normal brain, mutual facilitation would be expected to produce a positive correlation in arousal between hemispheres, but a certain degree of arousal asymmetry would be expected from the mutual inhibition occurring at lower levels. Under this model, right cortical damage would disrupt the inhibitory pathways to the ipsilateral limbic areas and midbrain, resulting in increased limbic activation and euphoria. The effects of left cortical damage on emotion would be indirect. There would be a release of ipsilateral limbic and midbrain activity and, via the reciprocally inhibitory brain stem commissures, a decrease in ascending activity to the right hemisphere and dysphoria.

The findings of Sackeim et al. (1982) that ictal laughing occurs predominantly with left hemisphere epileptic foci could be explained as follows. During seizure activity, although cortical processing is totally disrupted, there would be a massive inhibition of ipsilateral limbic and midbrain areas, biasing arousal output toward the right hemisphere and releasing pathological laughing. With right hemisphere foci, the entire emotional processing system would be disrupted so that pathological affective behaviors would not occur. This could also explain why pathological ictal crying is almost never observed. Sackeim et al. (1982) offer no explanation for the much greater frequency of ictal laughing as compared with ictal crying; under their lateralized valence model, ictal laughing and crying should be equally common.

During interictal states, R. C. Gur (personal communication, June 1981) reports that a large area surrounding the epileptic focus is greatly depressed in metabolic activity, that is, the area can be considered to be functionally ablated and equivalent to a cortical lesion. This is congruent, under the present arousal model, with Bear and Fedio's findings (1977) that epileptic patients with left and right hemisphere foci differ in self-evaluations, the former magnifying socially negative characteristics and underplaying socially positive characteristics within themselves, and the latter doing the reverse. In other words, left focus patients have an unduly harsh self-view and right focus patients have an unduly positive self-view. Bear and Fedio describe the consequences of an epileptic focus as producing a "hyperconnection" between cortical and subcortical areas, with the implication that subcortical systems come to play a more dominant role in emotional regulation than is the case in the nonepileptic brain.

Supporting at least some aspects of the model, frontocortical destruction results in a disinhibition syndrome correlated with relief from depression (Hécaen, 1964; Lishman, 1968), Perris and Monakhov (1979) found that greater activation of right frontal cortex correlated with greater depression in psychiatric patients. If right frontocortical activity represents strong inhibitory and/or modulatory input to ipsilateral limbic and midbrain regions, this would be exactly what is expected under the arousal model. As Tucker (1981) discusses, there is evidence that catecholamine-mediated arousal from antidepressant medication is associated with a specific effect on the right hemisphere, that an increase in norepinephrine mediates the effects of electroconvulsive shock, and that ECT produces a selective arousal of the right hemisphere (Kronfol, Hamsher, Digre, & Waziri, 1978). The cognitive aftereffects of ECT suggest that it produces a transient functional destruction of cortical processes, implying a reduction in cortical inhibition. It does not seem unreasonable, therefore, to propose that, when the cortical inhibitory component of the emotional regulatory system of the right hemisphere predominates over the subcortical activating component, overall arousal is low and affect is dysphoric and that when the subcortical activating component of this regulatory system predominates, overall arousal is high and affect is euphoric. If this proposal has any validity, it means that arousal asymmetries between hemispheres would be a secondary index of right hemisphere arousal; an arousal asymmetry in favor of the right hemisphere would indicate overall high right hemisphere arousal, and an arousal asymmetry in favor of the left hemisphere would indicate overall low right hemisphere arousal (and, of course, high left hemisphere arousal). Higher arousal of the left hemisphere would not indicate reliance on a dysphoric left hemisphere for emotional experience but would, instead, indicate a dysphoria emerging from the right hemisphere, due to its low arousal level.

Both Tucker's model (1981) and the present one would predict that variations in personality/emotional dimensions would be associated with differences in arousal relationships between hemispheres, higher right hemisphere arousal correlating with positive affect, and higher left hemisphere arousal correlating with negative affect. However, Tucker would predict that a highly aroused left hemisphere would manifest dysphoria in people with a gloomy outlook, whereas the present model would predict that the right hemisphere in such people would manifest dysphoria, with the left hemisphere displaying neutral affect. Both models would predict that the highly aroused right hemisphere in people with a sunny outlook would display euphoria, and both yield predictions that are opposed to those derived from Sackeim et al. (1982).

Individual Differences in Personality and Cerebral Function

The direction of lateral eye movements in response to reflective questions has been employed by many investigators as an index of asymmetric hemispheric engagement/arousal, leftward eye movements being taken to indicate right hemisphere activation and rightward eye movements being taken to indicate left hemisphere activation. R. E. Gur and R. C. Gur (1975) compared left-movers and right-movers on defensive style, finding that left-movers, significantly more often than right-movers, dealt with conflict in a positive or neutral fashion, that is, they employed the defense mechanism of reversal, entailing repression, denial, negation, and reaction formation. Left-movers, in other words, did not allow negative affect into consciousness. Psychosomatic symptoms were also found to be more prevalent in left-movers than in right-movers, and Galin, Diamond, and Braff (1977) and Stern (1977) found that hysterical conversion reactions were more prevalent on the left side of the body than on the right. These observations support the view that asymmetrically high right hemisphere arousal is related to a tendency to block negative affect from consciousness, resulting in a conversion to bodily disorders. Smokler and Shevrin (1979) supported these conclusions by finding that individuals showing a strong hysteric cognitive style versus those with obsessive-compulsive tendencies differed in eye-movement directionality, the former having a predominance of leftward eye movements and the latter having a preponderance of rightward eye movements.

Shearer and Tucker (in press) had subjects view slides of aversive or sexual material and requested subjects either to facilitate or inhibit their emotional arousal. Ratings of subjects' cognitive strategies showed that verbal/analytic mechanisms were used to inhibit arousal, whereas global/imagistic mechanisms were used to facilitate arousal. In a second study (Tucker & Newman, in press), subjects were trained to use either a verbal/analytic or a global/imagistic strategy to inhibit arousal to aversive or sexual slides. Self-reports and measures of skin temperature indicated that verbal/analytic processes were more effective in inhibiting emotional arousal. Since it may be presumed that sexual arousal is positive in affective tone, while aversive arousal is negative in affective tone, these data suggest that, regardless of the valence of the affect, differential engagement of the right hemisphere serves to facilitate emotional arousal, whereas differential engagement of the left hemisphere cognitive (cortical) processes serves to reduce emotional arousal.

Neither lateralized-valence model can account for these data, although Tucker (1981) has suggested that the cognitive properties of the left hemisphere are well suited for the modulation and control of emotion and that those of the right hemisphere are well suited for their elaboration. He seems to propose that cognitive processing of the left hemisphere entails inhibition of limbically mediated affect and that right hemisphere engagement entails integration and elaboration of affective experience through a strong functional interconnection of cortical and subcortical regions within the right hemisphere. If so, one would expect that right cortical damage, because of disruption of the hypothesized integrative system, would never produce an exaggeration of affect, yet it is precisely such an exaggeration that Tucker suggests. There appears to be a basic inconsistency between Tucker's two proposals, and I am unable to perceive how they can be resolved.

Under the present arousal model, which attributes a predominant role to the right hemisphere in affective experience, there are complex relations among ipsilateral midbrain, limbic, and neocortical areas that regulate arousal at an adaptive level and between hemisphere pathways that tend to equalize arousal through neocortical commissures and that tend to produce arousal asymmetries through brain stem commissures. If the right hemisphere is differentially engaged in affective experience, it would be expected to participate in any task requiring an attempted regulation of emotional reactions, whether accomplished via verbal/analytic mechanisms or via global/ imagistic mechanisms. My intuitions are that Tucker (1981) is correct in his proposal that close corticolimbic integrations are involved in right hemisphere function, more so than in left hemisphere function, but I would guess that this integrative system is of central importance in both the elaboration and inhibition of emotion. The inhibitory functions over emotional reactions may depend upon a right hemisphere regulation of the left hemisphere, with the inhibitory actions accomplished via facilitation of the left hemisphere. These notions are purely speculative and will probably require careful studies of regional cerebral metabolism and/or blood flow through tomagraphic methods as subjects engage in tasks such as those presented by Tucker, before they can be evaluated.

Tucker, Antes, Stenlie, and Barnhardt (1978) examined performance of high-anxious and low-anxious subjects on lateralized tachistoscopic tests of verbal and nonverbal function and on perception of loudness of tones played to the left and right ears. High-anxious subjects showed a specific deficit in RVF performance on both tachistoscopic tasks and perceived tones played to the right ear as louder than those played to the left ear, indicating overarousal of the left hemisphere in high-anxious subjects, sufficient to interfere with performance. This result is consistent with Tucker's proposal that the left hemisphere has negative affect, as well as with the arousal model that would attribute the high anxiety to the low arousal level of the right hemisphere, which fails to inhibit negative experience.

Tucker, Roth, Arneson, and Buckingham (1977) found that leftward eye movements increased for emotional as compared with nonemotional questions, confirming Schwartz, Davidson, and Maer (1975), but they also found that leftward eye movements were increased when questions were presented in a stressful context that had been determined in pretests to increase subjective anxiety. This result raises the question as to why trait anxiety, as measured by Tucker et al. (1978), should be associated with indications of greater left than right hemisphere arousal, while state anxiety, as induced by Tucker et al. (1977), should be associated with indications of greater right than left hemisphere arousal. Possibly, confrontation with a stress-inducing situation produces engagement of the right hemisphere as the individual attempts to reduce the anxiety reaction, that is, as mechanisms of repression and denial come into play, entailing right hemisphere arousal.

That dysphoric/euphoric personality traits are related to the direction of eye movements is given further weight by data from Dawson, Tucker, and Swenson (1981). They found positive associations between leftward eye movements and favorable self-descriptions, extraversion, responses to whole inkblot configurations rather than details, and lack of depression, while rightward eye movements, in contrast, were associated with critical self-evaluations, introversion, responses to inkblot details, and depression.

Although not directly measuring tendencies toward dysphoria or euphoria, Charman (1979) compared subjects who were at the extremes on an introversion/extraversion dimension for visual-field asymmetries on a letter-matrix task. As noted earlier (Eysenck, 1967), introversion is associated with a depressive, pessimistic personality style and extraversion with a sunny, optimistic personality style. A 3 row × 4 column matrix was flashed to the LVF or the RVF, with simultaneous presentation of the letters T, M, or B at the center fixation to designate reporting of the top, middle, or bottom row. In spite of the small sample size (4 subjects/group), there was a highly significant group × field interaction ($p < 0.0001$), with all introverts showing an RVF advantage and all extroverts showing an LVF advantage. The Charman data are not only important in helping to clarify the relationship between personality dimensions and aspects of lateralization, but also in showing that standard indexes of laterality can be strongly affected by personality characteristics of right-handed subjects.

Another characteristic that is likely to be related to the introversion-pessimism-critical versus extraversion-optimism-uncritical dichotomy is hypnotic susceptibility. Hypnosis entails an ability of subjects for an imaginative involvement in external events, trust of the hypnotist, reduced testing of reality, and an uncritical acceptance of suggested ideas (Hilgard, 1970), all of which contrast with the personality traits of individuals with the critical, depressive, inward-looking attitudes of introverts but conform to the uncritical, optimistic, outward-looking attitudes of extroverts. Bakan (1969) and R. C. Gur and R. E. Gur (1974) found that left-movers were more susceptible to hypnosis than right-movers. Frumkin, Ripley, and Cox (1979) investigated linguistic asymmetry of the two ears on a dichotic listening test, in relation to hypnotic susceptibility and the effects of hypnotic induction. The right ear advantage was significantly reduced during hypnosis, as compared to pretest and posttest conditions, and a significant correlation was found between the laterality scores obtained during all three conditions and hypnotic susceptibility. The greater the hypnotic susceptibility, the smaller was the linguistic advantage of the right ear. Like the Charman (1979) data, the Frumkin et al. findings reveal the importance of personality in right-handers in affecting standard laterality indexes.

The normative investigations would seem to offer support for the view that individuals who tend toward introversion and are characterized by anxiety, depression, critical evaluations of self and others, and a generally pessimistic outlook are biased toward left hemisphere reliance, contrasting with individuals who tend toward low anxiety, absence of depression, uncritical evaluations of self and others, and a generally optimistic outlook and who are biased toward right hemisphere reliance. Tucker (1981) would say that this conclusion supports his hypothesis that the right hemisphere has a positive affective tone and that the left hemisphere has a negative affective tone. However, as suggested, it could be that differential reliance on the left hemisphere reflects asymmetrically low right hemisphere arousal and that the dysphoria results from this low right hemisphere arousal.

A recent study (Levy, Heller, Banich, & Burton, submitted) examined 32 right-handers on a lateralized tachistoscopic test of syllable identification; 24 of these subjects were also given a free-vision test indexing right hemisphere engagement in face processing. The Phi coefficient was computed as a laterality measure for each subject on the syllable test, and subjects were divided by a median split according to the magnitude of the asymmetry. The strong-asymmetry group (Group S) all had an RVF advantage of 14% or greater, and the weak-asymmetry group (Group W) displayed no overall asymmetry, with 8 subjects having a weak RVF advantage, 1 subject having no asymmetry, and 7 subjects having a weak LVF advantage.

We first sought to determine whether the two groups differed in overall performance level, summed across fields, since this was a critical question in determining whether variations among subjects in the degree of asymmetry reflected random error, differences in hemispheric specialization, or diversities in asymmetric hemispheric arousal. If random factors account for the differences among subjects in asymmetry, performance levels for Groups S and W should be the same. If subjects in Group W actually had bilateral representation of language function, whereas subjects in Group S had language functions specialized to the left hemisphere, Group W should have outperformed Group S since they would equal Group S for the RVF and surpass Group S for the LVF. If all subjects had language specialized to the left hemisphere, but Group W had asymmetrically high right hemisphere arousal, which counteracts the hemispheric specialization effect, Group S should have outperformed Group W; Group W would have been at an advantage for the right hemisphere initial encoding of LVF syllables but at a disadvantage in the subsequent left hemisphere linguistic processing of those syllables. The two factors would tend to cancel, so that the groups would perform equally for the LVF. However, the quality of initial encoding and the subsequent linguistic analysis would be positively related for the RVF, so that Group S should have outperformed Group W for RVF syllables, yielding an overall superiority for Group S. Statistical analysis on overall performance scores strongly supported the arousal-variation model. Planned comparisons showed no group difference for the LVF and an extremely large superiority of Group S for the RVF.

On each trial of the tachistoscopic test, subjects supplied a rating on a six-point scale, estimating whether they thought their syllable identification had been correct or incorrect. From the ratings, two independent indexes were derived for each visual field—index D, which reflected how well subjects could actually discriminate their own performance (a metacognitive judgment), and index B, which measured the extent to which subjects were pessimistically or optimistically biased in rating performance. The B and D indexes were uncorrelated. On the D index, Groups S and D did not differ for the LVF, but Group S showed a significant RVF advantage and was superior to Group W for the RVF; Group W showed no asymmetry in D.

Of greatest interest was the B index since this was a measure of affective outlook for each visual field. There was a very strong group x field interaction. The groups did not differ for the RVF, both groups showing zero bias and suggesting neutral affect for the left hemisphere. There was a very large group difference for the LVF, Group S being pessimistic and Group W being optimistic. Thus, on syllable identification and on the D index, the groups differed only for the RVF, but on the B index, they differed only for the LVF. Bias for the LVF significantly predicted RVF syllable performance, with no additional predictive capacity being given by bias for the RVF. A B-asymmetry score $(B_{LVF} - B_{RVF})$ was calculated for each subject. This strongly predicted asymmetry for syllable identification; the greater the optimism for the LVF relative to the RVF, the smaller the RVF advantage for syllable identification.

We also found that leftward asymmetries on the free-vision face test were correlated with asymmetry on the syllable test; the greater the leftward asymmetry on the face test, the smaller the RVF advantage on the syllable test. In addition, the B-asymmetry score was correlated with asymmetry on the face test; the larger the leftward asymmetry on the face test, the greater the optimism for the LVF relative to the RVF. The set of data strongly supports the conclusions that variations among right-handed subjects in perceptual asymmetries on either verbal or face-processing tasks are predominantly due to variations in arousal asymmetries between hemispheres, and that asymmetrically high right hemisphere arousal (reducing RVF advantages on verbal tests to zero and magnifying leftward asymmetries on face-processing tests) is associated with an optimistic bias for the LVF (right hemisphere), whereas asymmetrically high left hemisphere arousal (magnifying RVF advantages on verbal tests and reducing leftward asymmetries on face-processing tests) is associated with a pessimistic bias for the LVF (right hemisphere). I believe that these results add considerable weight to generally held views that the right hemisphere is predominant in affective experience and that they disconfirm lateralized valence models. Subjects showing strong RVF advantages for the syllable test and reduced leftward asymmetries on the face test did not manifest pessimism for the RVF but instead, pessimism for the LVF.

In conformance with other studies discussed in this section, our research shows that there are real variations among right-handers in standard laterality indexes, which have important associations with dimensions of personality and emotional perspective. Discrepancies among different studies of lateralization in right-handers and failures to find expected asymmetries might often be due to sampling variations in the personalities and outlooks in subject populations. Discriminations among groups or among effects of manipulated experimental variables in laterality experiments would very likely be improved if relevant information regarding personality characteristics of subjects were available.

Cognitive Variations and Cerebral Organization

Much of the discussion on the appropriate laterality index has centered around methods of controlling for performance variations among subjects so that "pure" measures of laterality, uncontaminated by performance differences, could be derived. However, one danger of removing performance variations from laterality indexes is the possibility of removing real associations between patterns of differential hemispheric functioning and ability for the task under assessment. As noted in the preceding section, right-handed subjects who displayed weak or no asymmetries for syllable identification were significantly poorer in overall performance than were subjects showing strong RVF advantages. This observation shows that asymmetry variations were not random and that they did not represent error variance but, instead, reflected real individual differences among subjects in patterns of hemispheric usage. Further, had language functions been bilaterally represented in weak-asymmetry subjects, their overall performance should have been superior to strong-asymmetry subjects, since performance of the two groups should have been equal for the RVF (because, in both groups, language functions would be present in the left hemisphere), but the weak-asymmetry group should have surpassed the strong-asymmetry group for the LVF (because language functions would be present in the right hemisphere of the weak-asymmetry group but not in the strong-asymmetry group). The actual outcome was highly revealing in pointing to the conclusion that both groups of subjects had language functions specialized to the left hemisphere but that they differed in patterns of asymmetric hemispheric arousal that either counteracted the hemispheric-specialization effect (for the weak-asymmetry group) or that magnified it (for the strong-asymmetry group).

Thus, covariations between asymmetries of performance and overall level of performance reflect psychologically meaningful relationships and are highly informative, with respect to the mechanisms underlying the covariation. We have recently obtained evidence (Burton and Levy, in preparation) that the same asymmetry/performance relations hold for a tachistoscopic face-recognition test with RT as the dependent variable. Twenty right-handed male subjects were given the free-vision test of face processing as well as the tachistoscopic test of face recognition. In this latter task, full-face photographs were presented in the center of the visual field for inspection. At the offset of the center face, a face of one of the two posers, shown in three-quarter profile, was flashed to the LVF or to the RVF. Subjects were asked to judge whether or not the center and lateral face was the same individual by making a discriminated RT response.

The hypothesis that right-handers vary in asymmetric hemispheric arousal entails the prediction that performance on a face-recognition task should be related to visual-field asymmetries; high performance predicts a strong LVF advantage, and low performance predicts no significant asymmetry. High-performing subjects, by hypothesis, have differentially high right hemisphere arousal, which would promote reliance on the appropriately specialized hemisphere and an LVF advantage. Low-performing subjects, by hypothesis, have differentially high left hemisphere arousal, which would promote reliance on the inappropriate unspecialized hemisphere and would counteract the LVF advantage expected from hemispheric specialization.

Subjects were divided by a median split according to overall RT into a fast-responding group and a slow-responding group (RT was a direct measure of performance since error rates were very low and there was no speed/accuracy trade-off). There was a highly significant group difference in laterality scores, with fast-responding subjects showing a large asymmetry in favor of the LVF and slow-responding subjects showing a nonsignificant asymmetry in favor of the RVF. The laterality indexes from the free-vision and the tachistoscopic tests were strongly correlated; the greater the leftward asymmetry on the free-vision test, the larger the LVF advantage on the tachistoscopic test. In addition, leftward asymmetries on the free-vision test were significantly correlated with overall RT on the tachistoscopic test; the larger the leftward asymmetry on the free-vision test, the faster were overall responses on the tachistoscopic test.

The results of our studies imply that, among right-handers, the degree of right hemisphere or left hemisphere engagement on either verbal or nonverbal tasks is closely related to the level of performance; asymmetric right hemisphere engagement diminishes tachistoscopic verbal performance and enhances tachistoscopic face recognition, with the opposite relations holding for those with asymmetric left hemisphere engagement. These results are consistent with findings from others. Rapaczynski and Ehrlichman (1979) tested 24 females who had been classified as field dependent or field independent, according to their performance on the Rod-and-Frame Test, for their lateralization and ability on a tachistoscopic face-recognition test.

For upright faces, field-independent subjects showed a 48 msec advantage for the LVF and field-dependent subjects showed a 45 msec advantage for the RVF. Additionally, the mean RT for field-independent subjects was 1406 msec, while the field-dependent subjects had a mean RT of 1543 msec. Although this difference did not reach statistical significance, the groups did differ in terms of errors, with field-independent subjects being more accurate, in spite of their faster reactions.

Oltman, Ehlichman, and Cox (1977) investigated perceptual asymmetries for comparing a normal face with two symmetric face composites, one composed of two right-half faces and one composed of two left-half faces. Subjects were asked to judge which composite looked more like the original. A significant correlation was found between field independence and a leftward asymmetry, consistent with the relationships observed by Rapaczynski and Ehlichman (1979) and also suggesting that subjects in the Burton and Levy (in preparation) experiment, having an LVF advantage on the tachistoscopic test and a leftward asymmetry on the free-vision test, were more field-independent than others.

Gur and Reivich (1980) examined regional cerebral blood flow as subjects engaged in a verbal (Miller Analogies items) and a nonverbal (Gestalt Completion items) task. As compared with baseline measurements, there was a significant asymmetric increase in left hemisphere flow during verbal processing, with no correlation between asymmetry of flow and accuracy on the verbal task. However, there was no significant blood flow asymmetry for the group as a whole on the nonverbal test, but a significant correlation was found between asymmetry of flow and performance—the greater the asymmetry in favor of the right hemisphere, the better was performance on the Gestalt Completion task. Blood flow asymmetry scores were computed for each subject by averaging over baseline, verbal, and nonverbal conditions. Subjects who had been classified as left-movers (for eye movement directionality in response to reflective questions) showed asymmetrically high right hemisphere flow, whereas right-movers had a nonsignificant tendency toward greater left hemisphere flow. These data raise the interesting possibility that the cognitive dimensions associated with eye-movement directionality might have an intimate association with the personality dimensions related to this factor, that is, that ability for right hemisphere tasks, correlated with asymmetric reliance on the right hemisphere, might be related to personality dimensions of extraversion, optimism, and susceptibility to hypnosis.

Observations supporting the findings of Gur and Reivich (1980) have been reported by Dabbs and Choo (1980) and by Dabbs (1980). These studies measured blood temperature either over the ophthalmic arteries above each eye or at the tympanic membrane of each ear, taking the asymmetry in temperaure between the left and right sides as an index of asymmetry of blood flow to the two hemispheres. Dabbs (1980) compared honors English with honors architecture students, finding that there was greater inferred blood flow to the left hemisphere in the former and to the right hemisphere in the latter. Dabbs and Choo (1980) administered standardized tests of verbal and spatial ability to a large number of right-handed subjects, computed the verbal/spatial difference scores, and selected two groups of subjects from opposite extremes of the distribution. Those with higher verbal than spatial ability had greater inferred blood flow to the left hemisphere, and those with higher spatial than verbal ability had greater inferred blood flow to the right hemisphere.

The physiological indexes of hemispheric asymmetry employed by Gur and Reivich (1980), Dabbs (1980), and Dabbs and Choo (1980) are concordant with behavioral data in showing that differential right or left hemisphere engagement is associated with ability on nonverbal tasks, verbal tasks, or both, and also suggesting that individual variations in performance measures do not merely reflect differences in momentary changes in hemispheric activation but, instead, are related to stable characteristics of asymmetric hemispheric arousal. If so, the question of whether or not cerebral laterality variations among right-handers are most accurately described as static organizational properties or, alternatively, as dynamic arousal properties, may be moot. Whether the latter are secondary consequences of the former or not, individuals might be quite inflexible with respect to changing their habitual modes of hemispheric engagement.

Samar (1981) examined a group of right-handed subjects for lateralization on two tachistoscopic verbal tests (three-letter words and nonsense syllables) and on two conditions of a spatial task (line-slope comparisons for "match" trials and line-slope comparisons for "mismatch" trials) and simultaneously recorded the evoked cortical potentials to tachistoscopic stimuli.

The averaged evoked responses were factor analyzed, and significant hemispheric asymmetries were observed for certain components. When the various factor components were used to predict performance asymmetries, the multiple correlations ranged from 0.82 to 0.98, depending upon sex of subjects and the tachistoscopic task under consideration. Subjects were also given the Verbal Reasoning and Spatial Relations subtests of the Differential Aptitude Test battery (DAT), and performance on both tests for females and the Verbal Reasoning test for males had correlations ranging from 0.93 to 0.97, with multiple aspects of electrocortical asymmetries. Thus, cognitive ability, as assessed on standardized tests, is not only related to the inferred blood flow asymmetries, as described by Dabbs and Choo (1980), but also to electrophysiological asymmetries.

It becomes increasingly apparent that the classical descriptions of "the brain of the right-hander" are great oversimplifications that may be accurate only for a modal minority of dextrals. There is a fairly good consensus regarding group-typical patterns of lateral specialization but little understanding of or agreement about the various functional organizations related to arousal asymmetries and their relationships with personality or cognitive dimensions. Laterality research has now reached a stage where it is justified in moving beyond descriptions of invariances among right-handers, while tossing diversities in the "wastebasket" of "error variance." Serious attention needs to be devoted to the nature of variations in differential hemispheric involvement, their causes, and their behavioral/psychological consequences.

SUMMING UP

Until relatively recent years, laterality researchers have focused on trying to understand the characteristics of cerebral lateralization as they pertain to some idealized "typical individual," with some attention also directed to the effects of handedness, sex, or other organismic variables, such as eye or foot dominance. However, for the most part, variations among right-handers in the degree and direction of ear asymmetries on dichotic tests or visual-field asymmetries on tachistoscopic tests have rarely been considered except when various pathological or learning-disabled populations have been compared with normal controls. For normal right-handers, homogeneous with respect to sex, individual differences in behavioral asymmetries are often so little noted that tables and figures depicting data may show only measures of central tendency, with no indication of variance. Even when both means and measures of variation are given, it is unusual for authors to describe frequency distributions of subjects. Quite probably, this tendency to ignore variation has derived from the belief that there is no way to decide whether the observed variance was due to random error of measurement or to real individual differences in the underlying dimension of interest, and no way to surmount the problem of choosing a laterality index giving an appropriate ordering of subjects with respect to asymmetric functioning of the brain.

I hope that it has been made apparent that there is good reason for concluding that real differences do exist among right-handers in both the direction and degree of hemispheric engagement that are predictive of personality and cognitive characteristics, and that there are rational ways of dealing with questions of reliability, the choice of the laterality index, and validity. That powerful relationships have been found between measures of laterality and important psychological characteristics, in spite of the problems of reliability being quite imperfect, the laterality index itself not being ideal, and the measure employed picking up not only aspects of hemispheric functioning but also extraneous factors, strongly suggests that, with improvements in experimental and statistical techniques, even clearer relations will appear.

The central aim of the neuropsychological endeavor is to discover how properties of neurological organization generate behavior and psychological function. One wishes to make statements of the sort, "Given certain conditions, the neurological structure, organization, and/or dynamic property called A is both necessary and sufficient for the behavioral/psychological characteristic called B." Such statements imply that, when non-A obtains, then non-B will obtain. Thus, if one posits that Broca's area is necessary for speech (and sufficient, given certain other conditions of neurological and organismic function), one implies not only that speech will be normal if Broca's area is normal (given certain assumed organismic conditions), but also that speech will be defective if Broca's area is damaged. In other words, whenever any causal conclusion is reached, relating a cause A to a consequence B, it must necessarily be assumed that there are conditions when neither A nor B obtains. Variance in both the causal and outcome dimensions is essential if casual relationships are to be specified.

In clinical investigations, variations in the causal dimension are usually produced by lesions; covariations are observed in behavior, and a causal inference is drawn. In normative studies, it is necessary to be sensitive to the same logical limit, and this means that the variations among subjects in both psychological and neurological dimensions offer one of the richest sources of information for breaking the brain/behavior code. As the experimental techniques improve, as statistical methods become more sophisticated, and as the conceptual foundations of the research enterprise are better understood, it is hoped that the rich diversities among people in values, outlooks, propensities, interests, personalities, and in cognitive structure and abilities can be mapped onto similar diversities in neural organization.

ACKNOWLEDGMENTS

The support of The Spencer Foundation, for studies from my laboratory discussed in this chapter and for preparation of this manuscript, is gratefully acknowledged. I deeply appreciate the thoughtful and helpful comments of my students, Marie Banich, Leslie Burton, and Wendy Heller, whose time and effort surely improved the clarity and quality of this contribution. Any deficiencies of presentation, ideas, or logic are, however, entirely my own.

REFERENCES

Alford, L.B. Localization of consciousness and emotion. *American Journal of Psychiatry*, 1933, *12*, 789–799.

Bakan, P. Hypnotizability, laterality of eye movements, and functional brain asymmetry. *Perceptual and Motor Skills*, 1969, *28*, 927–932.

Bear, D.M., & Fedio, P. Quantitative analysis of interictal behavior in temporal lobe epilepsy. *Archives of Neurology*, 1977, *34*, 454–467.

Birkett, P. Measures of laterality and theories of hemispheric process. *Neuropsychologia*, 1977, *15*, 693–696.

Buchtel, H.A., Campari, F., De Risio, C., & Rota, R. Hemispheric differences in discriminative reaction time to facial expressions. *Italian Journal of Psychology*, 1978, *5*, 159–169.

Burton, L., & Levy, J. Lateral differences among right-handers for face recognition and judgement of facial emotion as a function of processing speed, in preparation.

Campbell, R. Asymmetries in interpreting and expressing a posed facial expression. *Cortex*, 1978, *14*, 327–342.

Charman, D.K. Do different personalities have different hemispheric asymmetries? A brief communiqué of an initial experiment. *Cortex*, 1979, *15*, 655–657.

Chaurasia, B.D., & Goswami, H.K. Functional asymmetry in the face. *Acta Anatomica*, 1975, *91*, 154–160.

Cicone, M., Wapner, W., & Gardner, H. Sensitivity to emotional expressions and situations in organic patients. Unpublished manuscript, Boston V.A. Hospital, 1979. Cited in Tucker, 1981.

Colbourn, C.J. Can laterality be measured? *Neuropsychologia*, 1978, *16*, 283–289.

Dabbs, J.M., Jr. Left-right differences in cerebral blood flow and cognition. *Psychophysiology*, 1980, *17*, 548–551.

Dabbs, J.M., Jr., & Choo, G. Left-right carotid blood flow predicts specialized mental ability. *Neuropsychologia*, 1980, *18*, 711–713.

Dawson, S.L., Tucker, D.M., & Swenson, R.A. Lateralized cognitive style and self-description. Unpublished manuscript, University of North Dakota, 1981.

Eysenck, H.J. *The biological basis of personality*. Springfield, Ill.: Charles C. Thomas, 1967.

Frumkin, L.R., Ripley, H.S., & Cox, G.B. A dichotic index of laterality that scores linguistic errors. *Cortex*, 1979, *15*, 687–691.

Gainotti, G. Réactions catastrophiques et manifestations d'indifférence au cours des atteintes cérébrales. *Neuropsychologia*, 1969, *7*, 195–204.

Gainotti, G. Emotional behavior and hemispheric side of lesion. *Cortex*, 1972, *8*, 41–55.

Galin, D., Diamond, R., & Braff, D. Lateralization of conversion symptoms: More frequent on the left. *American Journal of Psychiatry*, 1977, *134*, 578–580.

Gur, R.C., & Gur, R.E. Handedness, sex and eyedness as moderating variables in the relationship between hypnotic susceptibility and functional brain asymmetry. *Journal of Abnormal Psychology*, 1974, *83*, 635–643.

Gur, R.C., & Reivich, M. Cognitive task effects on hemispheric blood flow in humans: Evidence for individual differences in hemispheric activation. *Brain and Language*, 1980, *9*, 78–92.

Gur, R.E., & Gur, R.C. Defense mechanisms, psychosomatic symptomatology, and conjugate lateral eye movements. *Journal of Consulting and Clinical Psychology*, 1975, *43*, 416–420.

Hall, M.M., Hall, G.C., & Lavoie, P. Ideation in patients with unilateral or bilateral midline brain lesions. *Journal of Abnormal Psychology*, 1968, *73*, 526–531.

Harshman, R., & Krashen, S. An "unbiased" procedure for comparing degree of lateralization of dichotically presented stimuli. UCLA, *Working Papers in Phonetics*, 1972, *23*, 3–12.

Hécaen, H. Clinical symptomatology in right and left hemispheric lesions. In V.B. Mountcastle (Ed.), *Interhemispheric relations and cerebral dominance*. Baltimore: Johns Hopkins University Press, 1962.

Hécaen, H. Mental symptoms associated with tumors of the frontal lobe. In J.M. Warren & K. Akert (Eds.), *The frontal granular cortex and behavior*. New York: McGraw-Hill, 1964.

Heilman, K.M., Scholes, R., & Watson, R.T. Auditory affective agnosia: Disturbed comprehension of affective speech. *Journal of Neurology, Neurosurgery, and Psychiatry*, 1975, *38*, 69–72.

Heller, W., & Levy, J. Perception and expression of emotion in right-handers and left-handers. *Neuropsychologia*, 1981, *19*, 263–272.

Hier, D.B., LeMay, M., Rosenberger, P.B., & Perlo, V.P. Developmental dyslexia: Evidence for a subgroup with a reversal of cerebral asymmetry. *Archives of Neurology*, 1978, *35*, 90–92.

Hilgard, J.R. *Personality and hypnosis: A study of imaginative involvement.* Chicago: University of Chicago Press, 1970.

Hochberg, F.H. & LeMay, M. Arteriographic correlates of handedness. *Neurology*, 1975, *25*, 218–222.

Krashen, S., & Harshman, R. Lateralization and the critical period. UCLA, *Working Papers in Phonetics*, 1972, *23*, 13–21.

Kronfol, Z., Hamsher, K. deS., Digre, K., & Waziri, R. Depression and hemispheric functions: Changes associated with unilateral ECT. *British Journal of Psychiatry*, 1978, *132*, 560–567.

Kuhn, G. The phi coefficient as an index of ear differences in dichotic listening. *Cortex*, 1973, *9*, 450–457.

LeMay, M. Morphological cerebral asymmetries of modern man, fossil, and nonhuman primate. *Annals of the New York Academy of Sciences*, 1976, *280*, 349–366.

LeMay, M. Asymmetries of the skull and handedness. *Journal of Neurological Science*, 1977, *32*, 243–253.

LeMay, M., & Kido, D.K. Asymmetries of the cerebral hemispheres on computed tomograms. *Journal of Computer Assisted Tomography*, 1978, *2*, 471–476.

Levy, J., Heller, W., Banich, M., & Burton, L. Inferential evidence for variations among right-handers in patterns of asymmetric hemispheric arousal: Effects on lateralized performance and consequences for the emotional tone of the right hemisphere, Submitted.

Lishman, W.A. Brain damage in relation to psychiatric disability after head injury. *British Journal of Psychiatry*, 1968, *114*, 373–410.

Luchins, D.J., Weinberger, D.R., & Wyatt, R.J. Schizophrenia: Evidence for a subgroup with reversed cerebral asymmetry. *Archives of General Psychiatry*, 1979, *36*, 1309–1311.

Luchins, D.J., Weinberger, D.R., & Wyatt, R.J. Reversed cerebral asymmetries in schizophrenia. Paper presented at the 134th Annual American Psychiatric Association Meetings, New Orleans, 1981.

Magnusson, D. *Test theory.* Reading, Mass.: Addison-Wesley, 1967.

Marshall, J.C., Caplan, D., & Holmes, J.M. The measure of laterality. *Neuropsychologia*, 1975, *13*, 315–321.

McRae, D.L., Branch, C.L., & Milner, B. The occipital horns and cerebral dominance. *Neurology*, 1968, *18*, 95–100.

Moscovitch, M., & Olds, J. Asymmetries in emotional facial expressions and their possible relation to hemispheric specialization. Paper presented at the International Neuropsychology Society, Holland, 1979.

Oltman, P.K., Ehrlichman, H. & Cox, P.W. Field independence and laterality in the perception of faces. *Perceptual and Motor Skills*, 1977, *45*, 255–260.

Perris, C., & Monakhov, K. Depressive symptomatology and systematic structural analysis of the EEG. In J.H. Gruzelier & P. Flor-Henry (Eds.), *Hemisphere asymmetries of function and psychopathology*. Amsterdam: Elsevier, 1979.

Rapaczynski, W., & Ehrlichman, H. Opposite visual hemifield superiorities in face recognition as a function of cognitive style. *Neuropsychologia*, 1979, *17*, 645–652.

Richardson, J.T.E. How to measure laterality. *Neuropsychologia*, 1976, *14*, 135–136.

Ross, E.D., & Mesulam, M.M. Dominant language functions of the right hemisphere? Prosody and emotional gesturing. *Archives of Neurology*, 1979, *36*, 144–148.

Rossi, G.F., & Rosadini, G. Experimental analysis of cerebral dominance in man. In C.H. Milliken & F.L. Darley (Eds.), *Brain mechanisms underlying speech and language*. New York: Grune & Stratton, 1967.

Sackeim, H.A., Greenberg, M., Weiman, A. et al. Hemispheric asymmetry in the expression of positive and negative emotions: Neurological evidence. *Archives of Neurology*, 1982, *39*, 210–218.

Sackeim, H.A., & Gur, R.C. Lateral asymmetry in the intensity of emotional expression. *Neuropsychologia*, 1978, *16*, 473–481.

Safer, M.A. Sex and hemisphere differences in access to codes for processing emotional expressions and faces. *Journal of Experimental Psychology: General*, 1981, *110*, 86–100.

Safer, M.A., & Leventhal, H. Ear differences in evaluating emotional tones of voice and verbal content. *Journal of Experimental Psychology: Human Perception and Performance*, 1977, *3*, 75–82.

Samar, V. Multiple determination of visual half-field asymmetries and differential aptitude test scores by independent components of cerebral specialization. Paper presented at the International Neuropsychological Society, Atlanta, 1981.

Schenkman, M., Butler, R.B., Naeser, M.A., & Kleefield, J. The relationship of cerebral hemispheric asymmetries to functional recovery from hemiplegia. Paper presented at the National Meeting of the American Physical Therapy Association, Washington, D.C., 1981.

Schwartz, G.E., Davidson, R.J., & Maer, F. Right hemisphere lateralization for emotion in the human brain: Interactions with cognition. *Science*, 1975, *190*, 286–288.

Shankweiler, D., & Studdert-Kennedy, M. A continuum of lateralization for speech perception? *Brain and Language*, 1975, *2*, 212–225.

Shearer, S.L., & Tucker, D.M. Differential cognitive contributions of the cerebral hemispheres in the modulation of emotional arousal. *Cognitive Therapy and Research*, in press.

Smokler, I.A., & Shevrin, I. Cerebral lateralization and personality style. *Archives of General Psychiatry*, 1979, *36*, 949–954.

Stern, D.B. Handedness and the lateral distribution of conversion reactions. *Journals of Nervous and Mental Disease*, 1977, *164*, 122–128.

Teng, E.L. Dichotic ear differences is a poor index for functional asymmetry between the cerebral hemispheres. *Neuropsychologia*, 1981, *19*, 235–240.

Trevarthen, C. Functional relations of disconnected hemispheres with the brain stem, and with each other: Monkey and man. In M. Kinsbourne & W.L. Smith (Eds.), *Hemispheric disconnection and cerebral function*. Springfield, Ill.: Charles C. Thomas, 1974.

Tucker, D.M. Lateral brain function, emotion, and conceptualization. *Psychological Bulletin*, 1981, *89*, 19–46.

Tucker, D.M., Antes, J.R., Stenslie, C.E., & Barnhardt, T.N. Anxiety and lateral cerebral function. *Journal of Abnormal Psychology*, 1978, *87*, 380–383.

Tucker, D.M., & Newman, J.P. Verbal and imaginal cognitive strategies in the inhibition of emotional arousal. *Cognitive Therapy and Research*, in press.

Tucker, D.M., Roth, R.S., Arneson, B.A., & Buckingham, V. Right hemisphere activation during stress. *Neuropsychologia*, 1977, *15*, 697–700.

Wechsler, A.F. The effect of organic brain disease on recall of emotionally charged versus neutral narrative text. *Neurology*, 1973, *23*, 130–135.

14

The Measurement of Hemispheric Asymmetries in Children with Developmental Reading Disabilities

Francis J. Pirozzolo

Keith Rayner

George W. Hynd

INTRODUCTION

The cause of developmental reading disability (or developmental dyslexia) continues to elude researchers despite over three-quarters of a century of research on this disorder. Morgan (1896), who is credited with the first clinical observations of children with reading disability, provided speculation that the angular gyrus was underdeveloped in these children. Later, Orton (1937) hypothesized that there was a connection between hemispheric specialization (cerebral dominance for language) and reading failure. When neuropsychological research techniques for examining the behavioral correlates of hemispheric specialization were devised, researchers quickly recognized their utility for evaluating hypothetical constructs such as Orton's. This chapter will review the extensive literature on two such techniques for studying children with reading disability.

DICHOTIC LISTENING RESEARCH WITH READING AND LEARNING-DISABLED CHILDREN

Since Broadbent (1952a, 1952b) first introduced the procedure now known as dichotic listening to investigate memory processes, it has become one of the most favored clinical-experimental techniques in the study of children with learning disorders. Initial studies sought to determine the utility of this procedure in assessing cerebral laterality with both normal and clinical populations. It was Kimura (1961a, 1961b), however, who first demonstrated that the differential recognition of simultaneously presented auditory stimuli revealed underlying structures of functional cerebral lateralization. Thus, in a normal population, dichotic stimuli of a linguistic nature presented to the right ear should be reported with greater accuracy than those presented to the left ear, as contralateral auditory pathways are known to be prepotent in signal transmission (Kimura, 1967). This concept has received support from a variety of sources (e.g., Doehring, 1972; Frankfurter & Honeck, 1973; Milner, 1962; Milner, Taylor, & Sperry, 1968; Rosenzweig, 1951). (See also Porter & Hughes in this volume.)

Studies with young normal children using a number of different linguistic dichotic stimuli (e.g., digits, words, sentences, consonant-vowel syllables) typically reveal that a right ear advantage (REA) is manifested in children between the ages of two and one-half to five (Gilbert & Climan, 1974; Hynd & Obrzut, 1977; Ingram, 1975; Kimura, 1963; Nagafuchi, 1970). Furthermore, performance on a dichotic listening task does not seem to be related to sex or socioeconomic level of the subject (Davidoff, Done, & Scully 1981; Hynd & Obrzut, 1977). While the REA may be established at an early age, controversy exists as to whether or not the magnitude of the dichotic ear effect and hence, functional lateralization, increases with development. Various investigators report an increase in the ear effect with age (e.g., Bakker, Satz, Goebel, & Van der Vlugt, 1973; Berlin, Hughes, Lowe-Bell, & Berlin, 1973; Bryden, 1973; Nagafuchi, 1970; Porter & Berlin, 1975; see also Porter & Hughes, this volume). Other investigators using a similar approach find no developmental parameters in the dichotic ear effect in subjects ranging in age from five through late adolescence (e.g., Hynd & Obrzut, 1977; Schulman-Galambos, 1972). The reconciliation of these two positions regarding the development of cerebral dominance probably lies somewhere between these two extremes. For instance, there exists good evidence that the magnitude of REA does vary according to age level, especially when the dichotic stimuli require more advanced processing strategies (e.g., Van Duyne, Bakker, & De Jong, 1977). Those studies that find no development effect (e.g., Geffen, 1976, 1978; Hynd & Obrzut, 1977; Schulman-Galambos, 1972) can be criticized for using stimuli that produce a ceiling effect, especially at the older age levels where developmental variation is most likely to be manifested. While these authors might argue, in their defense, that this criticism is not valid since total accuracy rarely exceeds 50% at any age level (Hynd, Obrzut, Weed, & Hynd, 1979), it does seem that several conclusions are warranted regarding research with normal children. First, an REA and presumed left cerebral hemisphere lateralization for speech is evident for subjects at a very young age. This finding is contrary to the developmental hypothesis of Lenneberg (1967) and is interpreted as implying that the brain is "prewired" for speech and language processing. Second, if developmental variation exists, it probably is only manifested in those dichotic paradigms that use stimuli requiring more complex processing strategies (e.g., paired digit strings) and, hence, may tap abilities more related to attention or auditory short-term memory (see Geffen, 1978). Finally, the evidence strongly suggests that the vast majority of subjects report an REA, presumably indicating a left cerebral hemisphere specialization for speech and language processing.

By far the greatest application for the dichotic listening paradigm has been in examining differences in performance between reading- and learning-disabled children and normal children. The hypothesis has been that, if reading- and learning-disabled children are truly delayed in the establishment of cerebral dominance for language, their REA will be either nonexistent or inferior to that of normal children. While most of these studies have examined matched populations of normals and reading-disabled children (e.g., Bakker, 1969; Bakker, Teunissen, & Bosch, 1976; Fennell, Satz, & Morris, 1980; Hynd et al., 1979; Leong, 1975; Obrzut, Hynd, Obrzut, & Leitgeb, 1980; Satz, Rardin, & Ross, 1971; Sparrow & Satz, 1970; Witelson & Rabinovitch, 1972; Yeni-Komshian, Isenberg, & Goldberg, 1975; Zurif & Carson, 1970), a noted few have attempted to differentially examine subgroups of reading- and learning-disabled children, in an attempt to identify underlying cognitive factors related to functional cerebral lateralization (e.g., Ayres, 1977; Bakker, Licht, Kok, & Bouma, 1980; Cermak, Cermak, Drake, & Kenney, 1978; Obrzut, 1979). As each of these approaches has much potential to offer in terms of contributions to existing knowledge, a representative few will be discussed critically.

Studies Examining Matched Groups of Reading Disabled and Normal Children

Witelson (1976) conducted an investigation with dyslexic children using a dichotic listening task. Over a 5-year period, 113 children were identified who demonstrated a Performance Scale Intelligence Quotient (PSIQ) of 85 or greater on the Wechsler Intelligence Scale for Children (WISC), had demonstrated reading difficulty over a period of years, and were reading at least one and one-half years below their present grade placement. In agreement with other studies examining incidence rates (e.g., Critchley, 1970), there was a six to one ratio in favor of boys to girls in the dyslexic population. A sample of children who were normal readers was also included. In addition to other measures, a dichotic task was administered and consisted of the presentation of digit pairs (the numbers one to ten excluding seven, a two-syllable numeral). An analysis of variance including group, age, and ear revealed significant main effects for group, age, and ear but no interactions. Approximately 70% of each group demonstrated an REA, although the dyslexic children clearly performed more poorly in both ears when compared with the normals. Furthermore, total accuracy increased with age. Witelson (1976) interprets her data as indicating that dyslexic children suffer a deficit in linguistic processing but have normal lateralization.

A more common approach in research has been to examine groups of matched-reading retarded and normal children, representative of one age group. Leong (1976), for instance, identified 58 dyslexic children (male) and matched them with a control population. A dichotic tape prepared by the author used three sets of digits (0 to 9) presented in two to four digit series. Examining both attempted order of report as well as ear, Leong (1976) found both reading group and the two (ear order) report condition main effects to be significant, but there were no interactions with the reading group. Consequently, similar to Witelson (1976) and others (e.g., Bakker et al., 1976; Hynd et al., 1979; Leong, 1975; Witelson & Rabinovitch, 1972; Zurif & Carson, 1970), he interprets the data as implying that both normal and reading-disabled children are lateralized for language function, but the better readers demonstrate more proficient processing strategies. He concludes that his results constitute evidence of a lag in functional cerebral development of the disabled readers. The Leong (1976) study is suspect on several accounts, but obviously his greatest error is in assuming that degraded performance at one age level is indicative of developmental delay. His results could be equally indicative of neurological deficit.

By far the most methodologically sound research has been conducted by Satz and his associates with the Florida longitudinal project (Darby 1974; Fennell et al., 1980; Satz, Bakker, Tennissen et al., 1975; Satz, Friel, & Rudegeair, 1974; Satz et al., 1971; Satz, Taylor, Friel, & Fletcher, 1978). In this project all of the white male children entering school in one county were evaluated with a variety of measures, including a dichotic task. Longitudinal analysis of the performance of these children, including those later identified as having reading problems, indicates a developmental trend in stimulus recall on the dichotic task. According to theory, this increased asymmetry should be related to reading achievement. However, in reality, regression analysis consistently demonstrates no relationship between these variables. The reported developmental changes in ear difference are apparently more related to handedness than to reading disability (Fennell et al., 1980). While the Florida project has contributed to our knowledge of the predictors of reading disability, its results using the dichotic listening paradigm are difficult to interpret since its methodology differs so considerably from other studies. One conclusion that does seem supported, though, is that, in reading-disabled children, a delay or deficit in stimulus recall (both ear advantage and total recall) of a dichotic task exists. This is in general agreement with most other dichotic studies.

Research Investigating Subgroups of Disabled Readers

Another approach in dichotic research is to use subgroups of disabled learners. The logic of this line of research suggests that subgroup differences may emerge that heretofore were masked when using undifferentiated groups of disabled children. Two studies have been conducted in this fashion.

Cermak et al. (1978) examined three groups of learning-disabled children defined according to their WISC IQ scores and a normal control population. The three learning-disabled groups included those with VSIQ< PSIQ (> 15 points), PSIQ< VSIQ, and those with no difference (5 points) between their VSIQ and PSIQ. Based on the dichotic task results (using digit strings), the authors concluded that the children with the largest disparity between their VSIQ and PSIQ (in either direction) failed to show a significant REA. However, those who had no differences between their VSIQ and PSIQ did demonstrate the expected REA. Unfortunately, the authors offer little interpretation of their data. It seems reasonable to conclude that those with the greatest IQ discrepancies are going to be deficient in some aspect of neuropsychological functioning. Differentiating groups on the basis of IQ scores poses problems, however, as it is well known that Verbal and Performance IQ scores on the WISC are not factorially pure (Kaufman, 1979).

Obrzut (1979) separated 216 normal and reading-disabled male children into four groups, based on Boder's (1971, 1973) conceptualization of developmental dyslexia. The groups were dysphonetic, dyseidetic combined and equal readers. Using dichotically presented digit strings of varied lengths, he reported that the dyseidetic readers performed best and that those with linguistic processing deficits did poorest. Similar to the studies using undifferentiated samples of reading-disabled children, Obrzut (1979) found that the reading-disabled children generally did less well on the dichotic task than did the normals.

The results of the Cermak et al. (1978) and Obrzut (1979) studies shed some light on the neuropsychological processes involved in subgroups of disturbed readers. Most importantly, they demonstrate the utility in using clinically differentiated subgroups of disabled learners. The research by Bakker et al. (1980) presents another approach that may also provide valuable insight into the cognitive factors involved in reading disability.

Rather than separate subjects into groups on the basis of some performance not necessarily related to cerebral lateralization, Bakker et al. (1980) examined event-related potentials (ERPs) in right and left "eared" normal and reading-disturbed children. Bakker (1979, 1980) has proposed that right and left "eared" children may be equally good readers but may use different reading strategies. Right ear dominant readers, he proposed, read fast but inaccurately, while left ear dominant (presumably right hemisphere dominant for speech) readers tend to read slowly but without many errros. He believes these reading types reflect the differential use of the two hemispheres. Sixteen normal children and 11 reading-disturbed children participated in this study. These groups of children were separated on the basis of the ear score that they obtained on a dichotic task. Consequently, half the children in each group were identified as being either right or left ear dominant. Interestingly, in examining the ERPs for both groups, differential activation of one cerebral hemisphere seemed apparent only with the normal subjects. The reading-disturbed children failed to show the ear × side interaction found in the normals. Bakker et al. (1980) interpret this finding as supporting the notion that reading is a multistage cognitive process and that this phenomenon is reflected in the performance of the normal children. However, the reading-disturbed children seem to process information bilaterally and, hence, fail to differentiate preferred reading strategies. Using performance on a dichotic listening task as an independent variable rather than as a dependent variable may be a promising line of research.

Interpreting the Dichotic Research

What can be concluded about the enormous volume of research conducted, using a dichotic listening paradigm with reading- and learning-disabled children? In drawing conclusions it may be useful to evaluate the results as they relate to theoretical issues.

Dichotic listening was originally believed by Kimura (1963) to be an excellent noninvasive tool for the examination of functional cerebral lateralization. While the procedure seems to be generally reliable in test-retest and intertest measures (Bakker, Van der Vlugt, & Claushius, 1978), there are some significant problems in interpreting a one-to-one correspondence between demonstrated ear effect and the degree of cerebral specialization for language. As Satz (1976) has pointed out, using a Baysean analysis, a strong REA is an extremely probable predictor of left hemisphere specialization for speech and language function. However, a left ear effect, which was originally thought to indicate right hemisphere lateralization for language abilities, in reality may accurately predict such a condition only 10% of the time. This may be the reason that Bakker et al. (1980) found a nonsignificant interaction between ear and side among their reading-disabled children.

Other problems with the dichotic task relate to adequate screening of subjects prior to inclusion in the subject pool, stimulus onset criteria, type of stimuli used, procedural constraints (Bryson, Mononen, & Yu, 1980), and the effects of varied acoustical parameters on dichotic performance (see Cullen, Thompson, Hughes et al., Porter & Hughes, this volume). If the results of dichotic listening experiments do not reflect the degree of cerebral dominance, then what do they reflect? Kinsbourne (1974, 1980) has offered an attentional explanation and argued that perceptual asymmetries reveal attentional biases.

Noting that children with learning and reading disorders may have attentional problems, Hynd et al. (1979) corrected the raw scores obtained from a dichotic task with learning-disabled children. They reported that it was the increased rate of guessing on the dichotic task that caused the disabled readers to perform more poorly than their matched normal controls. They concluded that children with anomalous lateralization on a dichotic task are probably "wired" the same as normal children but apply inappropriate processing strategies. Furthermore, they suggest that differential trends in attentional deficits may have been erroneously interpreted as developmental trends in the establishment of functional cerebral dominance. A recent investigation using a directed dichotic condition, where subjects were told to attend a given ear, with normal and learning-disabled children revealed that learning-disabled children could dramatically alter their performance according to ear effect, whereas the normals could not (Obrzut, Hynd, Obrzut, & Pirozzolo, 1981). Additional evidence for the validity of these findings was obtained in a follow-up study in which it was found that the directed left attention condition accounted for more than 86% of the variance in separating the two groups of subjects, even when a number of other neuropsychological tests were included (Obrzut, Hynd, & Obrzut, in press).

It is apparent that the initial enthusiasm that researchers had for the dichotic listening task and its ability to assess the in vivo status of the human brain has dimmed considerably. Recent investigations have begun to sort out the important methodological issues. Future investigations that examine memory and attentional variability and their relationship to ERPs in reading-

or learning-disabled children may hold the greatest promise for future research.

VISUAL HALF-FIELD RESEARCH WITH READING- AND LEARNING-DISABLED CHILDREN

In 1952 Mishkin and Forgays used a tachistoscope to present English words to the right and left parafoveal regions. When these words were exposed briefly, that is, at exposure durations shorter than that necessary to program and launch a saccadic eye movement, they were more easily recognized when they appeared in the right visual field than in the left visual field. Using bilingual subjects, they also showed that, when Hebrew words were presented in a similar way, a left field superiority was found. These investigators attributed half-field effects to left-to-right scanning habits for English words and right-to-left scanning habits for Hebrew words. Heron (1957) used bilateral linguistic and numerical stimuli and found consistent left field advantages. He argued that these laterality effects were the result of directional scanning of a rapidly decaying memory trace. Numerous other early studies found similar effects seemingly in support of a postexposural scanning mechanism (e.g., Harcum & Finkel, 1963). In 1965, however, Barton, Goodglass and Shai discovered that the right visual field superiority for recognition of English words was independent of this horizontal scanning effect. Using both English and Hebrew words arranged vertically, Barton found that bilingual subjects had a significant right visual field advantage for words in both languages. These effects, as those of the dichotic listening right ear effect, were attributed to the more direct pathway running from the right side to the language center in the left cerebral hemisphere. While some investigators still maintain that postexposural scanning habits are responsible for visual half-field effects, most are convinced that hemispheric specialization plays the greater role, although exactly by what mechanism is far from clear (see Pirozzolo, 1977a). For further discussion of visual half-field methodology, see also Hardyck, this volume, and Zaidel, this volume.

If visual half-field studies are a second-order reflection of the linguistic specialization of the left hemisphere, they make for excellent research techniques in evaluating the nature of neuropsychological deficits in children with developmental reading disability. Orton (1937) first suggested that poor reading achievement may be related to poorly established cerebral dominance for language functions. Forgays (1953) provided the first experimental data to test this hypothesis, in part. He studied the developmental effects on right visual field superiority in normal readers. Using children as young as grade two and readers at all levels through college, he found that right field superiority is not established until grade eight. This finding has not been supported in more recent studies. Studies of normal children (e.g., Miller & Turner, 1973; Olson, 1973; Reitsma, 1975) show establishment of right field superiority in much younger children. In agreement with studies of dichotic listening, it appears that, while younger readers do show right visual field superiorities, there may be age by visual field interactions in cross-sectional studies of the phenomenon. It is tempting to infer from these data that cerebral dominance develops pari passu with language development. Better tests of the presence of hemispheric specialization are: incidence of language deficit following lateralized focal cerebral damage in young children, and evoked responses. In both cases, recent studies have overwhelmingly supported the notion that language may be genetically preprogrammed to the left hemisphere and that cerebral dominance may be detectable at very early ages (Pirozzolo, Campanella, Christensen, & Lawson-Kerr, 1981).

There have been numerous studies of visual half-field effects in disabled readers during the past several years. McKeever and Huling (1970) found that poor readers show a right visual field superiority for recognition of words. Similarly, McKeever and Van Deventer (1975) found a right visual field superiority in adolescent disabled readers. Olson (1973), however, was unable to find a right visual field superiority for verbal stimuli in her early study of disabled readers. Marcel, Katz, and Smith (1974) and Marcel and Rajan (1975) found a reduced right field superiority in their disabled readers and, curiously, argued that this represented, not a left hemisphere dysfunction, but a linguistic superiority of the disabled readers' right hemispheres. In direct contrast to these results, Yeni-Komshian et al. (1975) showed that disabled readers have increased right visual field superiorities. These investigators argued that the causal pathophysiology may thus reside with the right hemisphere (or the corpus callosum) and not with the left. The right hemisphere deficit in reading disability, according to this line of reasoning, would reflect itself in the inability to analyze the physical, visual, and featural characteristics of letters and words. Most investigators have tended to focus upon the linguistic nature of the visual half-field task and, therefore, also concern themselves with the left hemisphere. Clearly, the visual analysis stage of reading is a possible site of difficulty for disabled readers. Studies of normal readers show that the right hemisphere may play a role in word recognition, especially at the early stages of feature analysis (Pirozzolo & Rayner, 1977).

Contrary to the foregoing, most studies do find depressed right visual field performance on the part of disabled readers. Pirozzolo and Rayner (1979) showed that disabled readers have no visual half-field asymmetry, either in unilateral or bilateral studies of this effect. Kershner (1977) found a continuous relationship between reading ability and visual field asymmetry.

Using three groups of readers (disabled, normal, and gifted), he demonstrated a correlation between increasing right field superiority and increasing reading ability. While this study was the first to fully test the role of reading ability on visual half-field performance by the addition of a group of gifted readers, the conclusion that the latter group is characterized by "superlateralization" must be avoided.

Young and Ellis (1981) have argued that different strategies of accomplishing the aforementioned tasks may underlie the differences in visual half-field performance. Among other factors that influence findings in tachistoscopic studies are: viewing conditions, ocular dominance, handedness, report instructions, fixation control, eye movements, preexposural attention sets, type and arrangement of displays, and stimulus characteristics.

Young and Ellis (1981) have criticized several standard methods of conducting visual half-field studies. Of particular pertinence are fixation control, which has been employed by only a small number of studies, and characteristics of verbal tasks. It is well known that disabled readers have more difficulty maintaining fixation (Pirozzolo, 1977b).

Some disabled readers have (Gross, Rothenberg, Schottenfeld, & Drake, 1978) been observed to have longer thresholds for identifying words. Since standard procedure is to present stimuli for less than the time it takes to make an eye movement (arbitrarily set at 200 msec in most studies), the presentation of stimuli can approach the time necessary to make an eye movement. Gross et al. (1978) found threshold durations approaching 150 msec in some subjects; this duration is critically close (and in some cases less than that necessary to launch an eye movement) to saccadic latency (e.g., Pirozzolo & Rayner, 1980; Rayner, 1978).

A final problem concerns the selection of subjects and the diagnosis of developmental reading disability. It is now widely accepted that developmental reading disability is not a single homogeneous clinical entity (see, for example, Mattis, 1981; Satz & Morris, 1981). Numerous studies of groups of disabled readers have found that several subtypes exist (Kinsbourne & Warrington, 1963; Mattis, French, & Rapin, 1975; Pirozzolo, 1979). A strong case can be made for the existence of two main subtypes that differ from each other in a variety of important ways. Auditory-linguistic dyslexics are disabled readers with poor language skills, while visuospatial dyslexics are disabled readers with poor spatial and visual perceptual processing (Pirozzolo, 1979) (see Table 14-1).

As in many other areas of neuropsychological performance, auditory-linguistic disabled readers differ from visuospatial-disabled readers on visual half-field examination (Pirozzolo, 1979). When words were projected in the fovea, there were no differences between groups or between disabled readers and normal readers. When words were projected into the right visual field,

TABLE 14-1.
Two Types of Dyslexia

Some Neuropsychological Criteria for the Differential Diagnosis of Visuospatial Dyslexia	Some Neuropsychological Criteria for the Differential Diagnosis of Auditory-Linguistic Dyslexia
1. 1½-2 years delay in reading acquisition after age 8	1. At least 1½-2 years delay in reading acquisition
2. Right-left disorientation	2. Developmentally delayed language
3. Spatial dysgraphia (e.g., poor handwriting, micrographia, poor use of space allotted)	3. Expressive speech defects (e.g., developmental articulation disorders)
4. Finger agnosia	4. Anomia, object-naming, or color-naming defects
5. Spelling errors predominantly involving the visual aspects of text (letter and word reversals, confusions, omissions, and substitutions)	5. Spelling errors, predominantly involving the phonological aspects of written language, i.e., phoneme-to-grapheme translation
6. Reading errors predominantly involving the visual characteristics of written language	6. Reading errors predominantly involving the phonological aspects of written language, i.e., grapheme-to-phoneme translation errors
7. Faulty eye movements during reading (e.g., inaccurate return sweeps)	7. Low verbal IQ (relative to performance IQ)
8. Early evidence of preference for mirror- or inverted-writing	8. Average or above-average performance IQ
9. Low performance IQ (relative to verbal IQ)	9. Relatively intact visuospatial abilities
10. Average or above-average verbal IQ	10. Normal eye movements
11. Relatively intact oral language abilities	11. Letter-by-letter decoding strategy
12. Phonetic decoding strategy	12. Agrammatism

Table 14-1

auditory-linguistic dyslexics showed poor performance relative to normals and visuospatial dyslexics; in the left visual field, the groups did not differ significantly. Thus, normal readers showed a strong right visual field advantage, as did the visuospatial dyslexics, while auditory-linguistic dyslexics showed no asymmetry. At the more eccentric retinal locations, visuospatial dyslexics' performance decreased significantly, a finding supporting the notion that these disabled readers may have problems with the initial registration and visual analysis stages of word recognition. It is, therefore, reasonable to conclude that the selection of subjects for entry into the disabled reader group is an important factor that influences group performance data.

CONCLUSION

The measurement of hemispheric asymmetries in children with developmental reading disabilities is a popular research topic among neuropsychologists, experimental psychologists, and educational psychologists. It derives its importance from suggestions that these children do not read on a level expected of them because of faulty cerebral dominance. The concepts and methods of cerebral dominance research are marked by considerable oversimplicity. Important confounds characterize many, if not all, studies in this area. While children with developmental reading disabilities seem to perform consistently differently from normal readers in most studies, it is unclear what the causal mechanism is in their poor performance and whether or not it derives from a common underlying etiologic factor causing reading retardation. Techniques such as dichotic listening, visual half-field, and other divided sensory field studies seem well suited for describing the important neuropsychological deficits that disabled readers experience. A better elucidation of each of the factors that influences these tests is imperative in order to improve the understanding of developmental reading disability.

REFERENCES

Ayres, J.A. Dichotic listening performance in learning-disabled children. *The American Journal of Occupational Therapy*, 1977, *31*, 441–446.

Bakker, D.J. Ear asymmetry with monaural stimulation: Task influences. *Cortex*, 1969, *5*, 36–42.

Bakker, D.J. Hemispheric differences and reading strategies: Two dyslexias? *Bulletin of the Orton Society*, 1979, *29*, 89–100.

Bakker, D.J. Cerebral lateralization and reading proficiency. In Y. Lebrun & O. Zangwill (Eds.), *Lateralization of language in the child*. Lisse, Belgium: Swets & Zeitlinger, 1980.

Bakker, D.J., Licht, R., Kok, A., & Bouma, A. Cortical responses to word reading by right- and left-eared normal and reading-disturbed children. *Journal of Clinical Neuropsychology*, 1980, *2*, 1–12.

Bakker, D.J., Satz, P., Goebel, R., & Van der Vlugt, H. Developmental parameters of the ear asymmetry: A multivariate approach to cerebral dominance. Paper presented at the 1st Annual Meeting of the International Neuropsychological Society, New Orleans, 1973.

Bakker, D.J., Teunisson, J., & Bosch, J. Development of laterality-reading patterns. In R.M. Knights & D.J. Bakker (Eds.), *The neuropsychology of learning disorders*. Baiitmore: University Park Press, 1976.

Bakker, D.J., Van der Vlugt, H., & Claushuis, M. The reliability of dichotic ear asymmetry in normal children. *Neuropsychologia*, 1978, *16*, 753-757.

Barton, M., Goodglass, H., & Shai, A. Differential recognition of tachistoscopically presented English and Hebrew words. *Perceptual and Motor Skills*, 1965, *21*, 431-437.

Berlin, C.I., Hughes, L.F., Lowe-Bell, S.S., & Berlin, H.L. Dichotic right ear advantage in children 5-13. *Cortex*, 1973, *9*, 372-402.

Boder, E. Developmental dyslexia: A diagnostic screening procedure based on three characteristic patterns of reading and spelling. In B. Bateman (Ed.), *Learning disorders*. Seattle: Special Child Publications, 1971.

Boder, E. Developmental dyslexia: A diagnostic approach based on three atypical reading patterns. *Developmental Medicine and Child Neurology*, 1973, *15*, 663-687.

Broadbent, D. Listening to one of two synchronous messages. *Journal of Experimental Psychology*, 1952a, *44*, 51-54.

Broadbent, D. Speaking and listening simultaneously. *Journal of Experimental Psychology*, 1952b, *43*, 267-273.

Bryden, M.P. Dichotic listening in the development of the linguistic process. Paper presented at the 1st Annual Meeting of the International Neuropsychological Society, New Orleans, 1973.

Bryson, S., Mononen, L.J., & Yu, L. Procedural constraints on the measurement of laterality in young children. *Neuropsychologia*, 1980, *18*, 243-246.

Cermak, S.A., Cermak, L.S., Drake, C., & Kenney, R. The effect of concurrent manual activity on the dichotic listening performance of boys with learning disabilities. *The American Journal of Occupational Therapy*, 1978, *320*, 493-499.

Critchley, M. *The dyslexic child*. London: Heinemann, 1970.

Cullen, Jr., J.K., Thompson, C.L., Hughes, L.F. et al. The effects of varied acoustic parameters of performance in dichotic speech perception tasks. *Brain and Language*, 1974, *1*, 307-322.

Darby, R. Ear asymmetry phenomenon in dyslexic and normal children. Unpublished master's thesis, University of Florida, 1974.

Davidoff, J.B., Done, J., & Scully, J. What does the lateral ear advantage relate to? *Brain and Language*, 1981, *12*, 332-346.

Doehring, D.G. Ear asymmetry in the discrimination of monaural tonal sequences. *Canadian Journal of Psychology*, 1972, *26*, 106–110.

Fennell, E.B., Satz, P., & Morris, R. The development of handedness and ear asymmetry in good and poor readers: A longitudinal study. Paper presented at the Annual Meeting of the International Neuropsychological Society, San Francisco, 1980.

Forgays, D.G. The development of differential word recognition. *Journal of Experimental Psychology*, 1953, *45*, 165–168.

Frankfurter, A., & Honeck, R.P. Ear differences in the recall of monaurally presented sentences. *Quarterly Journal of Experimental Psychology*, 1973, *25*, 138–146.

Geffen, G. Development of hemispheric specialization for speech perception. *Cortex*, 1976, *12*, 337–346.

Geffen, G. The development of the right ear advantage in dichotic listening with focused attention. *Cortex*, 1978, *14*, 169–177.

Gilbert, J.H.V., & Climan, I. Dichotic studies in 2 and 3 year-olds: A preliminary report. *Speech communication seminar* (Vol. 2). Stockholm, Uppsala, Sweden: Almquist & Wiksell, 1974.

Gross, K., Rothenberg, S., Schottenfield, D., & Drake, C. Duration thresholds for letter identification in left and right visual fields for normal and reading-disabled children. *Neuropsychologia*, 1978, *16*, 709–715.

Harcum, E.R., & Finkel, M.D. Explanation of Miskin and Forgay's result as a directional reading conflict. *Canadian Journal of Psychology*, 1963, *17*, 224–232.

Heron, W. Perception as a function of retinal locus and attention. *American Journal of Psychology*, 1957, *70*, 38–48.

Hynd, G.W., & Obrzut, J.E. Effects of grade level and sex on the magnitude of the dichotic listening advantage. *Neuropsychologia*, 1977, *15*, 689–692.

Hynd, G.W., Obrzut, J.E., Weed, W., & Hynd, C.R. Development of cerebral dominance: Dichotic listening asymmetry in normal and learning disabled children. *Journal of Experimental Child Psychology*, 1979, *28*, 445–454.

Ingram, D. Cerebral speech lateralization in young children. *Neuropsychologia*, 1975, *13*, 103–105.

Kaufman, A.S. *Intelligent testing with the WISC-R*. New York: Wiley, 1979.

Kershner, J.R. Cerebral dominance in disabled readers, good readers, and gifted children: Search for a valid model. *Child Development*, 1977, *48*, 61–67.

Kimura, D. Cerebral dominance and the perception of verbal stimuli. *Canadian Journal of Psychology*, 1961a, *15*, 166–171.

Kimura, D. Some effects of temporal lobe damage on auditory perception. *Canadian Journal of Psychology*, 1961b, *15*, 156–165.

Kimura, D. Speech lateralization in young children as determined by an auditory test. *Cortex*, 1963, *3*, 899–902.

Kimura, D. Functional asymmetry of the brain in dichotic listening. *Cortex*, 1967, *3*, 163–178.

Kinsbourne, M. Mechanisms of hemispheric interaction in man. In M. Kinsbourne & L. Smith (Eds.), *Hemispheric disconnection and cerebral function*. Springfield, Ill.: Charles C. Thomas, 1974.

Kinsbourne, M. Mapping a behavioral cerebral space. *International Journal of Neuroscience*, 1980, *11*, 45–50.

Kinsbourne, M., & Warrington, E.K. Developmental factors in reading and writing backwardness. *British Journal of Psychology*, 1963, *54*, 145–156.

Lenneberg, E. *Biological foundations of language*. New York: Wiley, 1967.

Leong, C.K. Laterality patterns in disabled and non-disabled nine-year-old readers. Paper presented at the Boerhaave International La France on Lateralization of Brain Functions, Leiden, The Netherlands, 1975.

Leong, C.K. Lateralization in severly disabled readers in relation to functional cerebral development and synthesis of information. In R.M. Knight & D.J. Bakker (Eds.), *The neuropsychology of learning disorders*. Baltimore: University Park Press, 1976.

Marcel, T., Katz, L., & Smith, M. Laterality and reading proficiency. *Neuropsychologia*, 1974, *12*, 131–139.

Marcel, T., & Rajan, P. Lateral specialization for recognition of words and faces in good and poor readers. *Neuropsychologia*, 1975, *13*, 489–497.

Mattis, S. Dyslexia syndromes in children: Toward the development of syndrome-specific treatment programs. In F.J. Pirozzolo & M.C. Wittrock (Eds.), *Neuropsychological and cognitive processes in reading*. New York: Academic Press, 1981.

Mattis, S., French, J., & Rapin, I. Dyslexia in children and young adults: Three independent neuropsychological syndromes. *Developmental Medicine and Child Neurology*, 1975, *17*, 150–163.

McKeever, W., & Huling, M.D. Lateral dominance in tachistoscopic word recognition of children at two levels of ability. *Quarterly Journal of Experimental Psychology*, 1970, *22*, 600–604.

McKeever, W., & Van Deventer, A.D. Dyslexic adolescents: Evidence of impaired visual and auditory language processing associated with normal lateralization and visual responsivity. *Cortex*, 1975, *11*, 361–378.

Miller, L.K., & Turner, S. Development of hemifield differences in word recognition. *Journal of Educational Psychology*, 1973, *65*, 172–176.

Milner, B. Laterality effects in audition. In V.B. Mountcastle (Ed.), *Interhemispheric relations and cerebral dominance*. Baltimore: John Hopkins Press, 1962.

Milner, B., Taylor, L., & Sperry, R.W. Lateralized suppression of dichotically presented digits after commissural section in man. *Science*, 1968, *161*, 184–186.

Mishkin, M., & Forgays, D.G. Word recognition as a function of retinal locus. *Journal of Experimental Psychology*, 1952, *43*, 43–48.

Morgan, W.P. A case of congenital word blindness. *British Medical Journal*, 1896, *2*, 1378.

Nagafuchi, M. Development of dichotic and monaural hearing abilities in young children. *Acta Ota Laryngologica*, 1970, *69* 103–105.

Obrzut, J.E. Dichotic listening and bisensory memory skills in qualitatively diverse dyslexic readers. *Journal of Learning Disabilities*, 1979, *12*, 304–314.

Obrzut, J.E., Hynd, G.W., & Obrzut, A. *Neuropsychological assessment of learning disabilities: A discriminant analysis*, in press.

Obrzut, J.E., Hynd, G.W., Obrzut, A., & Leitgeb, J.L. Time sharing and dichotic listening asymmetry in normal and learning disabled children. *Brain and Language*, 1980, *11*, 181–194.

Obrzut, J.E., Hynd, G.W., Obrzut, A., & Pirozzolo, F.J. Effect of directed attention on cerebral asymmetries in normal and learning disabled children. *Developmental Psychology*, 1981, *17*, 118–125.

Olson, M.E. Laterality differences in tachistoscopic word recognition in normal and delayed readers in elementary school. *Neuropsychologia*, 1973, *11*, 343–350.

Orton, S.T. *Reading, writing and speech problems in children*. New York: Norton, 1937.

Pirozzolo, F.J. Lateral asymmetries in visual perception: A review of tachistoscopic visual half-field studies. *Perceptual and Motor Skills*, 1977a, *45*, 695–701.

Pirozzolo, F.J. *Visual-spatial and oculomotor deficits in developmental dyslexia: Evidence for two neurobehavioral syndromes of developmental reading disability*. Unpublished doctoral dissertation, University of Rochester, 1977b.

Pirozzolo, F.J. *The neuropsychology of developmental reading disorders*. New York: Praeger, 1979.

Pirozzolo, F.J., Campanella, D., Christensen, K., & Lawson-Kerr, K. Effects of cerebral dysfunction on neurolinguistic performance on children. *Journal of Consulting and Clinical Psychology*, 1981, *43*, 771–787.

Pirozzolo, F.J., & Rayner, K. Hemispheric specialization in reading and word recognition. *Brain and Language*, 1977, *4*, 248–261.

Pirozzolo, F.J., & Rayner, K. Cerebral organization and reading disability. *Neuropsychologia*, 1979, *17*, 485–491.

Pirozzolo, F.J., & Rayner, K. Handedness, hemispheric specialization and saccadic eye movement latencies. *Neuropsychologia*, 1980, *18*, 225–229.

Porter, R.J., & Berlin, C.I. On interpreting developmental changes in the dichotic right ear advantage. *Brain and Language*, 1975, *2*, 186–200.

Rayner, K. Eye movement latencies for parafoveally presented words. *Bulletin of the Psychonomic Society*, 1978, *11*, 13–16.

Reitsma, P. *Visual asymmetry in children*. Paper presented at the International Conference on Lateralization of Brain Functions, Leiden, The Netherlands, 1975.

Rosenzweig, M.R. Representations of the two ears at the auditory cortex. *American Journal of Physiology*, 1951, *167*, 147–158.

Satz, P. Developmental parameters in the lateralization of brain functions. Paper presented at the Boerhaave Conference on Lateralization of Brain Functions, Leiden, The Netherlands, 1975.

Satz, P. Laterality tests: An inferential problem. *Cortex*, 1977, *13*, 208–212.

Satz, P., Bakker, D.J., Tennissen, J. et al. Developmental parameters of the ear asymmetry: A multivariate approach. *Brain and Language*, 1975, *2*, 171–185.

Satz, P., Friel, J., & Rudegeair, F. Some predictive antecedents of specific reading disability: A two-, three-, and four-year follow-up. In *Hyman Blumberg symposium on research in early childhood education*. Baltimore: Johns Hopkins Press, 1974.

Satz, P., & Morris, R. Learning disability subtypes. In F.J. Pirozzolo & M.C. Wittrock (Eds.), *Neuropsychological and cognitive processes in reading*. New York: Academic Press, 1981.

Satz, P., Rardin, D., & Ross, J. An evaluation of a theory of specific developmental dyslexia. *Child Dvelopment*, 1971, *42*, 2009–2021.

Satz, P., Taylor, H.G., Friel, J., & Fletcher, J. Some developmental and predictive precursors of reading disabilities. In A.L. Benton & D. Pearl (Eds.), *Dyslexia: An appraisal of current knowledge*. New York: Oxford University Press, 1978.

Schulman-Galambos, C. Dichotic listening performance in elementary and college students. *Neuropsychologia*, 1972, *15*, 577–584.

Sparrow, S., & Satz, P. Dyslexia, laterality and neuropsychological development. In D.J. Bakker & P. Satz (Eds.), *Specific reading disability: Advances in theory and method*. Rotterdam: Rotterdam University Press, 1970.

Van Duyne, H.J., Bakker, D.J., & De Jong, W. Development of ear-asymmetry related to coding processes in memory in children. *Brain and Language*, 1977, *4*, 322–334.

Witelson, S.F. Abnormal right hemisphere specialization in developmental dyslexia. In R.M. Knight & D.J. Bakker (Eds.), *The neuropsychology of learning disorders*. Baltimore: University Park Press, 1976.

Witelson, S.F., & Rabinovitch, M.S. Hemispheric speech lateralization in children with auditory-linguistic deficits. *Cortex*, 1972, *8*, 412–426.

Yeni-Komshian, G., Isenberg, D., & Goldberg, H. Cerebral dominance and reading disability: Left visual field deficit in poor readers. *Neuropsychologia*, 1975, *13*, 83–94.

Young, A.W., & Ellis, A.W. Asymmetry of cerebral hemispheric function in normal and poor readers. *Psychological Bulletin*, 1981, *89*, 183–190.

Zurif, E.B., & Carson, G. Dyslexia in relation to cerebral dominance and temporal analysis. *Neuropsychologia*, 1970, *8*, 351–361.

Index

age: and dichotic listening, 199–200, 444; and manual activity, 281–285, 297–299, 314–315; as a variable in clinical studies, 48–51

Alzheimers's dementia, 59

anatomical diversity in the human brain, 465–467

anatomical locus models, 220–222, 471–474

angular gyrus, 401

anxiety, 483–484

aphasia: Broca's, 14, 26, 34–38; case study approach, 28–31; classification by locus of damage, 24–25; classification by syndrome type, 25–26; and cognitive processes, 19–22; group/case study method, 32–33; group research methods, 22–27; and neuropsychological theory, 19–22; and right hemisphere language, 82–83, 143; Wernicke's, 14, 33, 38–42

arousal, 474–477

attention: and brain potentials, 343; in dichotic listening, 177–185; and localized blood flow, 400, 407–408; and manual activity, 9, 255–326; in reading disorders, 504; in spiit-brain patients, 133, 157–160; (see also attention gradient model, dual process model, functional cerebral distance)

attention-bias explanations of perceptual laterality (see attention gradient model)

attention gradient model, 7, 224–225, 415–416

bias, 486–487

binomial distribution, 450–453

binomial response experiments, 453–454

brain damage, 2–4; left hemisphere (see aphasia); right hemisphere, 46–94; and split-brain studies, 101–103

brain potential: dynamic spatial patterns, 369; methodological issues, 345–346, 348, 349;

origin and significance, 341; signal processing, 341; (see also electroencephalogram, evoked potential)

callosal connectivity, 104–105

callosal relay model: definition, 105–107; tests of, 108–121, 127–139

case-study approach, 28–31

ceiling effects: in blood flow studies, 394; in developmental studies, 500; and interactions, 11, 420, 470

cerebral neoplasms: diffuse, 59–61; focal, 58–59

cerebrovascular infarction, 57–58

cognitive style, 487–491

commissurotomy (see split-brain)

computerized axial tomography, 55

contingent negative variation, 344

corpus callosum and transfer of information, 104–105, 152–157, 224

developmental reading disability, 498–509; and the corpus callosum, 506; dichotic listening studies, 499–505; visual laterality studies, 504–508

dextrals, 465–466

dichotic listening: and age, 199; asynchronous presentation, 180, 188–189; individual differences in, 198–210; Kimura's model of, 7, 177–179; limited capacity, 182–185; in normals, 177–210; procedures and methods, 185–195; in split-brain patients, 123–130

difference models, 220

difference score, 190, 430, 445, 467–469

direct access model, 7, 106–121; disconnection syndrome (see split-brain)

disinhibition, 392–393, 402, 478–479

double cancellation, 439

double dissociation, 69, 70–72, 413

dual processor models, 229–231, 241–245